W9-ANJ-687

WHAT TO EXPECT®
BEFORE YOU'RE EXPECTING

2nd EDITION

By Heidi Murkoff
and Sharon Mazel

Foreword by Charles J. Lockwood, MD
Professor of Obstetrics and Gynecology and Public Health
Dean, Morsani College of Medicine, University of South Florida

Workman Publishing • New York

To Erik, my everything

To Emma and Wyatt, for making me a mom
and Lennox for making me a grandmom

To Arlene, my first partner in What to Expect and my most important one—
you'll always be loved and always be remembered

To moms, dads, and babies everywhere—
and to all who care for and about them

———————

Copyright © 2009, 2017 by What to Expect LLC
What to Expect is a registered trademark of What to Expect LLC.

Library of Congress Cataloging-in-Publication Data is available
ISBN 978-1-5235-0150-2 (paperback)
ISBN 978-1-5235-0151-9 (hardcover)

Cover design: Vaughn Andrews
Cover photo: © MattBeard.com
Cover quilt photo: Gregory Case, gregorycase.com
Cover quilt design: Anna Sutton, bunnyhilldesigns.com
Book design: Lisa Hollander and Barbara Peragine
Interior illustrations: Karen Kuchar

Workman books are available at special discounts when purchased in bulk for premiums and sales promotions as well as for fund-raising or educational use. Special editions or book excerpts can also be created to specification. For details, contact the Special Sales Director at the address below, or send an email to specialmarkets@workman.com.

Workman Publishing Co., Inc.
225 Varick Street
New York, NY 10014-4381

workman.com

WORKMAN is a registered trademark of Workman Publishing Co., Inc.

Printed in the United States of America
First printing October 2017
10 9 8 7 6 5 4 3 2 1

Thanks Again

So, here I am again, about to deliver a book—more precisely, a new edition. As I've pointed out once or twice before, books (whether new or new editions) and babies have a lot in common—they're a lot of work, they keep you up at night and get you up way early in the morning, they bring both joy and stress. (One key difference being babies update themselves. Books, not so much.)

Needless to say, you can't create a book—or a baby—solo, at least strictly speaking. My human babies, Emma and Wyatt, were created with the most wonderful man in the world—my husband, best friend, soulmate, and partner in all things, Erik.

My book babies, well, that takes a team effort with a much bigger team—and this new baby is no exception. Some members are new to the What to Expect team, but many have been by my side since book one. With that, I'd like to thank:

Suzanne Rafer, my forever editor (it may actually be longer than forever by now) and forever my favorite. Many xo's.

Peter Workman, who created the house we live in, and Dan Reynolds, who preserves and improves our home. And everyone else at Workman who has contributed to this latest WTE baby, including the creative Vaughn Andrews and the artistic Lisa Hollander. Karen Kuchar, for clearly and beautifully illustrating the art and science of conception (and for making reproductive parts look so pretty!). Beth Levy, for coordinating all those editing passes. Barbara Peragine, for fitting in more boxes than ever. Julie Primavera and Monica McCready, for those phenomenal production values. Suzie Bolotin, David Schiller, Page Edmunds, Selina Moore, Moira Kerrigan, and Lily Kiralla. The women who make special markets so special (and are so special to me), Jenny Mandel and Emily Krasner. And everyone in digital, ebooks, and the entire book sales team. (Books don't sell themselves, after all!)

Phenomenal photographer and friend Matt Beard, for having us covered yet again—with beautiful cover photos of Emma and Lennox.

Sharon Mazel, who has been (virtually) by my side for pass after pass of edition after edition of book after book, surviving (no, thriving!) under deadline after deadline, and maintaining a type A+ personality to match my own, while somehow raising 4 girls (women!) and occasionally (hopefully) dating her husband, Jay.

Dr. Charles Lockwood, trusty and trusted medical adviser, for delivering the most accurate, up-to-date, and carefully curated information on all matters mom—and all matters that matter to moms (and their partners). Thanks for your wisdom, wit, insight, care, compassion, and the endlessly invaluable contributions you've made to What to Expect. Drs. Stephanie Romero, Shayne Plosker, and Anthony Imudia—many thanks for your RE expertise. And of course, Dr. Howie Mandel, for delivering compassionate care—and Lennox.

ACOG, for being passionate advocates of women and their reproductive rights, and leaders in health care policy. And thanks to all the ob-gyns, fertility specialists, midwives, and nurses who believe that delivering preconception care can deliver a healthier future. To the CDC, for your dedication to the health and wellbeing of our global family, shared commitment to preconception health, and most recently, for the up-to-the-minute facts on Zika virus.

Our always awesome WhatTo Expect.com team, lovingly led by Michael Rose, Kyle Humphries, and Siobhan Adcock, plus our new Ziff/ Davis family, including Jimmy Yaffe, for being the web partners of our dreams– and believing in the power of moms, dads, babies, purple, and #BumpDay. And for helping create a truly amazing community of moms, Sara Stefanik.

International Medical Corps, first responders, humanitarian heroes and our passionate partners in maternal child health and #BumpDay, with extra love to Margaret Traub and to all the humanitarian health workers who care for the most vulnerable members of our human family, especially Amazing Grace Losio, my personal midwife hero in South Sudan.

The USO, our partners in the Special Delivery program—and all the military moms, dads, and babies I've gratefully hugged already, and those I've yet to hug (can't wait).

Marc Chamlin, for always being there for me, always protecting me, always caring for me, and Alan Nevins, for managing the unmanageable (is there anything you can't put on a spreadsheet?), putting out fires, cleaning up messes, and picking up pieces—in short, for being the best agent a girl could ever have.

Erik, the love of my life—I can't remember having a life before you, and couldn't imagine one without you. Emma and Wyatt, for making me one very happy and proud mama. I love you both so much. And of course, the latest love of my life, Lennox.

Contents

Foreword
to the Second Edition

By Charles J. Lockwood, MD

Professor of Obstetrics & Gynecology and Public Health
Dean, Morsani College of Medicine
Senior Vice President USF Health
University of South Florida

Would you undertake the most exhilarating, exhausting, and expensive trip of your life without knowing where you were going, how to get there, and how much it was going to cost? I thought not. Well having a baby is all of that and much more. *What to Expect Before You're Expecting* is your tour-guide, travelogue, and guidebook to achieving a successful pregnancy. It provides solid, evidence-based recommendations that, if followed, should help you get pregnant, stay pregnant, and have a healthy baby.

The book begins, appropriately enough, with preconception care—how to get your body (and brain) ready to conceive and carry a pregnancy to term. It provides a practical set of steps to help ensure that you will start your pregnancy in the best possible shape for success. Information is provided on what your ideal body weight should be, and how to get there through diet, exercise and sleep—yes, getting enough sleep will help optimize your reproductive potential (and general health). Practical advice is also provided on how to stop smoking, cut down on caffeine and alcohol, and ensure that the prescription, over-the-counter, and herbal medications you are taking are baby-safe. Critically important advice is provided on working with your physician to optimize management of any preexisting medical conditions you might have, what preventive care you should receive before your conceive (for example, vaccinations, Pap test, dental care, genetic testing), how to avoid work-related and environmental toxins, and even how to avoid Zika and other infection risks. The finances of establishing a family are also discussed—a crucial but frequently overlooked topic by many couples—as well as vital information on health insurance and what it may cover (and not cover).

Two chapters are devoted to optimizing your weight and nutrition—critical aspects of both getting pregnant and having a successful pregnancy. Moreover, achieving your optimal pre-pregnancy weight is not only important for conception and pregnancy, it will also reduce your risk of obesity and related medical complications later in life (so you can take great care of that baby) and it will help prevent obesity and chronic medical problems for your child!

While many couples conceive without much effort (or sometimes planning), others have challenges. There are multiple chapters devoted to basic reproductive biology, predicting ovulation, assessing your fertility potential, "activities" to optimize the chance of getting pregnant, and then how to best test whether you are pregnant. For those who aren't so lucky, there are several outstanding chapters that detail the causes of both female and male infertility in clear, cogent, yet in-depth ways. The tests that might be needed to assess fertility potential and the full range of treatments available to achieve a pregnancy are described in detail. The book also covers one of the most challenging problems on the road to making a baby:

recurrent miscarriage. It covers the causes, workup, and treatments of this stressful problem, and offers both hope and a realistic assessment of prognoses. The book ends with a handy fertility planning "count-down" that summarizes steps to maximize your chance of conceiving and successfully carrying a pregnancy.

As with *What to Expect When You're Expecting*, Heidi Murkoff's *What to Expect Before You're Expecting* packs in a truly extraordinary amount of much needed information in a highly readable format with her usual and funny, positive and optimistic tone and style. While it is a must-read for all women thinking about having a baby, it will also help future dads optimize their own reproductive health and better understand what their partner is going through. I recommend it to everyone thinking about having a baby.

What Can You Expect Before You're Expecting

(And why does it matter, anyway?)

....

Pregnancy, as you probably know, is 9 months long (or 38 weeks from conception, if you're really serious about keeping count). And if you've ever been pregnant before, you probably think that's plenty long enough. Maybe even a little too long, especially once your belly's the size of a prize-winning watermelon and your breasts have worked their way through the cup alphabet . . . twice. But is 9 months really long enough? Does that time-honored baby-making timetable really stand up to the latest science?

According to experts, no. From the CDC to the American College of Obstetricians and Gynecologists, the March of Dimes, American College of Nurse Midwives, the American Academy of Pediatrics, and the American Academy of Family Physicians—that traditional 9-month timeline has been bumped by this recommendation: It's time to add more months to pregnancy.

That's right, more months. At least 3 more, in fact, for a full 12. But before you panic (3 extra months of not seeing my feet? Of passing on the sushi? Of waiting to hold that bundle of joy?), here's what you need to know: Those extra months aren't meant to be spent being pregnant, but getting ready to be pregnant.

The truth is, a healthy pregnancy begins before sperm and egg meet up. Before the home pregnancy test announces the good news. Before the queasies kick in and your waistline checks out. Even before you ditch your diaphragm or peel off your patch. A healthy pregnancy begins before you're expecting—which is why, if you're planning to get pregnant, you might want to start planning (and prepping) ahead.

What's New About Getting Pregnant?

Sure, getting pregnant isn't considered rocket science. It's biology—for most of us, the really fun kind of biology. And the basic mechanics of baby making aren't only, well, basic (insert part A into part B, repeat as needed and desired), but they haven't changed much over the history of human reproduction. And certainly, they haven't changed much over the 8 years since I delivered the first edition of *What to Expect Before You're Expecting*.

That said, there's plenty that's new about getting pregnant—especially when it comes to couples who aren't able to get pregnant the basic way—and that's why I'm delivering a brand new 2nd edition. In it you'll find the latest his-and-hers advice on getting ready to get pregnant: from diet (why high protein may lower your fertility) and weight (how it affects fertility and your future baby) to the workplace (how your 9 to 5 job may impact your baby-making job, especially if you work the night shift) and lifestyle (which habits to kick before you get busy). What checkups and vaccines to get, what screenings you'll need (including up-to-date information on expanded genetic carrier screening), and how to make sure your health insurance has you covered. What medications might need adjusting (including antidepressants), and what supplements you'll need to stop (or start) popping.

Yes, you'll find the fertility basics (when and how often to have sex, in what positions, with what lubricants). But this edition goes way beyond those basics—from new tests to assess your ovarian reserve to high-tech ways to track your ovulation (with wearables that sync with smartphones) and check your partner's sperm count at home (there's an app for that, too).

There's a new chapter on the fertility workup: when and how to seek help if you're having trouble conceiving, distinguishing between subfertility and infertility, a comprehensive section on fertility challenges (from elevated prolactin to PCOS to low sperm count to unexplained infertility). And a brand new chapter devoted to fertility treatments, including the most cutting-edge technology, advanced procedures, and the newest medications. Frozen embryos vs. fresh for IVF, 3-day embryos vs. 5-day, why ICSI is edging out standard IVF, when to consider preimplantation genetic screening, everything you'll need to know about donor sperm and donor eggs, embryo donation, and surrogacy. How to finance it all. And, if you've experienced pregnancy loss, a chapter to help you start over, including treatments for recurrent loss.

Are you a same-sex couple hoping to become a pair of parents? All your conception and pregnancy options are covered, too.

Wondering how Zika virus might affect your baby-making plans? You'll find out everything you and your partner need to know about protecting the baby you're hoping to make.

And here's how. *What to Expect Before You're Expecting*—a complete, start-to-cuddly-finish guide to getting pregnant—is everything you need to know to get your body and your partner's body into the best baby-making shape possible before you start trying to conceive. What baby-friendly foods to order up often, and which fertility-busting foods—and drinks—to keep off the menu. (Hint: Get your sushi while you can, but can the fresh tuna.) How to get your weight where it needs to be for maximum fertility and optimum pregnancy health (packing on too many pounds—or too few—can compromise conception and complicate pregnancy). Which medications need to be shelved (including some surprises, like antihistamines), when to toss your birth control, why your partner should put hot tubs (and spinning classes) on ice, why kicking your smoking habit now can give fertility a boost (while protecting your future baby's health).

Once you've prepped for pregnancy, it's time to get pregnant. Sounds like the easy (and fun) part—and usually it is. But a little conception know-how can help you fast-track your fertility and make those baby dreams come true sooner. You'll find out how to pinpoint ovulation, when to schedule in sex, how sex toys and lubes fit in, why wet isn't wild when it comes to baby-making sex, how to keep on-demand sex spicy— plus the lowdown on sex positions and conception. Have you heard a few conception tales already, or read them on the internet? Fertility fiction and fact are sorted out here, too.

What if you encounter a bump on the way to baby? Fertility challenges— and how to overcome them—are covered, as well as the latest in fertility treatments. You'll also find out when to let nature take its course, and when to seek help.

Whether you've begun your conception campaign already, or you're just starting to think about getting pregnant, it's never too late—or too early—to start optimizing your preconception profile. So put time on your side, and add a few months to your baby-making calendar. More pregnancy, it turns out, is more.

May all your greatest expectations come true!

Heidi

PART 1

Getting Ready to Get Pregnant

Prepping Before You're Expecting

Are you gearing up for a pregnancy? Preparing for baby making isn't only about tossing your birth control (though you'll need to do that), charting your ovulation (you'll probably want to do that), and heading to bed (you'll be happy to do that). It's also about getting your body—and your partner's body—into tip-top baby-making shape. From the drinks you and your partner-in-procreation sip to the medications you take, from the habits you're best off kicking to the supplements you're best off popping (and not popping)—taking charge of your preconception prep will start you off on the right foot, making conception easier (hopefully) and pregnancy safer and more comfortable (ditto). So before you dive into bed to make that baby, dive into this chapter to find out what steps you should consider taking first.

Your Health Prep

It stands to reason that your overall health has a lot to do with your overall fertility. After all, it takes a healthy body (make that 2 healthy bodies) to make a healthy baby. Which means there's no better time than now—when that baby-to-be is just a gleam in your hopeful eyes—to make sure that you and your partner are healthy overall.

Just about every aspect of your health—from the medications you take to the immunizations you should have to the chronic conditions that need controlling and the dental work that needs doing—can have an impact on your fertility and on your healthy pregnancy to come. So check it all out, starting with those checkups.

Talk the Talk

Are you TTC? You probably are if you're reading this book—yet you may not have the slightest idea what "TTC" means (it's short for "trying to conceive"). Lots of fertility acronyms have become part of preconception-speak (check out any fertility website or online support group and you'll see), and they pop up occasionally in this book, too. Feel a little out of the preconception lingo loop? Here's a list of some of the acronyms you may encounter during your conception adventure:

2WW .... 2-Week Wait (until you can take a pregnancy test)

AF .... Aunt Flo(w), your period

BBT .... Basal Body Temperature

BC .... Birth Control

BD .... Baby Dance (aka sex)

BFN .... Big Fat Negative (pregnancy test result)

BFP .... Big Fat Positive (pregnancy test result)

BMS .... Baby-Making Sex

BT .... Blood Test

CD .... Cycle Day

CF .... Cervical Fluid

CL .... Corpus Luteum

CM .... Cervical Mucus

CP .... Cervical Position

CY .... Cycle

DI .... Donor Insemination

DP .... "Dancing" Partner; spouse, partner, or significant other

DPO .... Days Past Ovulation

DTD .... Doing the Dance; Do the Deed (aka sex)

EWCM .... Egg White Cervical Mucus (re: consistency of)

FTTA .... Fertile Thoughts to All

FMU .... First Morning Urine

hCG .... Human Chorionic Gonadotropin (pregnancy hormone)

HPT .... Home Pregnancy Test

IF .... Infertility

IUI .... Intrauterine Insemination

IVF .... In Vitro Fertilization

LH .... Luteinizing Hormone

LMP .... Last Menstrual Period

LP .... Luteal Phase

O/Big O ..... Ovulation

OPK .... Ovulation Predictor Kit

POAS .... Pee on a Stick (aka pregnancy test)

PCOS .... Polycystic Ovarian Syndrome

PG .... Pregnancy; Pregnant

SA .... Sperm/Semen Analysis

TTC .... Trying to Conceive

Preconception Checkups

"I'm young and in good health, and my periods are regular. Do I really need to see a doctor before I start trying to get pregnant?"

The best prenatal care starts long before conception—and it doesn't stop at your reproductive parts. So now's a great time to schedule that full-body tune-up. Even if you've never had a sick day, it's easier to tackle health issues before baby's on board than to play catch-up after your body is already baby building (and this preconception prep is even more essential if you're overweight or underweight or living with a chronic condition). To make sure all systems are go, make an appointment with your gynecologist (who, by the way, doesn't have to be your eventual prenatal care practitioner)—and believe it or not, with your dentist, too—for complete pre-prenatal checkups.

See your gynecologist. Your preconception checkup will include a lot of the same tests and screenings you get at your regular annual—plus a lot of pre-pregnancy-specific ones. Here's what you can expect:

- A Pap test and all the standards of your annual visit, such as a pelvic, breast,

---

Preconception Prep and Chronic Conditions

If you have a chronic health condition (such as diabetes, asthma, a heart condition, epilepsy, high blood pressure, celiac disease, or depression), deciding to start trying to conceive isn't always as easy as pulling the plug on birth control and getting busy. It's likely both your preconception prep and your pregnancy care will be a little more involved. But there's lots of good news—especially since you're planning ahead.

Though it's true that there are sometimes risks to fertility, as well as risks for a pregnancy (and baby) if a mom's chronic condition isn't well controlled, those risks can be minimized or even eliminated entirely by bringing the condition under control, preferably before sperm meets egg. With the right care and precautions, most chronic conditions are compatible with getting pregnant and having a healthy pregnancy.

But first things first. And your first step on the road to pregnancy should be at your specialist's office (or at your internist's, if that's who oversees your condition) for a preconception appointment. He or she will evaluate how you're managing your condition and determine whether you're ready to TTC or need to make some changes before you get going. Maybe you'll need to tweak your diet (or get more serious about sticking to dietary restrictions), lose or gain some weight, or finesse your fitness. Maybe you'll need to be weaned off medications that aren't fertility friendly or may be harmful during pregnancy (including opioids for chronic pain), or switched to meds that are TTC and pregnancy safe. Or alternative therapies may be integrated into your care, such as acupuncture or meditation to relieve stress or pain, or help lower your blood pressure. Maybe you'll be referred to a high-risk ob (known as a maternal fetal medicine doctor) for your pregnancy care, or maybe you'll find that your usual ob-gyn will be able to team up with your chronic-condition specialist to offer all the care you need.

and abdominal exam. Get ready to stick out your arm for a blood pressure reading, too.

- A screening for, or a followup of, any gynecological conditions that might interfere with fertility or pregnancy, such as irregular periods, polycystic ovarian syndrome (PCOS), uterine fibroids, cysts, or benign tumors, endometriosis, pelvic inflammatory disease (PID), or recurrent urinary tract infections. Now—before you get started on baby making—is the time to get any gynecological conditions diagnosed and treated, because certain ones may prevent you from getting pregnant in the first place, and others can complicate pregnancy.

- A weight check. Because your pre-pregnancy weight has a lot more to do with your fertility, your future pregnancy health, and even your yet-to-be conceived baby's future health than you might think, you'll be stepping right up to the scale for a baseline weight check. If that bottom line isn't where it should be (close to the ideal weight for your size and body type), your doctor can help you set some goals to get your weight conception-ready. See Chapter 2 for more on your weight and fertility.

- A urine test to screen for a urinary tract infection and kidney disease.

- A blood test. Nobody's favorite part of the checkup, but a blood draw is typically standard at a preconception visit to get a read on your current state of health. You'll likely need many of the following tests once you get pregnant anyway, so you might as well get a head start on them now—they may not need to be repeated if you conceive within a few months of this workup:

It Takes Two

Making a baby is always a 2-person production (one from column Mom, one from column Dad). But as is often the case with pregnancy, preconception can be pretty female-centric. It shouldn't be. Both partners in conception have their work cut out for them before sperm meets egg. Though this entire book will be enlightening for prospective parents of both sexes, the dark shaded "For Dads-to-Be" boxes throughout provide tips, advice, and information specifically geared to wannabe dads. So if you're looking to become a father, look for these just-for-you boxes.

- Hemoglobin or hematocrit to use as a baseline during pregnancy and to test for anemia (many women have lower iron stores than they think, thanks to that monthly flow).

- Vitamin D level. Your doctor may test for vitamin D deficiency (some women are deficient) and recommend supplementation as needed.

- Rh factor, to see if you are positive or negative. If you are Rh-positive, you don't have to give Rh factor another thought. If you are negative, your partner should be tested to see if he is positive. If he's positive, then any baby you conceive has a chance of being Rh-positive, and you may end up developing antibodies to your baby's blood during pregnancy (not a problem in a first pregnancy, but it can result in an Rh-incompatability in a subsequent pregnancy). That's important information to have, since Rh-incompatibility can be easily prevented.

- Rubella titer, to check for immunity to rubella, and a varicella titer, to check for immunity to varicella (chicken pox); see page 8 for more on the important immunizations you should have before becoming pregnant. If you're not up to date on any of those vaccines, you should get them now.

- Tuberculosis (if you're at high risk for TB)

- Hepatitis B

- Cytomegalovirus antibody titers, to determine if you're immune to CMV (this test isn't routinely recommended, but you can ask for it). If you have recently had a CMV infection, it's generally recommended that you wait 6 months—when antibodies appear in the blood—before trying to conceive, since exposure to the virus could be dangerous to a baby-to-be.

- Toxoplasmosis titer, if you have a cat, regularly eat raw or rare meat, or garden without gloves. If you turn out to be immune (because you've been infected in the past), you won't have to worry about becoming infected during pregnancy and passing it on to your baby.

- Thyroid function. Because thyroid function can affect both fertility and pregnancy, preconception screening is recommended if you have a family or personal history of thyroid condition or have symptoms of or risk factors for a thyroid disorder. Some doctors do routine preconception screening for thyroid function.

- Sexually transmitted disease (STD)

■ A medication review. Whether it's over-the-counter or prescription, you and your doctor will discuss all the medications you take—including those you pop only occasionally. Depending on the medication (some are safe during pregnancy, others may not be), a change may be in the cards. You'll also review any vitamin and herbal supplements you take to see if they're preconception and pregnancy safe.

■ A discussion about:

- When to stop your birth control (your doctor will let you know how long you should ideally wait, if at all, before you can start trying to conceive; see page 115 for more)

- How to make sense of your cycle and figure out when you're most fertile (see Chapter 6 for more)

- What to eat and not eat while you're trying to conceive (see Chapter 3)

- Whether you should consider any lifestyle changes now that you're about to start TTC (see page 15)

- Whether you should consider genetic screening and/or counseling (see page 13)

- How your age might affect your fertility and impact pregnancy (see page 110)

- Any medical problems that should be treated before conception or will need to be monitored during pregnancy. Two examples: If you need allergy shots (or other allergy prevention treatment), the doctor will advise you to take care of them now (you'll be able to continue to get allergy shots during pregnancy if you start allergy desensitization before you conceive). If you were a PKU baby you'll need to protect your own future baby by beginning a phenylalanine-free diet 3 months

Shaking Your Family Health Tree

Time to call your folks. Not to tell them you're expecting (hopefully you'll make *that* call soon enough), but to get the scoop on the health history on both sides of the family tree—yours and your partner's. Dig as deeply as you can, and write down everything you unearth so that you'll be ready to answer the family history questions you'll be getting from your practitioner. It's especially important to find out if there's a history of any medical problems, such as diabetes, high blood pressure, celiac disease, or thyroid disease, and genetic or chromosomal disorders, such as Down syndrome, Tay-Sachs disease, sickle-cell anemia, thalassemia, hemophilia, cystic fibrosis, muscular dystrophy, Huntington's chorea, or fragile X syndrome in your immediate family or your partner's (including your children, mothers and fathers, brothers and sisters, grandparents, nieces and nephews, aunts and uncles, and first cousins).

Your family health tree may also clue you in on how your future pregnancy might play out. Are there twins in your future? Fraternal twins can run in families, so look for trends on your side of the tree. Also running in families are some pregnancy complications. Ask your mom and your partner's mom if she (or her mother) ever had preeclampsia. Research shows that sons and daughters born from pregnancies complicated by preeclampsia may carry genes related to the condition. Ask, too, about gestational diabetes, depression, or other disorders (during pregnancy, postpartum, or in general), and other complications—and have this information at the ready when your practitioner asks for it.

It'll also help to find out more about your mom's pregnancies with you and your siblings. That's because the apple often doesn't fall far from the mama tree when it comes to gynecological and obstetrical history, which means that a look at your mom's pregnancy history may give you a peek into your pregnancy future. Keeping in mind that every pregnancy is different (even for the same woman, 2 pregnancies may be very different), moms may predispose their daughters to any number of pregnancy or delivery scenarios—both good (no stretch marks) and not so good (lots of varicose veins). So ask your mother anything you might be wondering about, remembering that her pregnancy story may or may not predict yours: How long did it take you to get pregnant? Did you have morning sickness? Did your pregnancies go full term? How long were you in labor?

before you conceive, and continuing it throughout pregnancy.

◆ Recent travel. If you or your partner live in or have recently traveled to an area where Zika virus is prevalent, your practitioner will counsel you about the best conception plan, including whether you should wait before trying to conceive (see the box on page 10 for more).

▪ A family history check. When you're starting or building on a family, your family tree matters—which is why your doctor will want to check it out. For instance, if there's a family history of breast cancer, you're at high genetic risk, and you're over age 30, the doctor may suggest getting a baseline mammogram for a clear picture of what your breast tissue looks like before all the hormonal changes of pregnancy and breastfeeding begin. Your doctor will also ask about your family history of medical conditions (such as type 2 diabetes, celiac or thyroid disease, or hypertension) and pregnancy conditions (such as preeclampsia) that might affect your pregnancy. See the box on page 7 for more.

- A mental health screening. Because depression, an anxiety disorder, an eating disorder, or any other mental health issue can interfere with conception, lead to physical complications, and increase your risk of mood disorders during pregnancy and postpartum, it should also be treated before you begin your big adventure. (See page 12 for information on the use of antidepressants when trying to conceive.) If you normally see a therapist (or think you need to see one), a visit for a preconception screening is a good idea as well.

You can also take this opportunity to ask your practitioner any questions you might have.

See your dentist. Here's something to smile about: You're about to make a baby. But before that positive home pregnancy test has you beaming ear to ear, make sure your teeth and gums are ready for baby making by scheduling a checkup and teeth cleaning with your dentist. This may sound unrelated (after all, what do teeth have to do with making a baby?), but the fact is that gum disease is associated with pregnancy complications such as preterm labor, preeclampsia, and gestational diabetes. Gum disease also tends to get worse during pregnancy, so getting your mouth in shape now is more important than ever—especially since treating

TTC To-Do:

Before you start TTC in earnest, call for appointments with your gynecologist and your dentist (as well as any specialists and mental health providers as needed) to schedule thorough preconception checkups. If your gynecologist doesn't do ob or if you think you might want to go elsewhere for your prenatal care, start looking for an ob-gyn or midwife to copilot your pregnancy, and schedule that preconception checkup with your new practitioner. If you don't know where to start looking, check out *What to Expect When You're Expecting* for tips on choosing the pregnancy practitioner who's right for you.

gum disease before pregnancy may help reduce the risk of those complications. Be sure, too, to have any necessary work completed now, including x-rays, fillings, that crown you've been putting off, and gum or dental surgery, so you won't have to deal with it during pregnancy (or deal with an unpleasant infection from an untreated problem). If you know or suspect that you have dental problems that need treating, make sure you give yourself enough time to get the treatment finished up before you start TTC.

Immunizations

"Do I need to get any vaccines before I become pregnant?"

That depends on which ones you've already had, and when. So first, check out your vaccination records and be ready to share them with your practitioner. Did you get your full set of vaccines as a child? That's a good start, but doesn't mean you're off the immunization hook entirely. Some vaccines require boosters to keep immunities going strong. The blood tests (titers) taken at your preconception checkup will reveal if you already have all the antibodies against certain vaccine-preventable diseases needed to keep you and your baby-to-be healthy during pregnancy, and continue to offer some protection until your baby is old enough to be fully immunized (which, in the case of diseases like measles and chicken pox, won't be until your baby is at least 12 months old). If you do have the necessary levels of antibodies, you're probably good to go vaccine-wise. If your antibody levels are low or you have some immunization holes that need filling in, now—before your TTC campaign begins—is the time to roll up your sleeve for all necessary vaccinations (once you conceive, some vaccines will be off the table). Vaccines that might be on the preconception agenda include:

- Measles, mumps, rubella (MMR). If you know you've never had rubella, mumps, and measles or been immunized against this trio of serious childhood diseases, or if testing shows you are not fully immune (sometimes immunity wears off), get vaccinated now with the MMR vaccine and then wait 1 month before you start trying to conceive. If you do accidentally conceive sooner, don't worry—any risk is purely theoretical.

- Chicken pox (varicella). If testing shows that you don't have antibodies or if you've never had chicken pox (most women of childbearing age have either had it or been vaccinated against it), it's recommended that you be immunized against it prepregnancy, at least 1 month before you conceive. But once again, don't worry

if you get pregnant before the waiting period is up.

- Hepatitis B. If you're at high risk for hepatitis B and testing shows you're not immune, immunization for this disease is also recommended. The hep-B shots come in a series of 3, and if you don't finish up the series before you conceive, it's safe to continue it while you're expecting.

- HPV (human papillomavirus). If you're younger than 26, you should be vaccinated against HPV, but you'll need to finish the full series of 3 shots before trying to conceive. If you become pregnant before completing the full series, you'll have to resume the shots postpartum.

Whether or not you have to bare your arm for any vaccines now, keep in mind that you'll be advised to line up for your flu shot during pregnancy, and for a Tetanus-diphtheria-pertussis (Tdap) vaccine between weeks 27 and 36 (ideally, closer to 27 weeks) of each pregnancy, even if you've had the Tdap before.

Medications

"Will I have to stop using all medications once I'm trying to conceive, or can I wait until I get pregnant?"

It's time to take stock of your medicine cabinet, but not necessarily to clear it out. As you've already figured out, it won't be medications as usual once you're expecting. During pregnancy some of the drugs you occasionally or regularly reach for may be off limits, some may be limited, and still others may be yours for the taking, as needed. But what about the medications you take before you're expecting? Should you start thinking before you keep popping?

Zika and TTC

Something else to think about when prepping for conception: protecting yourself against Zika virus.

Zika virus is primarily spread through the bite of an infected mosquito. It can also be spread through unprotected vaginal, anal, or oral sex (as well as via sex toys) with a person who has Zika—and from an infected mother to her fetus during pregnancy. The symptoms of Zika virus are so mild that infection often goes undetected in those who have it, but sadly the same may not be true for a developing fetus exposed to the virus. When moms-to-be are infected with Zika virus during pregnancy, their babies could be born with microcephaly—a neurologic condition characterized by smaller than expected heads, incomplete brain development, and other severe brain defects. The infection may also be related to miscarriage and stillbirth.

How would you know if you contracted Zika virus? Chances are, you wouldn't. Although common symptoms of the virus include fever, rash, headaches, red eyes, and muscle and joint pain, many infected people do not experience noticeable symptoms, making an infection easy to miss. In other words, if you or your partner traveled to or live in an area where Zika virus is a risk, you might not know that you have the virus, and could potentially spread it to your baby during pregnancy.

But why worry about Zika now—before you even get pregnant? Here's why: From what is known about other infections (for example, rubella) during pregnancy, Zika virus may have the potential to stay in the blood system long enough to affect a fetus that hasn't even been conceived yet. That's why the Centers for Disease Control and Prevention (CDC) recommends that a woman who has been infected with or exposed to Zika virus (through travel to an area with a CDC-issued travel notice or through sex with an infected or exposed partner) wait at least 8 weeks after her symptoms start or after exposure before trying to conceive. And because Zika virus can stay in semen longer than it does in blood, it's recommended that men who have been infected with or exposed to the virus wait at least 6 months after their symptoms start or after exposure before trying to conceive. This means that if your partner has traveled (with or without you) to an area with a CDC Zika travel notice, you should wait at least 6 months after his return to start TTC. While in this holding pattern, he should use a condom for vaginal, anal, and oral sex to prevent spreading the virus to you.

Since the virus can also be spread by females to their sex partners, the CDC recommends that lesbian couples who are planning to conceive abstain from sex and postpone pregnancy for at least 8 weeks if one of the partners (or both) has traveled to or lives in an area with Zika virus or has Zika virus symptoms. A gay couple planning to conceive using sperm from one partner should also postpone those plans until 6 months after possible exposure to Zika

That'll depend on what you normally pop. Most over-the-counter and many prescription meds are considered safe while you're trying to conceive. Still, it's smart to get the green light on any medications or supplements (including vitamins and herbals) before you take them during the preconception period. That's because some (from opiods taken for chronic pain to herbals touted for fertility) may not only affect your future pregnancy, but also

6 months after possible exposure to Zika or 6 months after symptoms started, and use a condom in the meantime to avoid spreading the infection.

The CDC recommends that couples who are thinking about getting pregnant (or are pregnant) should avoid travel to any area where Zika virus is a risk. But what if you live in an area where Zika virus is a risk, or you can't postpone travel to an area with a CDC Zika travel notice?

The good news is there are ways to reduce the risk of getting bitten by Zika-carrying mosquitoes: Make sure that your home or hotel room has tight-fitting screens on windows to keep mosquitoes out, keep doors and windows closed, and run AC if you have it. Wear protective long-sleeved shirts and long pants, treat clothing with permethrin, and use an EPA-registered insect repellent with DEET, picaridin, IR3535, oil of lemon eucalyptus, para-menthane-diol, or 2-undecanone on exposed skin. When used as directed, these insect repellents are proven safe and effective, even for women who are TTC, pregnant, or breastfeeding. Since repellents with purified forms of plants such as citronella and cedar are not as effective as DEET or picaridin, don't rely on them if you're in an area at risk for Zika. Always apply repellent after you've applied sunscreen, and be prepared to reapply sunscreen more frequently because DEET decreases SPF. Products that combine repellent and sunscreen aren't recommended.

Wondering if you can be tested for Zika just so you can know for sure that it's safe to continue TTC? The CDC, several state and local health departments, and some commercial labs currently do blood testing for Zika virus. However, the CDC does not recommend Zika virus testing for TTC couples who might have been exposed to the virus but don't have any symptoms. One reason why: Because Zika virus can stay in some body fluids (like semen) for a longer time than it would show up in a blood test, testing a person who doesn't have any symptoms could provide falsely reassuring results suggesting no recent Zika infection—even when the person is actually infected. As of now, there's also no approved test for Zika in semen, and because semen can remain infected for 6 months, there's no way to know if a man is carrying the virus. Bottom line: There's no easy way to know for sure whether it's safe to TTC if you and/or your partner have traveled to or live in an area with a risk of Zika virus. To play it safe, the CDC suggests following the waiting period recommendations from health officials before trying for a baby. Not sure where that leaves you? Check with your doctor for more specific guidelines.

What if you (or your partner) has had a confirmed case of Zika in the past? From what is known about similar viruses (like measles and rubella), experts believe a past infection will likely confer lifetime immunity—which would mean that you couldn't contract Zika virus again if you've already had it. Again, check with your doctor.

For the latest information on Zika, check with your doctor and visit cdc.gov/zika.

your chances of getting pregnant in the first place. Even something as basic as antihistamines may compromise fertility, and for a very unexpected reason: As they dry out your nasal mucus, they could also dry out your cervical mucus.

Ask your gynecologist or prenatal practitioner (if you've chosen one) for help figuring out what's safe to take, what should be dropped while you're TTC and while you're pregnant (and, thinking way ahead, while you're breastfeeding), and what's fine while you're TTC but should be dropped or limited once you're officially expecting.

If you depend on prescription drugs to treat a chronic condition (like asthma, allergies, diabetes, depression, migraines, or any other), discuss your TTC and pregnancy medication options with the physician overseeing your care and with your gynecologist or ob-gyn. Together, you can come up with a plan that'll help keep you healthy, fertile, and ready to welcome a pregnancy. You might have to drop some drugs for as long as 6 months before conceiving (and, of course, while you're pregnant and while you're breastfeeding), but there are almost always safer alternatives you can switch to during your reproductive break.

For more information on vitamin supplements while you're trying to conceive, see page 69. For information on herbal medications, see page 133.

Antidepressants

"I've taken antidepressants for the past 5 years, and the meds have kept my depression under control. I worry about going off them, but I wonder if they're safe to keep taking while I'm TTC and beyond."

When it comes to life changes, there's probably no bigger one than having a baby—or even deciding to take the baby plunge. But if you suffer from depression or anxiety, you may be wondering not only how your baby plans might change your life, but how they'll affect your ability to handle life—especially if trying to become pregnant might mean giving up your antidepressants or anti-anxiety meds.

Happily, many safe options (including medication options) are available for expectant moms with depression, anxiety, and other mental health conditions, though your current treatment plan may need to be modified or changed entirely now that you're planning a pregnancy. In fact, stopping antidepressants or other meds that you really need—and slipping back into depression—can actually do you (and the baby you're hoping for) more harm than good. Being clinically depressed or extremely anxious during pregnancy can make you less likely to eat well, sleep well, or otherwise live a baby-friendly lifestyle. Studies show that women who suffer from untreated depression during pregnancy may have a greater chance of preterm delivery and are also at higher risk for postpartum depression, which can make it difficult for them to nurture, bond with, and enjoy their babies after they're born.

So before you consider tossing your meds, talk to both your prescribing doctor and your prenatal practitioner or gynecologist. Together, you can weigh the benefits of continuing medication against the potential risks. Some medications come with more risks, others with very few. Most SSRIs (selective serotonin reuptake inhibitors), such as Celexa, Prozac, and Zoloft, are generally considered good options during pregnancy. SNRIs (serotonin and norepinephrine reuptake inhibitors) such as Cymbalta and Effexor XR are also among the treatment options for moms-to-be. Wellbutrin isn't considered a first-choice medication during pregnancy but can be used if an expectant mom isn't responding to the other options.

Now, before you become pregnant, is definitely the best time to make any treatment changes. If you and your practitioners decide that you should wean yourself off your meds entirely, or gradually decrease your dose to a safer level, or try switching to a safer med, start at least 3 months before you begin trying to conceive so you've got plenty

Avoiding a Repeat

If you've had a previous pregnancy with any complications, or one that ended with a premature delivery or late-pregnancy loss, or if you've had multiple miscarriages, talk to your practitioner about any measures that can be taken now—before you start trying again—to head off a repeat. For example, weight loss, a healthy diet, and regular exercise can help prevent gestational diabetes, preeclampsia, and other pregnancy complications. Good preconception dental care may help avoid gum and tooth problems often aggravated by pregnancy hormones, and prepregnancy treatment of gum disease may reduce the risk of pregnancy complications. Staying on a gluten-free diet if you have doctor-diagnosed celiac disease may prevent pregnancy problems (as well as, possibly, fertility challenges) Taking progesterone supplements in the luteal phase (the second half) of your cycle if you have a history of early miscarriage may help prevent a future loss (see page 237 for more on preventing repeat miscarriages). In other words, there may be steps you can take now to help maximize the odds that your next pregnancy will be a healthy one.

of time to see how it goes—and how you're feeling. If you notice the signs of depression coming back—sleep and appetite changes, anxiety, inability to concentrate, mood swings, and lack of interest in sex (which definitely won't help your baby-making plans)—talk to your medical team again about trying a different approach. Also report to them any changes in your condition once you become pregnant. The hormonal upheavals of pregnancy trigger mood swings in every expectant mom, but depression or anxiety that's consistent and interferes with functioning isn't normal.

Keep in mind that there are plenty of alternative therapies—from psychotherapy (talk therapy) to bright light therapy, meditation to biofeedback to acupuncture—that can boost your emotional state naturally, and can be used instead of or in conjunction with medications. Experts also consider exercise an effective complement to other treatments for depression and anxiety, and a particularly healthy one, too, for women who are TTC or pregnant. Those feel-good endorphins released with a brisk walk, a swim, yoga, or another workout can do your body—and your mind—good. The right foods may boost your mood, too—including dark chocolate (the higher the cocoa content, the better the benefit) and walnuts (rich in omega-3 fatty acids). Ask, too, whether taking a pregnancy-safe omega-3 supplement might be helpful.

Genetic Screening

"Is genetic screening a good idea before we conceive—even if we don't have any reason to believe we're at increased risk?"

Every baby-to-be gets a set of genes from mom and dad, and just how those genes combine and reveal themselves helps determine whether a baby will have curly or straight hair, brown or blue eyes, athletic ability, musical mojo, a way with words, a flair for fashion, a knack for numbers. But something else that unique pairing of genes may determine: whether a baby will have a genetic disorder.

Checking Up on Dad

Making a healthy baby takes the participation of 2 healthy bodies. Sure, you're not going to be the one carrying the baby you're about to make together, but you will be contributing half of the essential genetic material that will make that baby. Your fertility will matter, too, when it comes to sealing the baby deal. To be sure your body is in prime baby-making condition—and to find out how to get it there if it isn't—make an appointment with your doctor for a top-to-bottom preconception checkup of your own. A thorough physical can detect any medical conditions (such as undescended testicles, testicular cysts or tumors, or depression) that might interfere with conception or a healthy baby, as well as ensure that any chronic conditions that might interfere with fertility (such as diabetes or celiac disease) are under control. While at the doctor's office, ask about the sexual side effects of any prescription, over-the-counter, or herbal drugs you are taking. Some of the commonly prescribed medications that could affect fertility, sperm count or quality, and/or libido include SSRIs like Prozac, beta blockers and other drugs for hypertension, some ulcer drugs, and some prescription painkillers (including opioids like oxycodone). Ditto for steroids and testosterone pills. They'll bulk you up but can significantly cut back sperm production. If any of the meds you take regularly are potentially fertility-unfriendly, talk to your doctor about changing your treatment plan to fit your baby plans. In most cases, a different medication will do the trick without tripping up your sperm. You should also join your partner for any genetic screening consultation (see page 13)—especially if you have a family history or other indication that calls for such testing.

Need to lose weight, get fit, start eating better, get blood pressure or blood sugar under control, catch up on immunizations, cut down on alcohol, or seek treatment for a condition that may stand between you and the baby you and your partner are planning—or even adversely affect that baby's future health? Now—before the baby making begins—is the time to do it all.

Just about everyone carries a gene for at least one genetic disorder. Fortunately, most disorders don't show up unless both parents contribute an identical abnormal gene—something that's statistically unlikely. Still, because knowing what your genetic carrier profile looks like before conception can offer not only a heads-up on potential problems but a broader range of options and more time to make decisions, experts recommend that one or both hopeful parents-to-be be offered genetic screening. Certainly if you or your partner have a family history of particular conditions, or are of certain ethnic backgrounds, screening is an extra-good idea—and a great way to put your mind at ease. Remember: Most genetic disorders are recessive. That means both you and your partner would have to test positive for your baby to be at any risk at all of being affected (so if one of you tests negative, there's usually no need for the other to be tested). Happily, screening results are almost always reassuring.

It's already recommended that all couples (regardless of ethnic background) be screened for cystic fibrosis, that African Americans be screened for sickle-cell anemia, that those of

Mediterranean and Asian descent be screened for thalassemia, and that those of French Canadian, Southern Louisiana Cajun, and Pennsylvania Dutch descent be screened for Tay-Sachs disease. For those of European Jewish (Ashkenazi) descent, routine screening is recommended for Tay-Sachs disease, Canavan disease, and familial dysautonomia (contact victorcenters.org or jscreen.org to learn more).

But new advances in genetic testing are enabling all couples, regardless of their genetic or geographical profile, to test for a broad array of genetic conditions before conceiving. Such so-called expanded carrier screening can screen for the carrier gene of more than 300 diseases, and it gives you the power of knowing whether you and your partner are at risk of passing along any genetic conditions to the baby you conceive together. Knowing in advance that you and your partner carry a significant risk of having a baby with a genetic disorder gives you the choice of using advanced reproductive techniques (like IVF with preimplantation genetic testing to screen embryos for the diseases before implantation; see the box on page 212) or considering sperm donation and other nontraditional routes to starting a family. Currently, the American College

of Obstetricians and Gynecologists (ACOG) and the American College of Medical Genetics and Genomics (ACMG) agree that all couples should be offered the option of having carrier screening before they start trying to conceive. But to reduce the potential emotional downside of screening, experts recommend that it be accompanied by counseling with a physician or geneticist who can explain exactly which disorders the expanded carrier screening panels test for. That way, couples can opt out of receiving test results they don't want to know about, that are not medically actionable (diseases for which there are no treatments or cures), or that have little clinical significance (genetic anomalies that don't have any health significance). ACMG adds that the carrier screen should test only for disorders that would be relevant for reproductive decision making and not include disorders that are adult onset (as some of the conditions in the 300 disease carrier screen are) unless the couple provides specific consent to screen for them all.

The best way to decide how to approach genetic screening is to talk over the options with your gynecologist or prenatal practitioner—and then to decide as a couple on the best screening strategy for you.

Your Lifestyle Prep

Next up in preconception prep: a look at your lifestyle. Now that you're talking baby, will you have to say "later" to your morning lattes—and "lights out" to your nightcaps? Will you have to work out less, or (shudder) more? Can you still spend time in hot water—or hot saunas and tanning beds? How about those highlights—will

making a baby send you back to your roots? In the case of some lifestyle choices, the choice will still be yours (at least until baby's on board). In the case of others (those 4-shot espresso drinks), some tweaking will definitely be on the menu (make half those shots decaf, and you're good to go TTC).

Caffeine

"Do I have to cut out coffee now that I'm trying to conceive?"

Crave that cappuccino? Must have that morning macchiato? There's no need to drop Joe from your life entirely now that you're making room for Junior. In fact, depending on how much coffee and other caffeinated beverages you depend on, you may be able to continue your caffeine habit as usual even as you're trying to conceive that baby, especially if you're a light coffee drinker.

Have a hefty habit? You'll probably have to trim it down to baby-making size. Not only because you'll have to cut back anyway once you're pregnant, but because keeping caffeine intake sensibly

moderate now may actually help you get pregnant—and stay pregnant. Some studies have linked too much caffeine consumption with lowered fertility and an increased risk of miscarriage.

What's too much caffeine when you're trying to conceive? Technically, more than 200 mg a day. Too technical for you? Here are some caffeine stats to help you see how your intake adds up. That 200 mg will buy you about 12 ounces of brewed coffee a day (that's a "tall" or 2 small cups), or about 2 shots of espresso (which is why 4-shot lattes will definitely put you over the top). A can of caffeinated diet cola will cost you an average of 45 mg, and a regular cola 35 mg. Tea contributes to that tally, too, with between 40 and 60 mg per cup (whether it's iced, brewed, or green), as do energy drinks (80 mg in a Red Bull), chocolate, and some over-the-counter cold, allergy, and pain meds. Even coffee ice cream or coffee yogurt packs a modest caffeine punch.

But here's some news that may lift your spirits, along with your sagging afternoon energy levels: You won't have to cut back any further on caffeine once baby's officially on board. Most experts believe that the same 200-mg-a-day limit is fine throughout pregnancy, when you'll need that energy more than ever.

If your calculations indicate that you'll need to do some cutting down on your caffeine, or if you'd like to cut it out altogether, slow is the way to go. Rather than shocking your system into extreme exhaustion (and lots of headaches and crankiness) by quitting abruptly, gradually lower your caffeine intake. Think baby steps. Substituting decaf for some of each cup you normally drink will start you on the weaning process. Keep reducing the amount of regular and increasing the amount of decaf until your ratio is where you'd like to see it. Or order your espresso

---

FOR DADS-TO-BE

Dear Joe

Wondering if you'll have to step away from the coffee bar now that you're stepping up to the baby-making plate? Some (happy) research suggests that a little caffeine in the hour or two before ejaculation may actually help sperm swim faster—and faster swimming sperm may be more likely to hit their target. But other research has found that wannabe dads who drink 1 or more energy drinks (or other caffeinated beverages, including coffee and soda) per day have a lowered chance of conception in any given cycle compared with men who skip energy and caffeinated drinks altogether. Want to give your baby-making efforts the best shot? Keep those shots of espresso to a minimum and your overall caffeine intake moderate (no more than 2 cups of Joe per day) until your conception mission is accomplished.

TTC To-Do:

Baby in your plans? Time to put less coffee in your cup. While you're TTC (and expecting, too), limit your caffeine intake to no more than 200 mg per day. That's equivalent to a daily total of about 2 small cups of brewed coffee or about 4 diet colas. A bonus of cutting down on caffeine: You'll be more relaxed—a definite plus when it comes to conception.

drinks with 1 shot of regular, another (or another 2) of decaf. Eyeing that large coffee? Order a small in a large cup, then fill it to the rim with milk. You'll cut down on your caffeine while scoring a calcium bonus (and calcium is something you'll need to be getting more of, anyway).

Eating smaller, more frequent mini-meals containing some protein and complex carbs will keep your blood sugar up—and that will help lift your energy level during this possibly challenging transition. Your daily prenatal vitamin (see page 69) will also help you fill in some of the energy blanks without a caffeine fix, as will regular exercise.

Herbal Tea

"I'm not a coffee drinker, but I love herbal tea. Is it okay for me to keep drinking it when I'm trying for a baby?"

That depends on what you're brewing. Most commercial herbal teas are considered safe to drink both during pregnancy and the preconception period (for instance, peppermint, citrus, and ginger), but others may not be.

How do you pick a brew that's right for you while you're trying to conceive? Since there aren't many studies on the safety of herbal teas, it isn't easy. Check with your prenatal practitioner or an herb-knowledgeable medical doctor who knows that you're trying to get pregnant for a list of herbs to avoid. Among those usually making the no-go list are red raspberry leaf, southernwood, wormwood, mugwort, barberry, tansy, mandrake root, juniper, pennyroyal, nutmeg, arbor vitae, and senna. Screen for those red flag ingredients—as well as any that you're just not sure about—by reading the packaging carefully before buying (or brewing) an herbal tea.

Teas that are touted as fertility or pregnancy brews should also get the screening. Because the Food and Drug Administration (FDA) doesn't regulate these claims, it's a case of drinker beware. If there isn't any packaging (as in bulk teas sold at health food markets) or list of ingredients, play it safe and skip it for now. For more on the safety of herbs when you're TTC, see page 133.

Thinking of Going Green?

That cup of green tea may be brimming with health benefits, but should you go green-crazy when you're trying to make a baby? Maybe not. Green tea (including the Matcha varieties) decreases the effectiveness of folic acid (ironically, found in green leafy vegetables), a vitamin that's vital to the healthy development of your soon-to-be baby and one of the nutrients that you should be getting your quota of during your baby-prep phase. So it's smart to limit yourself to a cup a day (or a glass of iced) while you're TTC, or to switch to a black brew.

No need to read the tea leaves—or the tea leaf boxes—if you choose a traditional black tea, like Earl Grey or English Breakfast. Those are safe to sip, as long as you keep an eye on your total caffeine tally—remember that each cup of caffeinated black tea will cost you 40 to 60 mg of your 200 mg daily limit.

Drinking

"I know I have to stop drinking once I get pregnant, but we just started trying—and holiday season is coming up. Can I keep drinking a little until I get pregnant?"

If you're planning for a baby, you're probably already planning to change your drink order from cocktail to mocktail. But when exactly should you start putting that new order in? There aren't any hard and fast rules about alcohol drinking when you're in the TTC stage like there are during pregnancy (when most experts recommend total teetotaling). It is known, however, that heavy drinking can mess with your menstrual cycle, possibly interfering with ovulation and making it more difficult for a fertilized egg to implant in the uterus—and that can definitely put a crimp in your conception plans. And the more alcohol you consume, some research suggests, the less likely it is that you'll become pregnant. In fact, research has shown that even modest use of alcohol (5 drinks a week or less) can increase the time it takes to achieve conception.

What about a glass of bubbly with your brunch or a beer with your barbecue? What if you can't imagine ending the day without a nightcap? How about that holiday eggnog, now that you've got a different kind of egg on your mind? And what if it takes a few months to conceive—wouldn't all that

---

FOR DADS-TO-BE

Booze and Your Boys

Hoping to toast some big baby news soon? Cheers to that. But while you're waiting for that news to come through, you might actually want to taper off on your toasts. Too much alcohol (as you may have been disappointed to discover at one point or another) can impair a guy's sexual function—a function you're now counting on. But worse than that, research indicates that daily heavy drinking can damage sperm as well as reduce their number (in some men, even 1 or 2 beers or glasses of wine is enough to temporarily keep the number of boys down). Too many rounds on a regular basis can also alter testicular function and reduce testosterone levels (not a good scenario when you're trying to make a baby). Heavy drinking (equivalent to 2 drinks a day or 5 drinks in one sitting even once a month) by the dad-to-be during the month before conception could also affect a baby's birthweight. So for best baby-making results, your best bet is to drink only occasionally and lightly—or if you find that hard to do, cut it out altogether for now. And because the future mom in your life will also be laying off the libations as she gets her body ready for the long and happy baby haul ahead, those cutbacks will probably be easier to make (besides, no fair guzzling Guinness when she's sipping sparkling water).

preconception abstaining be kind of wasted (especially with 9 dry months ahead of you)?

Well, maybe. But here's the reason you might want to put in that mocktail order sooner rather than later. The timing of conception isn't a precise science. Since you won't be getting a "stop drinking" notification from your body the moment sperm and egg seal the deal—and chances are you won't have that fertilization heads-up for a couple of weeks after that momentous moment occurs—it's probably best to call it quits (or start cutting back a lot) once you're actively trying to get that baby on board. If you do opt to keep sipping in the meantime, sip with care. Drink only occasionally and lightly—preferably with a side of food to slow the absorption of alcohol into your system.

Smoking

"I'm planning to stop smoking once I become pregnant—but can I keep smoking until I do?"

Now's the time to kick butt. Smoking poses a whole pack of risks not only during pregnancy, but before—the most significant risk being that you'll have trouble getting and staying pregnant. Smoking can age your eggs (meaning that a 30-year-old smoker's eggs may act more like 40-year-old eggs), making conception more difficult, lowering the odds that a fertilized egg will implant in your uterus, and making miscarriage more likely. What's more, heavy smoking damages the ovaries as well as the uterus, potentially reducing fertility even further—and probably explaining why smokers are 4 times more likely to take longer than a year to become pregnant. A smoke-free womb is the very best gift you can give your baby-to-be, but kicking the habit now will make it

FOR DADS-TO-BE

Butt Out, Dad

Are you a sworn smoker? It's time to swear off smoking, once and for all. Not only can your smoking be harmful to your partner's fertility, but it can lower your sperm count, lower the quality of your sperm by damaging its DNA—and overall lower the chances that you'll make a healthy baby together. Plus, after baby's on board, secondhand smoke can hamper your little one's development. Same is true of e-cigarettes, vape pens, hookahs, and so-called thirdhand smoke (the kind that lingers on clothes and hair, even if you're doing your smoking outside). Once baby has arrived, your smoking can pose significant health risks to that precious new bundle.

If you both smoke, commit to quitting as a team. If you're the sole smoker in the house, call it quits now. Easier said than done? For sure, but you can do it—and the tips in the box on page 20 can help.

more likely you'll conceive that baby-to-be sooner.

Pretty much the same applies to e-cigarettes, vape pens, and hookahs. Electronic cigarettes, which claim to have significantly fewer toxins and lower nicotine than traditional cigarettes, still have enough nicotine to affect your eggs and your fertility. Even the additives and flavorings used in many e-cigarettes could be questionable when you're thinking about a baby. Ditto for hookahs. Smoking a hookah—in which the smoke from specially made tobacco passes through water and is then drawn through a rubber hose to a mouthpiece—is as toxic as smoking a cigarette.

Calling It Quits

Need to clean house of all your unhealthy habits now that you're planning to fill that house with a baby? A smoke-free womb is a very good place to start—but you may be wondering exactly how to get started, not to mention finished. Here's how:

Give yourself props. The first thing you need to do is pat yourself on the back—or on the belly you're dreaming of filling—for taking this momentous step, as daunting as it probably is. Accept that the road ahead won't be without its bumps, but try to remind yourself that the baby bump you'll hopefully be sporting soon will make your efforts more than worthwhile.

Choose your method. Will it be cold turkey or gradual tapering off? You know your body and your willpower best, so choose the method of withdrawal that you think you can live with.

Pick a day, any day . . . soon. Whether you're doing cold turkey or going gradually, pick a "last day" that you can stick to. Be realistic: Stay away from high-stress periods (say, performance review week at the office) or a time of the month when your willpower is typically challenged enough. But also don't put your last day of smoking too far off in the future—remember, the faster you quit, the faster you may be able to make your baby dreams come true. Mark the day on your calendar and make it count. Instead of thinking of it as the end of smoking, think of it as the beginning of a smoke-free life. Plan a busy schedule for that day, preferably full of fun activities you don't associate with smoking, in places that don't allow smoking. Involve nonsmoking family and friends, and treat the day as a celebration (which it is!).

Tell all your friends. It'll be easier to stay honest about quitting if you don't keep your plans a secret. So let everyone in your life who cares about you know that you're about to embark on your quitting campaign, and that they can help you stay on course by cheering you on and supporting you (read: not nagging).

Do a cleanse. Get rid of all the cigarettes, ashtrays, lighters, and other smoking supplies you have around the house, in your car, in your handbags, at your office. If you smoke in your car, get the interior deep-cleaned so it, too, gets a fresh start. Get your teeth cleaned (a smart idea in preconception, anyway). And clean up your act in other ways, too—start drinking lots of water and stock up on healthy snacks.

Beat back withdrawal. Since nicotine is an addictive drug, withdrawal symptoms are common, and can include irritability, anxiety, restlessness, tingling or numbness in the hands and feet, light-headedness, headaches, fatigue, trouble sleeping or focusing, and tummy troubles. Symptoms can start within just a few nicotine-free hours and usually get as bad as they're going to get by the second or third day, but they gradually ease up, and should be mostly gone after about 5 smoke-free weeks. Eating regularly and well (grazing on protein and complex carbs will keep you feeling your emotional and physical best), getting some exercise daily, and staying away from excesses of caffeine and sugar (which can make you more jittery) may help while your body adjusts.

Sublimate and substitute. Figure out what you can swap those cigarettes for. If it's about oral gratification, chew gum, crunch on carrot sticks, or suck on a straw, a lollipop, or even a cinnamon stick. If you smoke for stress relief, try other ways of chilling out during times of high anxiety—meditation, deep breathing, listening to music, a swim or a workout, a warm bath, a massage (and maybe some post-massage sex). If you smoke to keep your hands busy, hold a pen between your smoking fingers, fiddle with a fidget cube or worry beads, squeeze a stress ball or some play clay, doodle, knit, or open some game apps.

Be tough. Cheer yourself on, but also know when you need a kick in the butt, too. Try telling yourself that stopping smoking is nonnegotiable. When you were a smoker, you couldn't smoke in a movie theater or a restaurant or at the office—now you can't smoke at all, period.

Picture your baby. Whenever you feel like reaching for a cigarette (or whenever you're feeling sorry for yourself or sick from withdrawal symptoms), close your eyes and picture the baby of your dreams, cradled in your arms. Or browse baby sites. Another reminder of your mission might help, too—a special bracelet, for instance, or a locket you'll be able to fill later.

Don't play with fire (or smoke). Stay away from smokers and smoky locales—and even from places where you can buy cigarettes. For inspiration, visit with friends and family who don't allow smoking in their homes. If you associate a certain activity or a certain food or drink with smoking, keep them off the agenda and off the menu for now.

Enlist help. It'll be easier to take one for Team Baby if your team has plenty of support. Turn to friends who've felt your withdrawal pain. Look for empathy and advice from ex-smokers or co-quitters online, particularly on TTC message boards (check out WhatToExpect.com). If your partner also has to quit, join forces and quit together. If you're comfortable with a group approach to quitting, consider programs run by Nicotine Anonymous, the American Lung Association, the American Cancer Society, and SmokEnders, which have helped millions of smokers break the habit. Check out smokefree.gov or cdc .gov/tobacco/quit_smoking for more information and help.

CAM do. Lots of smokers have become ex-smokers with the help of such complementary and alternative (CAM) therapies as acupuncture, aromatherapy, and meditation. Hypnosis can be especially effective in conquering those cravings.

See your doctor. You may get more than a pep talk (though that could help, too). Your doctor can also prescribe a medication, such as Chantix or Zyban, or recommend a nicotine patch, gum, or lozenge (if you haven't already tried nicotine-replacement therapies) to fast-track your quitting campaign so you can start your TTC campaign sooner. All of these options work best when they're used as part of a smoking-cessation program (you'll find plenty of those online). To get one-on-one counseling, call 800-QUIT-NOW—you'll be routed to your state's quitline.

Don't overwhelm your willpower. Need to quit smoking, but also need to drop a few pounds before you begin baby-making? Don't try to take on both campaigns at once—that will only make you more likely to fail at both. Smoking is potentially more harmful to your fertility and your future baby than those extra pounds, so cut that out before you get serious about cutting calories. But do try to begin eating more healthfully, if you can—nutritious foods can help sustain you best when willpower gets wobbly.

Take one day at a time. Think about the weeks of withdrawal ahead of you, and you'll make yourself crazy. Instead, take 1 day—or even 1 hour—at a time. Each time you pass another 24-hour smoke-free day, commemorate it on your calendar or post about it on social media, and give yourself a nightly round of applause.

Try, try again. If you slip up and have a cigarette, put it behind you right away. Don't give a second thought to the cigarette you smoked—think instead about all the ones you passed up (and will pass up). Get right back on your program, knowing that every cigarette you don't smoke gets you closer to your goal. And whatever you do, don't give up. You can do it—and you've never had a better reason to!

Despite what you may have heard, the water in the hookah does not filter out the toxic ingredients (like tar, carbon monoxide, and heavy metals) in the tobacco smoke. And what's worse, hookah smokers may actually breathe in more nicotine than cigarette smokers do because of the large volume of smoke they inhale during a smoking session.

Does your partner smoke cigarettes (or any of the above)? It's time for him to quit, too—and it will be easier if you join forces and quit together. Exposure to secondhand smoke is just as hazardous to your fertility and your baby's future health as smoking is. In fact, just spending time in a smoky room or with smokers who have tobacco byproducts lingering on their clothes, hair, and skin (thirdhand smoke) can harm your health, your fertility, and your future family. To tip the conception odds in your favor, stay as far away from smoke as you can.

Marijuana

"I've heard that marijuana can affect a guy's sperm, but is there any reason why I can't use it while I'm trying to conceive?"

H is sperm, his responsibility? Actually, not always. Though they're created in your partner's body, once his sperm have entered your body, they can be impacted by conditions there. What that means in terms of your marijuana use, believe it or not: It can adversely affect the ability of your partner's sperm to fertilize an egg—even if he doesn't partake (or never did). That's because THC—the active ingredient in marijuana—shows up in your vaginal fluids and reproductive organs (including your vagina, fallopian tubes, and uterus). When the sperm arrive, they've got the urge to merge with your egg, but can fail on follow-through because the

TTC To-Do:

N ow that you've learned some of the major don'ts of the preconception period (don't overdo the caffeine, don't drink a lot or at all, don't smoke, don't use drugs), you may be feeling a little daunted by the work you do have ahead of you (especially if you have some significant quitting to do). Habits, especially long-standing or hefty ones, can be hard to break—no matter how motivating that healthy baby reward might be. If you're having an especially hard time breaking a habit (like smoking or taking prescription painkillers) that might impair your fertility or put the baby you've been hoping for at risk (or both), get the help you need as soon as you can. Talk to your doctor and ask for advice and a referral, if needed, to an addiction specialist. Join local support groups or online ones for the camaraderie and help. A little company might provide all the motivation you need.

THC they've been exposed to impairs their normal function, possibly making these under-the-influence sperm too sluggish to get the very challenging job of fertilization done. The THC stays in your system, too, which means that avoiding a slacker sperm problem isn't as easy as skipping a smoke just before you start trying to conceive.

Clearly, pot smoking (or vaporizing or use of edibles) and baby making don't mix. Though you may conceive even if you do continue to ingest THC while you're TTC, it's also possible that your fertility will be compromised. Plus, while the risks of continuing weed use during pregnancy aren't fully documented, there's some evidence that THC may affect fetal brain

Say No to Weed
Before You Say Yes to a Wee One

Thought you were the only one getting stoned when you smoked? Actually, your boys are, too. According to research, the sperm of pot smokers don't behave the way they're supposed to or the way they need to in order to be good little fertilizers. Though sperm normally get washed into the cervix, going along for the ride until they approach their target (when the strength they've saved up is used to swim to the egg and forcefully penetrate its hard shell), sperm under the influence of THC (the active ingredient in marijuana) swim frantically at first, then fizzle out by the time they reach Egg Land. Sluggish and unmotivated, they're less likely to get the job done—or even to be in the right place at the right time. Meaning they can get wasted—and then wasted.

What's more, THC can cut the total number of boys on your swim team, sometimes significantly. It lowers levels of testosterone, that all-important hormone of male reproduction, and can reduce sperm count as well as the amount of seminal fluid. Though it's definitely possible for weed users to conceive a baby (even without trying), it's clear that smoking (or vaporizing, or eating) weed does handicap fertility—which means THC could put a dent in a guy's TTC plans, especially if he already has a borderline fertility issue. Passing on pot just before you have sex doesn't alleviate these fertility challenges, since THC can stay in your system, stored in your body fat, for a surprisingly long time. So aim to quit entirely now—before your sperm start aiming for that egg. Say good-bye to weed so you can say hello to a healthy baby, and seek professional help if you have trouble doing it alone.

development. To be on the safe side—and the most fertile side—now's the smart time to start passing on pot.

It may go without saying, but it needs to be said anyway: Using any illicit drug, including cocaine, crack, or heroin, can make conception more difficult and pregnancy much more risky, for both mother and baby. So can abuse of some prescription drugs. If you need help breaking any addiction, seek it before you begin your baby-making efforts.

Exercise

"I'm a bit of a fitness fanatic, and I work out just about every day. Is it okay to keep that up while I'm trying to get pregnant?"

You don't have to be fit to be fertile (and lots of women conceive without ever putting in a single day at the gym), but it may help. In fact, research has suggested that some laps around the track—or in the pool, or even around the mall—can put you on the right preconception track. A moderate exercise program that promotes overall fitness (about 30 minutes a day of aerobic exercise, strength training, stretching, and/or daily activities that get your heart going) can boost fertility, just as being in overall good health can. This may be especially true if you're packing a few extra preconception pounds you're trying to lose to increase your odds of conception (and to improve your overall health). And that's not all: The right

TTC To-Do:

It's time to exercise your right to make a baby. And there's no better place to start than exercising. Aim for 30 minutes a day combined of aerobics (to get your heart pumping), strength training (to tone your muscles), and stretching (to get yourself in shape for the pregnancy to come). No need to become an Olympic athlete, but the better shape you're in, the better your chances for conception and a healthy pregnancy.

kind of exercise helps release those feel-good endorphins, making your mind and body feel their relaxed best—which, in turn, can make baby-making efforts more productive (relaxation is a key component of any conception campaign; see page 30).

That said, you can get too much of a good thing when it comes to exercise and the conception connection. Take exercise to the extreme and your workouts may actually work against your fertility. Regular prolonged strenuous exercise can disrupt the delicate balance of hormones needed for ovulation and conception, especially if it reduces your body fat too much (some body fat is needed to keep those female reproduction functions functioning). While there are no hard-and-fast rules about how hard or fast you should exercise when you're trying to conceive, research indicates that more than 4 to 5 hours a week of vigorous exercise can lower your fertility by at least 30 percent. Clearly, if your exercise routine has been keeping you from having regular periods, conception will be challenging, at best. Even if your periods seem to be regular, a very strenuous workout routine may throw hormone levels off

enough to interfere with ovulation or implantation. If that appears to be the case with you, your body may need to slow down—and maybe trade in some of those cut muscles for a little maternal padding—before it can trade in those toned abs for a baby bump.

What's the best workout plan when you're planning a baby? Keep it moderate, keeping in mind that what's moderate for you might depend on your current fitness level. For a hard-core athlete, a 5-mile run may be like a walk in the park—but for a confirmed couch potato, even that walk in the park might be challenging for starters. Though many women maintain a rigorous routine and conceive easily, others find that they need to cut back a little, or a lot. Not sure whether your workout will work with your TTC plans? Check with your practitioner.

Keep it cool, too—avoid overheating when you work out (or anytime). Raising your core temperature excessively (to 102°F or above) isn't harmful to your fertility, but it can be harmful to your pregnancy—and when you're actively trying to become pregnant, you won't know right away when you've succeeded. It doesn't mean that you can't work up a sweat, just that you shouldn't exercise in hot environments (which means Bikram yoga is out for now).

And speaking of yoga, keep your workout relaxing. Choose one that's noncompetitive, that conditions your whole body and gets your heart pumping, that's stress reducing, and that's pregnancy appropriate (so that you'll likely be able to stick with it after you conceive). Yoga definitely comes to mind (and spirit)—and it seems to provide an especially beneficial pre- and post-conception workout because it focuses not only on relaxation breathing but also on body awareness (and this is definitely one time you want to be

FOR DADS-TO-BE

Your Workout and the Baby Race

Will your workout routine have to take a hit now that you're about to play in the baby-making big leagues? That depends. Participating in any kind of rough sports (including football, rugby, soccer, basketball, hockey, baseball, and horseback riding) without wearing protective gear to prevent injury to your genitals tops the list of must-don'ts, for obvious reasons (you'll need those genitals in their best operating order). Too much cycling (and that includes spin class or cycling on the stationary bike) also makes that list because the constant pressure from a bicycle seat on the genitals may, according to some experts, damage essential reproductive arteries and nerves. Occasional leisurely bike rides are probably not a problem, but more than 12 hours a week in the saddle (including the horseback-riding kind), especially if you're mountain biking—and you could be spinning your fertility wheels.

And though a regular workout routine probably boosts your fertility by boosting your testosterone levels (a good reason to hit the gym before you hit the sheets), it's probably smart not to take it to the max when you're trying to maximize your baby-making potential. Heavy-duty workouts that leave you exhausted can actually change your hormone levels and lower your sperm count—plus put you in the mood to collapse on the couch, not for love. Ditto for hot yoga or other workouts—and post-workout hot tubs, saunas, or steam rooms—that overheat you (and those precious family jewels).

Are spectator sports more your speed? You might want to jump in the game, or at least find your way to the gym or the running trails, now that you're trying to make a baby. Guys who don't work out at all—especially if they're also sporting plenty of extra padding—may be more likely to encounter fertility challenges than guys who are more fit.

---

aware of your body). It's good for overall body toning, but it's not physically draining—plus it's very low impact. What's more, the meditation you'll do during a yoga session may help you chill out, too. Finally, yoga can increase flexibility, so you'll be able to wrap yourself into some more interesting baby-making positions.

Yoga not your thing? Try swimming, dancing, Pilates, mild cardio workouts, light weight training, stationary bicycling, and other low-impact workouts—all of which are not only TTC appropriate but pregnancy appropriate, which means you'll likely be able to stick with the routine of your choice once you're exercising for two.

Hot Tubs

"I heard it's not safe to use a hot tub when TTC. Why's that?"

You heard right—sort of. The no-hot-tub recommendation is actually aimed at the hopeful dad in your life, because he needs to keep his nether regions cool to keep them reproductively functional (see box, page 26). As for you, it's safe to take the plunge before you've conceived (and the heat won't affect your chances of conceiving). But once baby's on board, you'll need to keep your cool, too, staying out of hot tubs, saunas, and other environments (like tanning beds) that can overheat. Because you never know for sure

Keep Your Cool, Dad

There's nothing more relaxing after a long day or a long workout session (and nothing more mood enhancing before a baby-making session) than a soak in a hot tub. But, sad to say, a hot tub can put your baby-making plans in hot water. Male fertility plunges with frequent dips in the hot tub, because sperm production is impaired when the testicles become overheated. That's why your testicles hang low—they prefer to be a couple of degrees cooler than the rest of the body. So hot tubs, steam rooms, and saunas (and even electric blankets or exercise that excessively raises your core body temperature) are off limits until mission conception has been accomplished. The same can be said about tanning beds, which send your body temperature soaring while they bake your skin (plus set you up for premature aging of the skin and a significantly increased risk of skin cancer—so who needs them, anyway?).

when that sperm and egg will actually get together, you might want to play it extra safe during the active TTC phase by sticking to warm tubs.

Skin Care

"Are there any skincare products I should stay away from while I'm trying to conceive?"

Face the happy face facts: There are very few skincare products or procedures (from the serums you slather on each night to the wrinkle injections you may be eyeing) that are off limits when you're TTC. In fact, you might as well indulge now—once baby's on board, many of your favorite treatments (including Botox and fillers, chemical peels, lasers, and a variety of skincare products) may need to be shelved.

But there is one very significant exception to this full-access skincare pass during the preconception period. The acne treatment Accutane can cause serious damage to a developing fetus. It's strictly off limits not only during pregnancy, but for at least a month before you begin trying to conceive

(stay on those 2 forms of birth control required with Accutane until that waiting period is over). Topical Retin-A, which is prescribed for both zit zapping and wrinkle smoothing, usually gets the red light during pregnancy and may, too, once you're officially TTC.

If pimples are your problem, you can try to keep your complexion all clear with over-the-counter and prescription-strength topical acne fighters (including some that may have to stay out of reach during pregnancy). It'll also pay to learn more about natural tactics for taming breakouts, since you'll likely be relying on them more once you're officially expecting: Eat well (a diet filled with fruits, vegetables, whole grains, and healthy fats may help keep your skin clear, while a diet high in sugar, refined foods, and saturated fat may make it more pimple-prone), keep your face clean, and follow every wash with an oil-free moisturizer.

As for those wrinkles you'd rather do without, treat away for now (some treatments will be tabled after you've successfully conceived). Just keep in mind that because fill-ups or followups won't be possible once you're expecting, the

Time for a Mommy Makeover?

Have your heart set on a new set of veneers? Or a brightened, whitened smile? Or maybe it's laser eye surgery you'd like—the better to see your baby with once he or she is a bundle on your lap and not just a gleam in your eye? Whatever elective procedure you've elected to try, you'll need to consider timing when you're TTC. Most cosmetic dentistry procedures (like veneers and whitening) aren't recommended during pregnancy—so you'll want to have your smile adjustment completed before baby's on board. As for laser eye surgery, not only isn't this procedure recommended during pregnancy, it's not recommended for 6 months before pregnancy and 6 months after giving birth. So if you're actively trying already, you'll need to stick with the glasses or contacts until halfway through baby's first year (or 6 months after you stop breastfeeding).

And just in case you're wondering, before-baby isn't the time to consider breast augmentation or reduction. After all, your breasts will be seeing enough changes in the 9 months after conception and then in the months after birth, especially if you'll be breastfeeding (and in fact, some breast surgery can impact your ability to breastfeed exclusively). If you're thinking about making any surgical adjustments, consider waiting until your baby-making days are behind you.

effects will likely wear off before you can safely repeat the procedures. Ask your practitioner about any that you're unsure of—and if you don't get the go-ahead, look at the bright side. Once you're pregnant, you'll be retaining enough fluid to fill in all those laugh lines—without a drop of collagen or Botox.

Hair Care

"What about hair coloring—do I have to quit that now, too?"

Ah, what moms won't do for their babies—even before they're moms. From giving up their favorite beverage to selecting a salad (when they'd really rather choose a large fries) to skipping their regular hair-coloring appointments, hopeful moms-to-be will do (or not do) just about anything it takes to get pregnant and have a healthy baby.

Fortunately, when it comes to hair maintenance, no preconception sacrifices are necessary. There's absolutely no reason why you have to revert to your roots or give up those straightening treatments or perms while you're trying to conceive. In fact, there isn't even any consensus about whether coloring or other chemical processes should stay off the salon menu once you're expecting (most doctors either green-light coloring or ask that you hold off until the second trimester).

If you feel more comfortable quitting your coloring once you're actively trying to conceive—because you never know when you're going to hit baby bingo—go ahead. You might want to change your routine anyway (based on your practitioner's advice) now that you're looking to get pregnant. Processes that are mostly natural or that don't come into contact with the scalp, such as highlights or lowlights, are widely considered safe. So rather than have roots to contend with in a couple of months, consult with your

A Preconception Day at the Spa

Looking for a way to chill out before baby making heats up in the bedroom? Melt tension and stress away with a good massage or another spa indulgence. There's nothing on the spa menu that's off limits while you're prepping for pregnancy, so detox and de-stress to your soul's content. A little relaxation might even bring you closer to your baby-making goal, since too much stress can actually hamper fertility.

Once you're actively TTC, you might want to play it extra safe by skipping treatments that raise your temperature significantly—just in case sperm and egg have already met up.

stylist about a prepregnancy hair color plan that will blend in with those pregnancy guidelines.

Tanning

"Can I continue going tanning while TTC?"

There is a dark side to preconception tanning. While there isn't any proof that tanning can keep you from reaching your fertility goals (no evidence exists on either side, actually), tanning beds can raise your body temperature to a level that can be dangerous to your developing baby when you do conceive—and there's no way of telling when you'll conceive once you begin actively trying. Plus, tanning beds aren't good for your skin or your health in general (think extra wrinkles and significantly increased risk for skin cancer).

Still a fan of the tan? Sunless tanning lotions and sprays are most likely a safe bet while you're TTC—check with your practitioner for specifics.

Stress

"I'm a stresser by nature, so naturally I'm already wondering whether stress is going to affect my chances of getting pregnant. Help!"

Don't stress about your stress. Scientists are still trying to make sense out of the stress-conception connection, but studies so far have linked only extreme stress to fertility difficulties—and that's not the kind of stress that most women have (even big-time stressers like you).

How exactly does excessive stress impact fertility? Potentially, in several ways. First, being under lots of stress can cause the brain to release neurotransmitters that affect the hormones controlling ovulation—which in turn can delay or disrupt ovulation. In fact, women who are under extreme emotional stress sometimes don't ovulate at all, even if they're getting their periods regularly. Second, extreme stress can cause fertile cervical mucus (the thin mucus that helps sperm swim to their target) to dry up altogether—making it difficult not only to pinpoint ovulation but also to conceive. And perhaps the most obvious reason why a super-stressed life can put a crimp in conception plans: Too much stress can keep couples from having frequent-enough sex, which is key, after all, to getting pregnant.

Fortunately, the body is really good at adapting to just about everything—including stress. Average everyday stress is probably something your body's already used to, which means that if your stress is manageable, it's not likely to be affecting your fertility. And even if the normal stress in your life—especially once it's combined with the potential stress of TTC—does seem to mess with your cycles (you don't seem to be ovulating on time, or your periods are less regular than usual), there's still no reason to stress over it. Chances are that as your body and mind learn to deal with the monthly challenge of TTC, they'll get used to this new, more stressed reality—and your cycles will normalize accordingly.

But that doesn't mean you should keep the stress up—at least not at levels that are stressing you out. Learning how to reduce stress now can help you in your conception quest and help you handle the (happy) stress that inevitably comes with pregnancy and parenting later. So relax, take a deep breath, and check out these de-stressing tips:

- Schedule in a chill pill. Yes, one of the reasons you're probably stressed is there's not enough time in the day (especially once you've added in all those TTC activities). Still, making time for occasional R&R breaks can really pay off, not only in helping you de-stress, but also in helping you be more productive in everything else you're doing—including all that baby-making sex. So take those breaks, and do whatever relaxes you. Read a few pages of a book you're enjoying, binge-watch your favorite TV series, play games on your phone, let loose on a fidget cube, or catch up on the latest celebrity shenanigans on a gossip site. Listen to music that soothes your soul—or to nature sounds, if that's what gets your calm to kick in. Take up knitting—a great way to unwind and hone your skills for those booties you may want to start whipping up soon. Start keeping a journal or scrapbooking or blogging your baby-making journey. Or just take a walk.

FOR DADS-TO-BE

Chill Out Before Things Heat Up

Stress can keep a good man down, at least when it comes to fertility. Too much stress can, as you probably already know, limit libido and bring down the curtain on performance—but it can also lower testosterone levels and sperm production. So after a busy day, and before you get busy—unwind a little (or a lot), using the tips on these pages or your own best stress busters. The less you worry about conceiving, the more easily you're likely to conceive.

- Cut back where you can. If you're like most women, you've probably got a lot on your plate—make that way too much. So try to cut back on those heaping servings of stressful activities, starting with those that aren't high priority (this is something you're going to have to do big time, anyway, once you have a new top priority: a new baby). Obviously, your baby-making activities are high on your to-do list now, so rather than trying to squeeze them into a too-tight schedule—which is only going to make doing them more stressful—decide which other responsibilities can be postponed or delegated to someone else. Learn to say no to new projects before you reach overload (another skill you're wise to cultivate pre-baby). If your job is adding to an unmanageable stress level and seems to be affecting your TTC plans, see if there are reasonable ways to reduce workplace stress. If not, a change to a less stressful job or career path might be something to consider now (finances and opportunities permitting), before pregnancy weighs you down. Just make sure there are no lapses in your health insurance coverage during that transition—definitely a stressful situation you'll want to avoid at any cost, especially when you're expecting to expect. You'll need maternity coverage to be in place before you TTC.

- Unload whenever you can. Of course, the TTC process can be an emotional roller-coaster ride—you're up (maybe we did it this time!), you're down (my period . . . again?). Letting those letdown feelings out is the best way to make sure they don't keep you down. So vent away. Start with your partner: Try to spend some time at the end of each day sharing feelings that need to find the nearest exit—you might be surprised to hear that he's feeling some of the same baby frustrations you are (just don't bring those feelings

TTC To-Do:

So you know you should lead a less stressful life, especially now that you want a baby in your life. One way to bring on the relaxation whenever and wherever: breathing exercises. Breathing is quick, it's free, and you have to do it anyway, so you might as well do it in a way that's relaxing. Pause a moment any time you're feeling hyped up (heck, pause a moment even when you're not) to do this exercise: Place one hand on your chest and one on your belly. Take a series of 3 deep, smooth breaths in through your nose and out through your mouth. Be sure that your diaphragm (your belly, not your chest) inflates with each breath, taking in enough air to stretch your lungs.

into the bedroom, where they could definitely derail your plans to get busy). Vent to anyone else who will listen, too, especially to those who best understand what you're going through. Possibly one of your best potential venting outlets: a TTC message board. There you'll find plenty of other hopeful moms who are riding that very same roller coaster at the very same time. Knowing that you've got lots of company won't necessarily make your stress go away, but it can definitely make it easier to cope with.

- Turn off. In the high-tech, fast-lane life most everyone's living, it's hard to find quiet time. So every now and then, unplug. Power off your cell, table your tablet, take a texting timeout and an Instagram break, and turn off the talk radio and TV. Get reacquainted with the sound of silence—and you're sure to regain some of the calm you and your body are craving.

- Sleep. Bringing stress to bed? Stress can keep you from sleeping, and not sleeping can make you more stressed. See the box on the facing page for more on getting the sleep you need.

- Walk it off. Or swim. Or run. Exercise relieves stress and boosts your mood, even when you're not in the mood for it. Plus it can help you work out some of those frustrations. Build some moves into your busy day every day.

- Hit the yoga mat. Or take on tai chi. Or Pilates. Any of these natural stress-relief techniques can help bring you that inner serenity you're seeking. Continue with them during pregnancy (and beyond) to stay relaxed and refreshed.

- Rub it away. Head to a day spa (budget permitting) for a soothing massage—or book your partner for a couple's

Sleeping Like a Baby to Make a Baby

Dreaming of a baby? Then you'll want to spend more time dreaming. Believe it or not, sex isn't the only in-bed activity that can contribute to conception. There's something else you should be taking care of when you hit the sack: getting sufficient shut-eye. Just like all those other well-known keys to overall good health (eating well, exercising, getting regular medical care), catching enough z's can help improve your chances of producing a little one. In fact, seriously skimping on sleep can mess with your hormones, which can lead to irregular periods—something a hopeful mom-to-be certainly doesn't need. Not spending enough time sleeping can step up stress, too, which can also undermine your fertility (via hormonal hijinks that can delay or prevent ovulation). Plus, if you're charting your basal body temperature to help better understand your cycle (you'll read more about that in Chapter 5), you need adequate, consistent slumber to get the best results. Need another reason to rack up those z's? Once you score a baby,

a good night's sleep will be but a pipe dream.

So take advantage of your still-baby-free home while you can, and seek the sleep your body craves. Nap when you can, turn in early, and stay in bed late (unless you're charting, in which case it's better to maintain regular nod-off and wakeup times), with the goal of catching 6 to 9 hours of shut-eye per night. If sleep proves elusive, turn to tried-and-true home remedies such as a consistent bedtime routine, an evening bath (add some lavender-scented bubbles), or a warm-milk or chamomile-tea nightcap. Avoid caffeine during the afternoon so you're not wound up when you're trying to wind down. And if it's stress that's keeping you up, check out the relaxation tips on these pages.

Thinking of popping a prescription, OTC, or herbal remedy to help you through your sleep slump? Check in with your practitioner first, since some sleep aids (including melatonin) can suppress fertility or affect a newly conceived baby.

massage (he kneads you, you return the favor). It'll de-stress you, and hopefully put you both in the mood for baby making.

- Consider CAM. Explore the many complementary and alternative medicine (CAM) therapies that can promise inner calm—among them biofeedback, acupuncture, and hypnotherapy. Meditation and visualization can melt the stress away, too—and you can try them at home or at your desk. Taking a couple of minutes to daydream about a place that makes you feel safe and soothed

can provide many of the benefits of actually being there. Close your eyes and visualize somewhere you've felt at peace—an ocean beach, a tranquil forest, a mountain trail, your grandma's kitchen. Mentally linger there, taking in the view, summoning up the smells and sounds—or even taking an imaginary bite of one of Grandma's warm-from-the-oven chocolate chip cookies—and relax.

- Have some scents. Your nose knows what scents you find soothing—so let it lead you to aromas that relax you (lavender is well known for its

Snooze Your Way to a Baby

Now that you're TTC, chances are you and your partner are already spending plenty of time in bed. But are you doing enough sleeping there? Research has found that too little sleep (less than 6 hours a night) or too much of it (more than 9 hours) can affect a man's fertility. In fact, one study found that men who slept less than 6 hours or more than 9 hours a night lowered their chances of conception by more than 40 percent in any given month. Another study found that men with poor sleep habits (they typically go to bed too late, for instance, or wake frequently during the night) have a lower sperm count and smaller testicles than men with healthy sleep habits.

What explains the too-little-sleep-fertility connection? Most of your daily dose of that all-important reproductive hormone, testosterone. Then why would too much sleep also possibly push "snooze" on fertility? That's unclear. But the research bottom line points to a sensible TTC sleep approach: When you're planning to make a baby, plan to get your 7 to 8 hours of sleep—not too much more, not too much less.

calming properties). Use an infused lotion (or infuse your own with a few drops of scented oil), and rub it onto your hands, shoulders, and arms. Or try an aromatherapy diffuser to fill the air around you with a soothing scent. Don't stock up on that scent, though: Once you do become pregnant, a relaxing fragrance can suddenly become a nauseating one.

▪ Wash it away. A warm bath is an excellent way to relieve tension. Try it after a hectic day or whenever you're stressed out. Add some soothing aromatherapy oil or salts to complete the spa experience. If there's enough room in your tub, invite your partner to join you for some romantic relaxation.

Stress still getting the best of you? Feeling unreasonably anxious? You might want to consider getting some professional counseling—learning some coping strategies can really help you relax and maybe even help you realize your baby dreams sooner.

Travel

"I travel often for work, and I'm wondering if that'll impact my fertility now that we're TTC."

No need to give up your frequent flier status now that you're trying to put a baby on board, but there are a few factors you might want to consider as you pack your bags . . . again. Certainly if you're out of town for work a lot, there's the potential for you and your partner not to be in the same place at the right time (when you're ovulating), making conception difficult if not impossible. But travel could present another, less obvious fertility challenge as well: For some women, it can mess with the menstrual cycle. That's because the body views travel as a stressor (yes, even if you've scored that upgrade), often leading to longer cycles or missed ovulation. That's especially true of travel that involves time changes: When your regular internal biological clock (the circadian rhythm) gets thrown off, all your important bodily functions—including the delicate balance of hormones responsible

PREPPING BEFORE YOU'RE EXPECTING

for the menstrual cycle—can also get thrown off. If your cycles aren't affected by your travel, there's no need to give your work schedule another thought (unless it's interfering with your baby-making schedule). But if you notice that you're not ovulating regularly when and/or after you travel, it might be a good idea to see if you can slow down your travel schedule so you can fast-track your conception plans.

There are a couple of other considerations when it comes to preconception travel. First, the CDC recommends that women hoping to become pregnant (as well as their partners) avoid travel to areas with known outbreaks of Zika virus or use enhanced prevention and followup if travel absolutely cannot be avoided (see the box on page 10 for more on Zika). Second, when traveling to destinations where food safety and water purity are questionable, take sensible precautions to be on the safe side.

BPA and Phthalates

"Should I be concerned about being exposed to all those chemicals in plastics now that I'm trying to have a baby?"

It's hard—even close to impossible—to live without plastics these days. But do the chemicals in plastics and other everyday products make it hard to conceive, too? They may. Studies have shown that excessive exposure to those chemicals, specifically BPA and phthalates, could have an adverse impact on both female and male fertility.

BPA (bisphenol-A), a chemical found in some plastic containers, cans, and even some store and ATM receipts, is believed to mimic the hormone estrogen and act as an endocrine disrupter, impacting cell division in the ovaries and altering the menstrual cycle. Too much BPA also affects male fertility, reducing

Fathers and Phthalates

Wondering whether you'll need to bag plastics now that you're trying to conceive a bundle of joy? You may be wise to. BPA and phthalates have a well-documented adverse effect on sperm and male fertility (see page 34). Possibly more concerning still, research has also found that a dad's preconception exposure to phthalates might have even more of a negative impact on a yet-to-be-conceived baby's health than a mom's preconception exposure. The research shows that higher preconception concentrations of phthalates in a dad (but not in a mom) are associated with significant decreases in a baby's birthweight. Help boost your odds of healthy baby making by reducing your exposure to BPA and phthalates: Choose "phthalate-free" products, opt for cloth bags instead of plastic, and use glass or stainless steel food and drink containers instead of plastic ones. You'll be doing the planet your baby will be growing up on a favor, too.

sperm quality, count, and motility. What's more, research has found that higher BPA levels in women undergoing fertility treatment lower their chances of becoming pregnant, while high levels in men affect embryo quality.

BPA is everywhere—in fact, the CDC estimates that 93 percent of all Americans have BPA in their bloodstreams. Fortunately, it's becoming easier to avoid. Here's how:

- Opt for canned foods that are "BPA-free," or choose food packaged in glass jars instead.

Cell Sense

Are you living the wireless life? Of course you are, and you wouldn't have it any other way. But even the smartest smartphone can come at a cost when you're a hopeful father, and we're not just talking roaming charges. Believe it or not, preliminary evidence links excessive cell phone use by a man with the potential for fertility difficulties. The more the guy uses his cell phone, the lower his sperm count is likely to be.

Researchers speculate that the electromagnetic radiation from a cell phone alters sperm cells, lowering their count and making them less healthy and less able to fertilize an egg. Stress might play some role, too (after all, wireless junkies tend to be . . . well, more wired). So what's a guy who wants to become a dad to do? Though moderate use of mobile technology is fine, you might want to consider cutting back if you're a certifiable addict. As much as you can, try to keep your phone out of your pants pocket (where it'll be closer to the package you're trying to protect), and hold any mobile device away from those jewels when you're using it.

- Select storage containers, cutting boards, and utensils made from BPA-free plastic or from glass, wood, or ceramic.

- Use stainless steel or "BPA-free" water bottles (those with recycle codes 3 and 7 are more likely to contain BPA).

- Eat soy. Interestingly, research suggests that soy (such as soy milk and soy-based tofu) may protect women against the harmful impacts of BPA.

What about phthalates? This widely used group of chemicals may also have a negative impact on fertility—most notably on male fertility, with studies showing lowered sperm counts in men with excessive exposure to phthalates. Studies have also shown that elevated levels of phthalates in women are associated with higher rates of implantation failure. In fact, researchers have found that phthalate levels are, on average, significantly higher in both infertile men and women than in fertile men and women.

Phthalates, sometimes known as plasticizers, come from compounds that enhance the flexibility of plastics. They're found in IV tubing, flexible PVC pipes used for plumbing, some flexible plastic bags (like single-use shopping bags), and some food and drink containers. Phthalates are also found in hundreds of personal care products, from fragrances to deodorants, shampoo to hair spray. You can reduce exposure by not only choosing products labeled "phthalate-free" but also watching out for the word "fragrance" (a blanket term that can hide phthalates) on the ingredient list of a product not labeled "phthalate-free." Using cloth bags instead of plastic and glass food and drink containers can further help reduce exposure. Not ready to give up on plastic storage containers altogether? Choose ones that are BPA- and phthalate-free—or at least be sure not to heat foods or drinks in regular plastic containers, since heating plastics allows the chemicals to break down and leach into the food.

Work and Fertility

"Could conditions at my job make it harder for me to get pregnant?"

You may have your work cut out for you making a baby, but that probably doesn't mean you'll have to cut out work to do it. Luckily, most 9-to-5 (or even 8-to-7) jobs are preconception compatible—and the vast majority of workplaces are perfectly safe when baby's on board, too. Even those jobs that might present some potential risks when it comes to conceiving and/or carrying a baby (x-ray technician, for example) can be made safer with some precautions. Here's how to play it extra safe when you're at work:

- Health care work. If you work in health care (including dentistry), you'll need to put your fertility health first. Check out what OSHA (Occupational Safety and Health Administration; osha.gov) says about job safety of health care work during pregnancy—the same will apply when you're TTC. Chances are, you already practice all of the recommended precautions (all mandated for health care workers anyway): keeping close track of daily radiation exposure, avoiding direct contact with potentially harmful chemicals, being scrupulous about handwashing and gloves, and staying up-to-date on immunizations. Just take precautions up a notch now that you're planning for pregnancy, and if necessary, look into changing any duties that might be fertility- or baby-unfreindly.

- Shift work. If you work nights or irregular shifts, see if you can get a more regular (daytime) schedule so that your circadian rhythms aren't being messed with (see page 31). If that's not possible, see if you can at least have the same hours each day so your schedule is regular for you.

- Airline work. Wondering if the friendly skies are fertility-friendly? What about the TSA screening you have to pass through each day to get to work? Pilots, flight attendants, and airline workers can breathe a sigh of relief. There is no evidence that the low levels of radiation airline workers are exposed to on flights impact fertility or the health of a pregnancy. Ditto for passing through security screenings. The low levels of electromagnetic waves emitted by metal detectors, security wands, and full body scans are perfectly safe for the hopeful mom- and dad-to-be. Lots of traveling to different time zones, however, could throw off your circadian rhythm and your menstrual cycle, sending your fertility plans into a tailspin (see page 32). If you're not ovulating regularly, consider requesting a same-time-zone travel schedule until mission conception is complete.

- Office work. Putting in a day at the office before you put in a night of baby making? No reason why not—even if your workday keeps you in front of a computer for hours at a time. Luckily computers don't pose a threat to fertility or fetuses. Laptops don't pose a risk to female fertility, either, because the ovaries are deep inside the body and any heat generated from a laptop sitting for long periods on your lap isn't enough to reach those precious eggs. (The same isn't true for men and their fertility. See the box, next page, for more.)

- Animal work. If you work with cats, you're probably aware that toxoplasmosis, an infectious disease that can be passed to humans through cat feces, is something pregnant women

Your Other Job

So how does your day job affect your nighttime (or early-morning) job of baby making? The answer: probably not much. The vast majority of workplaces are fertility-friendly for dads, so there's no need to give up your 9-to-5 just to make a baby. Studies show that most work conditions (including those involving high heat or noise levels or prolonged sitting) don't appear to affect sperm quality. Very physically demanding jobs may be linked to a lower sperm count—but doing strenuous work doesn't necessarily mean that you'll have a difficult time conceiving, just that it might be a factor to explore if you and your partner do end up having trouble.

Some jobs, however, are not as compatible with TTC, including those involving exposure to radiation and certain chemicals (such as lead, pesticides, and some organic solvents found in paints, glues, varnishes, and metal degreasers). Avoid or limit exposure to these as much as possible in preparation for conception, since they can damage sperm. Contact OSHA (Occupational Safety and Health Administration; osha.gov) to find out if your workplace poses risks to your fertility and how you can best play it safe.

Here's another preconception precaution you'll want to take on the job—even when you're working on the fly: Keep your laptop off your lap. Research has found that men who use a laptop on their lap have lower sperm counts. That's because the heat from a laptop (or another electronic device that can overheat) can raise the temperature in the testes, lowering sperm count and potentially reducing fertility. No need to pack up the laptop until baby's on board—just treat it like a desktop for now.

And one more thing to avoid on any job when you're in baby-making mode: excessive stress, which can take a toll on your fertility, too.

need to be concerned about. And that means pregnant-to-be women should be aware of it, too, since you never know when you might become pregnant, especially if you're already trying in earnest. If you're not sure whether you're immune to toxoplasmosis, ask your practitioner to test you. If you turn out not to be immune, stay gloved when changing cat litter and remember to wash up afterward. The same recommendations about toxoplasmosis hold true if you work with raw meats (in a restaurant kitchen, in a butcher shop, or in a meat-processing plant), since the disease can be spread that way, too. Be sure to wear gloves and not to touch your mouth, nose, or eyes when handling raw meat.

- Chemical exposure at work. Some chemicals (though far from all and usually only in very large doses) are potentially harmful to your eggs before conception, and later to a developing embryo or fetus. Though the risk in most cases is slight or even just hypothetical, play it safe by avoiding potentially hazardous exposure on the job. Take special care in certain fields (art, photography, transportation, farming and landscaping, construction, hairdressing and cosmetology, dry cleaning, and some factory work). Because elevated lead levels when you conceive could pose problems for your baby, you should be tested if you have been exposed to lead in the workplace or elsewhere. Contact OSHA for the latest information on job safety and pregnancy. In some cases, it may be wise to ask for a transfer to another position, change jobs, or take special precautions before trying to conceive.

- Heavy lifting at work. If your job involves heavy lifting on a regular basis, you may want to consider asking for a change of duties. That's because research shows that regular heavy lifting or other kinds of physically demanding duties on the job can diminish egg production and quality, especially in women who are overweight.

Whatever your workplace environment, common sense should always be your first order of business. Wash your hands frequently (hands down the best way to avoid infections, especially if you work where germs are an occupational hazard—as in a daycare or preschool, or a health care facility), don protective clothing as appropriate, and wear a mask or respirator when necessary. Talk to your doctor about your specific workplace circumstances. He or she will be able to let you know what might be dangerous and what you needn't be concerned about.

A final word on workplace issues and fertility: Extremely stressful work conditions, no matter what type of job you have, can contribute to fertility difficulties. For tips on how to try to minimize stress in your life, see page 28.

Nontraditional TTC

Most babies are made the old-fashioned way (boy meets girl, sperm meets egg). But what if you're a girl on your own? Or a couple of girls—or a couple of guys? Today's reproductive technology makes becoming a parent possible in just about any relationship scenario.

What should your preconception plans include if you're a same-sex couple (or single woman or man) pursuing parenthood? That all depends on the route you're planning to take. If one female partner will be carrying the baby-to-be, her preconception prep should mirror any other aspiring mama's. If one mom is going to use her egg that will be fertilized and transferred to the other mom for gestation (aka co-maternity or reciprocal surrogacy), both will need to get their bodies in tip-top baby-making shape. If intrauterine insemination (IUI) or in vitro fertilization (IVF) plus donor sperm will be involved, Clomid and/or hormone shots may be on the agenda (see page 220). If a pair of potential papas is planning to start a family using a surrogate and sperm from one of the partners (or both, if the plan is to create 2 separate batches of embryos—1 from each dad), preconception prep should be focused on getting his (or their) boys in the best possible shape before they go to work. Be sure to read all the dark shaded boxes in this chapter for info on getting yourself (and your sperm) ready for baby making.

You'll find more about the assisted reproductive therapies that can help make your baby dreams a reality beginning on page 181.

Your Financial Prep

Your body might be ready for a baby, but what about your wallet? Have you thought about how a baby is going to affect your bottom line (hint: a lot)? Or your career path or priorities? Planning now for the financial changes and business decisions that'll be coming your way long before your family officially expands (from the cost of prenatal care to the cost of a nursery, from health insurance to life insurance) is a smart component of your preconception prep. So open up the balance sheet, whip out the calculator, and start doing the baby math. And while you're at it, consider issues that can come up at your workplace, like maternity leave.

Baby Costs

"Every time we hear about the costs of raising a baby, we wonder if we can really afford it. Is there anything we can do now to prepare financially?"

Little babies do come with a hefty price tag. Factor in all the up-front big-ticket items (a crib, a stroller, and a car seat) plus the small ones you'll need to buy endlessly (like baby food and diapers), and that baby bottom line adds up faster than you'd think. Before you conceive is the perfect time to start getting your financial rubber duckies in a row and planning for the financial changes you'll experience once baby makes three.

No need to tackle every budgetary line item at once (don't stress out about how you'll pay those college bills—yet), but anything you can start taking stock of now (including your stocks) will make budgeting down the road easier on your wallet and your sanity. Start small:

Tally it up. Make a list of your current expenses and then make a list of items you'll be calculating soon—diapers, bottles and other feeding supplies, baby clothes, baby gear, baby food, baby toys, and so on—so you can get a clearer accounting of what your expenses really will be once your family starts to grow. Remember, there's a good chance you'll be getting plenty of those baby necessities and niceties as gifts, and others you'll be able to borrow from friends and family. Keep in mind, too, that the breast things in life are free—making breastfeeding a wise financial strategy, in addition to being the healthiest option for mom and baby (which will lower costs even more).

Rebalance the budget. Think of ways (big and small) to cut corners and generate savings. Cut back on luxuries you can live without (passing on that morning mocha can save you at least 20 bucks a week, bringing a sandwich to work instead of going out for one can save a lot more). Divert some of your current savings/investment dollars into an interest-bearing baby fund and get serious about saving even more. Look critically at monthly expenditures for cell phone plans, cable, gym memberships, and the like, and see if you can switch to cheaper ones (often just calling to threaten a switch will secure you a lower monthly cost). Negotiate discounts on whatever you can (more and more businesses and services are open to this option), and if you have a skill or a service that you can barter, save more cash by trading.

Crunch your credit. Still throwing away your hard-earned money on credit card interest payments? Stop (or at least slow down) the financial bleeding and reduce credit card debt by avoiding late fees, paying more than the minimum each month, and rolling balances onto low-interest cards. Once you get out of debt, consider staying that way. Pay your full balance each month and you'll save a yearly bundle on interest—a bundle you can invest, instead, in your bundle of joy. Living within your means definitely has its rewards (and may eventually help those means grow significantly). Reconsider your rewards cards, too—now may be the time to opt out of one that offers vacation perks (how practical will that trip to Bora Bora be when you're toting baby baby?) and swap it for one that'll help put cash back in your wallet (cash that can put you in the driver's seat of a family-friendly car or that'll score you savings on baby gear).

Start laying that egg. No, not *that* egg, but the egg that will keep your fledgling-to-be cozy and secure in the years ahead: your nest egg. If you've been saving up for something you'd love to have but can live without (that big-screen TV, perhaps), consider socking the cash away in a savings vehicle instead (stock or bond funds) so that your little nest egg can turn into a bigger one. Choose one that maximizes growth over the long term. If you haven't started saving yet, now's the time. Set aside a small amount from your monthly paycheck to start or add to your account (paid off by those skipped lattes or bagged lunches). If you're lacking in savings self-discipline, enrolling in an automatic savings program may give you the tough financial love you need. Almost all banks allow you to authorize monthly (or even weekly) deductions from your checking account to your investment account. Unexpected funds land in your lap (from a tax refund or a bonus—or a lucky scratch-off)? Sure,

Will Do

No one likes to contemplate mortality, especially when you're just about to begin a new life that's likely to be a very, very long and happy one. But planning for a baby should also mean planning for that baby's future security—and that includes planning for your baby's care in the highly unlikely event that you and your partner die. A will can provide for the financial security of your child (all your assets can go to your child and, depending on his or her age at your death, be managed by a responsible and trustworthy adult). But when a minor child is involved, there's more to your will than just money. If both of you die without a will (or if you're planning to have a baby on your own, if you die), it'll be up to the state to decide who will raise your child. And that could be a bad thing—especially if you have serious problems with your in-laws or your sister's husband and that's who the state chooses.

So think about drawing up that will soon—and definitely by the time your baby arrives. Choose a guardian who you believe will raise your child with values that best match your own, who will love your child as you would, and who will provide the healthiest and happiest environment for your precious one (and who is willing to take on the job—you definitely should ask first). And then don't give that will another thought.

that pair of strappy sandals would be a fun way to unload the windfall, but a smarter move would be to drop that spare change into your nest egg before you're tempted to hit the mall. Besides, once you're expecting, you won't be able to squeeze your swollen feet into those sandals anyway. And speaking of spare change, don't forget the oldest savings trick in the book: the jar. Drop those annoying pennies and other coins into a jar, convert them periodically at a supermarket coin changer, and add the found money into your savings account. Fattening up your piggy bank now will help you handle the bigger expenditures that are just around the corner. Plus, it'll get you in the savings habit (a habit that will definitely come in handy when you have a little someone else to save up for).

Be tax savvy. Look for tax-saving vehicles, such as a flexible health spending account at work. Such accounts allow you to sock away pretax dollars that can be used for medical expenses such as prenatal vitamins, ovulation kits, and practitioner and hospital co-pays. You can usually sign up only once a year for these plans (so plan ahead), though some will also allow you to start one with the birth of a baby.

Insurance

"Should I be changing anything about my insurance policies before I conceive?"

Now that you'll soon have more to protect than ever before (including that very precious bundle you're about to create), it's definitely time to take a critical look at (or sign up for) your health, disability, and life insurance policies. And chances are you'll find that some changes in coverage will be in order.

Health insurance. If you're like most healthy women of childbearing age, you haven't tapped into your health insurance coverage much up until now, beyond those annuals at the gyno and

TTC To-Do:

Health insurance? Check. Savings plan? Check. Balanced budget? Check. Sounds like a lot of financial planning to prepare for a baby you haven't even conceived yet—and pretty overwhelming if you're a finance newbie—but there's no better investment in your time right now than investing in your family-to-be's fiscal future and security. It's also a good way to avoid sticker shock down the road.

the occasional dragging-on cold that drags you to your internist. That's about to change—in a big way. You're about to discover how essential good health insurance coverage is, even if you, your pregnancy, and your baby are all completely healthy and complication-free. While the Affordable Care Act (ACA) mandates that health insurance cover prenatal care, birth, and well-baby care, not all policies are the same. Check out your medical plan choices at work to see how comprehensive the coverage is—for instance, are genetic screenings covered (coverage varies)? Fertility treatments (less commonly covered)? If you don't like what you see, consider making a preconception move if you can (even to your partner's plan, if it's better). Keep in mind that the opportunity to make this change may come only once a year at open enrollment time—if you've just missed this year's window, you may have a long wait ahead for another. But that wait might be preferable to having your pockets emptied by out-of-pocket expenses. If your employer or your partner's doesn't offer insurance or you're unemployed, you may be able to apply for a plan through the Health

Insurance Marketplace. Again, you must enroll during the open enrollment period (which happens on an annual basis) unless you're eligible for special enrollment for a qualifying life event such as marriage, divorce, or moving (pregnancy itself is not considered a qualifying life event). Find out more, including how to get in touch with a local marketplace representative, at healthcare.gov or 800-318-2596.

If you don't have health insurance and can't afford it, you may qualify for subsidies (available at open enrollment time) or Medicaid. If you don't qualify because your income is too high, there are low-cost health insurance programs that will cover your pregnancy as well as your child's health care after delivery. Your local Health Insurance Marketplace representative will let you know if you're eligible.

Disability insurance. Though you probably don't think of pregnancy as a disability (and it rarely is), you should be prepared for the very slim possibility that you might be put on precautionary bed rest or become too sick to work during pregnancy. If your family depends on your income, you might need disability insurance to protect that income in case you have to stop working earlier than planned.

Check with your employer first to see if you're covered under your state's short-term disability insurance, which would pay a portion of your salary if you get sick. In fact, short-term disability is what covers you when you take maternity leave, too, so it's important to have even if you're not put on bed rest. Short-term disability starts as soon as you need it, but covers you for only a very limited time (6 to 8 weeks) at a portion of your salary. When that time is up, long-term disability insurance—if you have it—takes over, usually kicking

in after a waiting period and then paying you some percentage of your salary (50 or 60 percent) for as long as you need it. Make sure you have both kinds—if your employer doesn't offer both, or if the benefits are skimpy, shop around for private coverage. Since you probably won't need these benefits (most pregnancies progress without a health hitch), the additional expense might seem like an extravagance. But disability insurance could help keep your family finances afloat in case the unexpected does happen. And that's what insurance is all about, after all—keeping you covered for that "just in case" scenario.

Life insurance. Again, nothing you've probably considered before—and something you've probably always associated with the much-older set. But there's no better time to think about a life insurance policy than when you're thinking about conceiving a new life. Although no amount of money will replace a lost parent or partner, every parent should be insured so that his or her surviving dependents will be financially protected. You don't need a policy with a huge payoff, but rather one that will cover costs of living and raising your child with one less salary. There's another reason (unfair as it may be) why shopping for a life insurance policy pre-pregnancy is worthwhile: Some insurance companies charge higher rates for pregnant women. It might be even harder to get a good premium later if you end up developing a complication during pregnancy that could develop into a chronic condition postpartum (for instance, preeclampsia could lead to chronic hypertension after delivery). Again, not fair, but a pretty common insurance practice.

Maternity Leave

"I have no idea what kind of maternity leave is available at my company—it's not something I ever thought about or looked into before. Should I now?"

Maternity leave may not be right around the corner (after all, you're not even pregnant yet), but now's actually a good time to take a peek around that corner—and find out everything you can about your company's maternity leave policy. The sooner you know what's in store for your career and your income once baby's born, the easier it will be to figure out your back-to-work plan and financial picture.

First, review your company's maternity leave policy. Ask someone at Human Resources, or if you'd rather be more discreet about your TTC plans, check the benefits handbook. Find out how long your company's maternity leave is, whether you'll be paid (and at what rate) during your leave, if you're allowed to add accumulated sick, holiday, or personal days, and if any other work conditions are required for you to qualify for maternity leave (such as being an employee for a certain amount of time before the benefits kick in). Find out, too, if you'll qualify for benefits under the Family and Medical Leave Act (FMLA), a federal program that enables employees who have worked for more than a year in a company with at least 50 workers to take up to 12 weeks per year of unpaid leave during and/or after pregnancy or a family illness.

Then decide as best you can at this point what your financial and career situation can bear, as well as what your preferences are, given a choice. Will your budget allow you to take a full 12 weeks if it's unpaid? If it's unpaid after that point, would you be able to consider taking more—and will your company allow that? Or will you be returning to work as soon as possible, either for financial reasons (the cost of childcare factored in) or career reasons? Will both of you have to work full-time, or will it make financial sense (given the high cost of childcare) for one of you to stay home? Are there other options such as flextime, job sharing, telecommuting from home, or working part-time that you can start exploring now (rather than right before your maternity leave is over and you're forced to make a decision you may not be happy with)?

Combining parenting (already a full-time job) with another full-time job will take plenty of juggling and, most likely, some shifting of priorities. But giving it some thought now, before the decision heat is on, can get you started on finding the happy (if not perfect) balance of work and home that will work for you and your family.

A Last Hurrah

Beyond excited about getting those baby plans under way, but feel like you have an adults-only vacation you need to get out of your system first? Pack your bags and go. Whether it's Sex on the Beach (the cocktail, that is) that you're craving, along with a couple of days of sun and sand, or a wine-and-cheese tasting in the Napa Valley, or that weekend in Vegas you never got around to before (enough said)—now, before conception efforts begin in earnest, is the best time for that last hurrah. Or turn your last hurrah into a conception-moon and start your baby-making efforts with some sex on the beach (minus the cocktail). One very important caveat when booking your getaway: stay away from any regions where the CDC has issued travel notices about Zika virus (see the box on page 10 for more).

Freezing Your Eggs

Are your eggs and your life having a scheduling conflict? As in, your eggs are ready for baby making, but your life definitely isn't?

You're far from alone if you're worried that your eggs will reach their use-by date before you're in any position to use them—more and more women are finding that their peak reproductive years aren't the perfect years to reproduce. After all, there's no way around it: 40 may be the new 30, and 30 the new 20—but female fertility hasn't evolved to keep pace. It can begin its gradual but steady decline while a woman's still climbing the corporate ladder, finishing up her fellowship, or searching for the ideal partner to make (and raise) a baby with.

Which is why you're also far from alone if you're thinking about egg freezing—a sort of reproductive insurance policy against age-related declining fertility. Egg freezing can be an option for women who aren't ready to get pregnant when their chances of getting pregnant are highest (in their 20s and early 30s). It can also be considered when a woman in her 20s has a family history of premature ovarian failure or early menopause—meaning her eggs may be aging and her reproductive clock ticking even faster than average, leaving her with an even smaller baby-making window. Same for women who have endometriosis or ovarian cysts, or women who are about to undergo a cancer treatment that might affect their eggs (see page 169). A hopeful mom undergoing IVF may also choose to freeze her eggs instead of freezing embryos.

Here's how egg freezing works:

- You'll undergo the same egg-retrieval process—including hormone injections—as a woman undergoing IVF (see page 202). About 10 to 20 eggs will be retrieved.

- Immediately after egg retrieval, your eggs will be frozen using a flash-freezing ultrarapid cooling process known as vitrification.

- The eggs can be frozen for a number of years (you'll pay a fee for storage). How long eggs can safely be stored isn't yet clear.

- When you're ready to become pregnant, one or more of the eggs will be thawed and assessed. The eggs that survive the freezing process will be fertilized with intra-cytoplasmic sperm injection (ICSI)—when a single sperm is inserted directly into the egg (see page 213)—with the hope that they become fertilized. The resultant embryo(s) will then be transferred to your uterus (see page 205).

There isn't a lot of data yet on egg freezing, but preliminary stats are promising, with some showing that frozen eggs may be as likely as fresh eggs to be fertilized and result in a healthy pregnancy and a healthy baby. So far, frozen eggs don't seem to be linked with an increased risk of pregnancy complications or birth defects. Still, since egg freezing doesn't come with guarantees but does come at a cost and with the same risks as any egg retrieval, it's a decision to make after careful consideration and discussion with your doctor. Factor in, too, that you may never be able to use the eggs you retrieve and store—or, on the happier flip side, that you may never end up needing them because you conceive naturally when the time comes.

Weighing In Before You're Expecting

So you probably figure that you'll be in for some weight changes once you're expecting, and maybe you're really looking forward to letting those numbers on the scale creep up, especially if you've spent your whole adult life trying to keep them down. But maybe you didn't realize that making some weight changes before you're expecting can actually help you expect sooner—and expect a healthier pregnancy, and even a healthier baby with a healthier future, too. That's right—getting your weight as close as you can to "ideal" should definitely top your preconception prep list. Whether you've got a little (or a lot) to lose, or a little (or a lot) to gain, weighing in before you're expecting can help you zoom in on conception and fast-track you to pregnancy.

Not sure where your weight should be, or how to get it where it should be in the most fertility-friendly way possible? Check in with your practitioner for some guidelines, and read on for tips on how to tip the scales in conception's favor.

Your Weight and Your Fertility

Are you overweight, underweight, or just the right weight to make a baby? There's a strong connection between weight and fertility, and it's much more than just a numbers game. Getting to the bottom of your bottom line is one of the most important steps you can take when you're getting your body ready for the baby-making big time.

Body Fat and Hormones

"My doctor mentioned that there's a connection between my weight and my hormones. What's that all about?"

Estrogen—the reproductive hormone responsible for helping eggs mature, building up the uterine lining, and providing conception-friendly cervical mucus—is produced primarily in your ovaries. But did you know that more than 30 percent of the estrogen in your body is created by your fat cells? It's true. The same cells you thought served no purpose at all (besides sitting around your butt and thighs) are closely tied to your fertility. And whether that's a good association or not is in the numbers. If you have about the right amount of fat cells (no need to count them, just take a look at your body mass index, or BMI; see the next question), then you're likely producing just the right amount of estrogen. If you have more than the normal amount of fat cells (because your BMI is high), those fat cells will be producing more estrogen than necessary. If you have far fewer fat cells than you should have (because your BMI is very low), your body may be estrogen starved. Because a delicate balance of hormones—which includes the perfect supply of estrogen—needs to be maintained for your reproductive cycle to work the way it's supposed to, too much or too little estrogen (from too many or too few fat cells) can throw your fertility off kilter. In fact, it's suspected that more than 10 percent of all fertility problems stem from weight issues.

Have too few fat cells, or too many? Give your hormones the best shot at conception by getting your weight on track. If you need to gain, see page 57; if you need to lose, see page 55.

Prebaby BMI

"How do I figure out whether I'm at the ideal weight for TTC?"

Bodies, in case you haven't noticed, come in all kinds of packages. Tall, thin packages; short, chubby packages; more muscular packages; more padded packages; top heavy; bottom heavy; nowhere heavy; everywhere heavy. And when it comes to figuring the "ideal" size for your TTC body, a lot really depends on the kind of package it comes in.

That's exactly why most practitioners don't rely on scale numbers alone in determining whether your weight is at or close to that preconception ideal, or whether you'll have some gaining or losing to do before you get busy TTC. They still use the scale (before you get excited about skipping that office weigh-in), but they factor it into a calculation known as body mass index, or BMI, which describes the relationship between weight and height and provides a better measure of body fat content than the scale alone. Remember, body fat is the key to fertility: Too little fat could mean too little estrogen, too much fat can mean too much estrogen. Either scenario could spell fertility trouble.

The formula for calculating your BMI is weight (pounds) ÷ height (inches)^2 × 700. For example, a woman who weighs 145 pounds and is 5 feet 5 inches (65 inches) will have the following BMI equation: 145 pounds ÷ (65 × 65) inches (4,225 inches) × 700, or 145 ÷ 4,225 × 700 = 24.

Once you've calculated your BMI (if you don't want to do the math, or

What's Your BMI?

BMI (kg/m²) Height (in.)	18	19	20	21	22	23	24	25	26	27	28	29	30	35	40
						Weight (lb.)									
58	87	91	96	100	105	110	115	119	124	129	134	138	143	167	191
59	90	94	99	104	109	114	119	124	128	133	138	143	148	173	198
60	93	97	102	107	112	118	123	128	133	138	143	148	153	179	204
61	96	100	106	111	116	122	127	132	137	143	148	153	158	185	211
62	99	104	109	115	120	126	131	136	142	147	153	158	164	191	218
63	102	107	113	118	124	130	135	141	146	152	158	163	169	197	225
64	105	110	116	122	128	134	140	145	151	157	163	169	174	204	232
65	109	114	120	126	132	138	144	150	156	162	168	174	180	210	240
66	112	118	124	130	136	142	148	155	161	167	173	179	186	216	247
67	115	121	127	134	140	146	153	159	166	172	178	185	191	223	255
68	119	125	131	138	144	151	158	164	171	177	184	190	197	230	262
69	122	128	135	142	149	155	162	169	176	182	189	196	203	236	270
70	126	132	139	146	153	160	167	174	181	188	195	202	207	243	278
71	130	136	143	150	157	165	172	179	186	193	200	208	215	250	286
72	133	140	147	154	162	169	177	184	191	199	206	213	221	258	294
73	137	144	151	159	166	174	182	189	197	204	212	219	227	265	302
74	141	148	155	163	171	179	186	194	202	210	218	225	233	272	311
75	145	152	160	168	176	184	192	200	208	216	224	232	240	279	319
76	148	156	164	172	180	189	197	205	213	221	230	238	246	287	328

have happily left those skills back in high school, just check the chart on the facing page), you can determine what category you fall into.

- Have a BMI lower than 18.5? You're considered underweight—and you'll probably need to put on some pounds before TTC.

- Have a BMI between 18.5 and 24? You're considered average weight—and at the ideal weight for TTC.

- Have a BMI between 25 and 29? You're considered overweight—and ideally, you should lose some weight before TTC.

- Have a BMI of 30 or higher? You're considered obese—and you should try to lose weight before you start trying for a baby.

Keep in mind that your BMI doesn't always tell the whole story when it comes to weight and body fat. For example, muscles are more dense than fat. So if your heavier-than-average weight is caused by a higher-than-average amount of fat cells, your BMI is probably pretty accurate—and those extra fat pounds may result in extra estrogen, which could undercut fertility. On the other hand, if you've been a regular on the training circuit (especially the weight-training circuit), all those dense muscles may weigh you down on the scale, placing you on the high end of the BMI chart even though you're not "fat." But as long as you're packing a normal amount of body fat atop those muscles, your body's likely to produce just the right amount of estrogen to keep your cycles regular and your fertility up to par.

Are you a lightweight on the BMI scale, falling under the ideal average? The same principle could apply on the flip side. You could be very thin but still have a light padding of fat. Chances are that the fat cells you have (as minimal as they might be, compared with a heavier woman's) will be enough to generate the estrogen your body needs to keep your reproductive cycle running smoothly. Thin but cut—all muscle, but virtually fat-free? Even if you weigh the same as someone who's thin but proportionately padded, you might produce much less estrogen, which could disrupt your cycles and undercut your fertility.

Overweight

"I'm overweight. Will that affect my fertility?"

Extra weight can definitely weigh you down when it comes to fertility—and it takes less extra weight than you might think. Obese women (those with a BMI over 30) with irregular menstrual cycles have a significantly lower chance of becoming pregnant compared with

---

What Fruit Are You?

Looking to the fruit bowl now that you're trying to shed preconception pounds? Take a look inside it, too, for a possible clue to your potential fertility. Researchers have found that, on average, overweight women who are apple-shaped (those with a high waist-to-hip ratio) have a harder time getting pregnant than overweight pear-shaped women (those with a low waist-to-hip ratio). It seems that when it comes to the fertility connection, where the excess fat is located on your body may be as important as—if not more important than—how much body fat you have.

Weighing In on Male Fertility

Extra weight doesn't impact just a woman's fertility—it can weigh heavily on a man's, too. Overweight and obese men tend to have more fertility problems than normal-weight hopeful dads. In fact, research suggests that a 20-pound overage increases a guy's chances of infertility by about 10 percent. That's because excess fat converts the male hormone testosterone into the female hormone estrogen, possibly suppressing sperm production and lowering overall sperm quality. It can also negatively impact libido (the more body fat you have, the higher your levels of a natural chemical that binds existing testosterone, making less available to stimulate desire)—and it almost goes without saying that libido is something you'll need in spades while you're TTC. What's more, obese men are more likely to have erectile dysfunction (vessel-clogging fatty deposits form in the tiny arteries in the penis, causing it to shut down), certainly a problem you don't want to bring to bed when there's baby making on the agenda.

To make sure you reach optimum fertility potential once you and your partner begin TTC, try to reach your optimum weight first (or as close as you can get to it). As with mom hopefuls who have preconception weight to shed, it's smart to go on a sensible diet plan—one that decreases calories and fat, but doesn't short change you on nutrients you'll need. If you have a lot of weight to lose, it might help to check in with your doctor first for some guidelines and suggestions, as well as to set a realistic goal. Getting some exercise, which boosts testosterone levels, can also boost both function and libido (a good reason to get busy in bed after you've just been busy at the gym).

If you're significantly overweight and haven't had any luck dropping the pounds through diet and exercise, you may have considered weight-loss surgery—but may also have wondered how such a procedure might affect your chances of becoming a dad. Good news: Research shows that a significant weight loss from bariatric surgery can actually improve fertility for obese men as well as for obese women. Many of the conception challenges often faced by obese guys may resolve post-op, often delivering a return of libido and sexual function.

average-weight women with regular cycles. But even being moderately overweight (with a BMI of 25 to 29) can slow down—or even put the brakes on—your baby-making efforts. Extra pounds (in the form of extra fat) trigger extra estrogen production. And though having extra female hormones sounds like a good thing when you're trying to make a baby (after all, isn't reproduction the most fundamental of biological female functions?), the opposite is actually true. Too much estrogen can keep you from ovulating regularly, or even ovulating at all (30 to nearly 40 percent of obese women have irregular menstrual cycles)—decreasing your chances of becoming pregnant.

Even if you're obese but have normal periods, you're still not out of the weight woods completely. Studies show that obese women have a harder time getting pregnant even if they have normal periods. That's because obesity (and even overweight) is associated with decreased ovarian function, anovulation (cycles that appear normal but are actually ones in which ovulation doesn't occur), and diminished egg quality.

Here's another reason why extra pounds can weigh fertility down: Being obese or overweight is associated with polycystic ovarian syndrome (PCOS), a fairly common cause of fertility problems (see pages 50 and 159). Too much weight can also cause insulin levels to rise—and too much insulin, in some women, can cause the ovaries to overproduce testosterone, a male hormone that definitely doesn't help in the female fertility department.

Plus, here's another weighty issue to contemplate while you're contemplating conceiving: Not only can being overweight compromise fertility, but it can also be problematic once you do become pregnant—even if you don't gain too much weight during pregnancy. Those extra pounds can increase the risk of miscarriage, gestational diabetes, gestational hypertension, preeclampsia, a longer labor, and a cesarean delivery. What's more, children born to moms who were overweight or obese at the time of conception are at increased risk of becoming obese or developing Type 2 diabetes during childhood and as adults. And prepregnancy obesity can also raise the risk of neural tube and other birth defects, especially if a woman wears much of her weight around her middle, rather than on her hips.

Clearly, getting to an ideal BMI (of 20 to 24, if possible) before you conceive is ideal—not only helping to speed baby-making success, but to boost your chances of having a healthier pregnancy, a safer delivery, and a healthy baby who has a healthier future. But any amount of weight loss in obese or overweight women can improve fertility and possibly egg quality. In fact, research shows that spontaneous ovulation reoccurs in 60 percent of women who reduce their body weight by as little as 5 to 10 percent. So if getting to your goal weight before you start your conception campaign isn't a realistic goal, just aim to lose what you can (see page 55 for tips how).

If you're considering weight-loss surgery to help you close in on that ideal BMI (or if you've already had the surgery), see page 54.

"I'm about 60 pounds overweight, and I know I'm supposed to get down to my ideal weight before I get pregnant, but I just don't want to wait that long. Can I just go ahead and try to conceive?"

Ideally, every woman would conceive when her weight was right about where it was supposed to be—giving her the optimum chances of conception and a healthy, comfortable pregnancy, a safe delivery, and a healthy baby. But conception doesn't always wait for the ideal circumstances, and sometimes waiting for conception isn't ideal, either, especially if you're over 35 (timing can be everything when you're planning a family).

It's possible that you'll have more trouble getting pregnant if you're significantly overweight (the statistics

TTC To-Do:

If you're overweight, aim to bring your weight down so your BMI is in the 20-to-24 range. Can't get that low—or get that low quickly enough for your preferred conception timetable? Even a weight loss of just 5 to 10 percent (that's about 8 to 16 pounds for someone who weighs 165 pounds) can help regulate your cycle and get you pregnant faster.

Couple Reasons to Lose Weight

Are you an obese couple trying to conceive? Though fertility can be compromised when just one of the partners is overweight, conception challenges multiply when both are packing extra pounds. In fact, making that baby can take 3 times longer for obese couples than for average-weight ones. To help ensure that you and your partner reach your baby-making goal together, try reaching your weight loss goals together first. After all, it's always easier to shed pounds as a team than solo (and when nobody's chowing down on Cheetos while you're nibbling on veggies and dip—or slumped on the sofa while you're trying to get motivated to take that morning walk). Eating right and exercising together will make it more likely that you'll both hit your goals (and the baby jackpot) faster. Go, Team Baby!

definitely support that possibility). But it's also possible that you won't. Though it's best to have a normal BMI when you are TTC, overweight women get pregnant all the time—just as underweight ones do. If your cycles run like clockwork, and if you appear to be ovulating regularly, your odds of conceiving may be pretty good.

Of course, improved fertility isn't the only reason why waiting for that ideal prepregnancy weight (or something approaching it) makes sense. Being overweight at the beginning of pregnancy poses a number of potential risks that can weigh down your pregnancy and even impact your baby-to-be's future health (see previous answer). Keeping your pregnancy weight gain to a minimum, under close supervision by your practitioner, can help reduce the risks significantly, if not eliminate them entirely. So can getting regular exercise (again, with your practitioner's input) and eating as well as you can. And, if you decide to move ahead with your TTC plans, don't wait to make those adjustments to your lifestyle. Getting on a balanced eating plan and an appropriate exercise program now can not only improve your fertility, but get your body

in the best possible shape for pregnancy. Who knows, maybe you'll even lose a good chunk of weight while you're waiting (or not waiting) to get pregnant.

Before you make any decisions about your TTC timing, though, talk to your practitioner about your plans and about ways to help optimize your conception and pregnancy success, even if you're not waiting for that optimum weight.

Polycystic Ovarian Syndrome and Overweight

"I have PCOS. Is that why I'm overweight and have so much trouble losing weight?"

It definitely could have something to do with it—or even everything to do with it. Polycystic ovarian syndrome, or PCOS, is a condition associated with irregular periods, lack of ovulation, elevated levels of male hormones, and, very often, obesity and/or persistent, sometimes unexplained weight gain. Women with PCOS may find that losing weight is a losing battle, even when they're giving dieting everything they've got. In fact, studies show that women with PCOS tend to gain more weight than women without PCOS, even if they eat the same foods and number of calories. Definitely unfair, but at least it explains what you're up against.

So what's the biological connection between PCOS and weight gain (and trouble losing weight)? First, women with PCOS often have insulin resistance. Normally, insulin transports glucose (sugar) out of the blood and helps convert it to energy. But with insulin resistance, the body is unable to use insulin properly. Thinking that there's not enough insulin to push sugar out of the blood and into the cells, the body reacts by producing even more insulin. Too much insulin, however, causes the glucose to be stored as fat instead of being converted to energy. Extremely high levels of insulin also turn off a fat-metabolizing enzyme, preventing you from burning stored fat—and making shedding the pounds frustratingly difficult. Second, some women with PCOS are hypothyroid (they don't make enough thyroid hormone). This thyroid dysfunction causes a lower metabolic rate (the rate at which you burn calories), and it makes losing weight tougher still. A thyroid imbalance can also throw your reproductive hormones off kilter, whether you're overweight or not.

Even with all the weight-loss cards seemingly stacked against you, there are treatments that can help you in your efforts, so that you can lose weight and regain your fertility. Some women with PCOS are prescribed metformin, an insulin-resistance medication that seems to help reduce the effects of PCOS, often making weight loss possible. A diabetes-friendly low-glycemic type of diet—your doctor (and perhaps a dietitian) can put one together for you—plus exercise can also help get your weight under control, giving your fertility a much-needed boost. And if you haven't yet been screened for thyroid dysfunction, ask your doctor about testing now. Treatment for a thyroid condition is simple (as easy as taking thyroid replacement hormone) and effective. For more on PCOS, see page 159.

Diabetes and Weight

"I have type 2 diabetes and I'm overweight. My diabetes is under control, so do I have to worry about my weight?"

Pat yourself on the back for getting your diabetes under control—no cakewalk (as you're no doubt reminded every time you walk away from a cake), and yet such an important step to take when you're hoping to get pregnant. But it's not the only step you should take. Being overweight—whether those extra pounds have triggered your diabetes or not—is still a risk factor for decreased fertility and increased pregnancy problems. Which is why your next step should be a concerted effort to get your weight down to where it should be (or close to that ideal).

And that goal may be easier to reach now that your diabetes is under control. It's true that having insulin-resistant diabetes makes you more prone to extra pounds because the excess blood sugar in your body is stored as fat. Excess insulin also turns off a fat-metabolizing enzyme, not allowing stored fat to be burned off and creating a double weight-loss whammy. But controlling your diabetes may help you get your weight under control, which may help you keep your diabetes under control. With well-controlled blood sugar, a good diet (usually low-glycemic, which keeps blood sugar level), and regular exercise (shoot for a minimum of 30 minutes a day of cardio, strength training, and stretching), you should be able to get your weight down. Yes, it'll take plenty of effort, loads of dedication, and more than a little sweat and sacrifice, but the rewards don't get any better. Not only will this strategy help put conception within reach, but if you continue it after conception, it'll help deliver an uncomplicated pregnancy and a healthy baby.

Underweight

"I'm underweight. Will that make it harder to get pregnant?"

Thin may be in, but here's the skinny on being really skinny. Women who have a very low BMI—usually under 18.5, though that benchmark can be a little higher or a little lower—tend to have very little body fat. Too little fat can mean too-low estrogen levels and possibly an imbalance of other reproductive hormones, which can lead to irregular ovulation or periods (or even no ovulation or periods). Irregular (or nonexistent) cycles can—stating the obvious here—make conception tricky or impossible. And if that's the case with

you, you may have to get some extra pounds on board before you can get that baby on board, too.

There are other reasons to consider filling out your frame before filling up your uterus, besides avoiding conception pitfalls. Women who are underweight when they become pregnant have an increased risk of severe nausea and vomiting during the early months of pregnancy, and extreme underweight (a BMI of less than 18) is linked to a higher risk of miscarriage. Extremely underweight expectant moms also run a higher risk of having a premature baby or one who's born too small, though excellent nutrition and good weight gain before and during pregnancy can definitely reduce those risks.

Talk to your practitioner about whether you should pack on some pounds before beginning your baby-making efforts—and how many pounds you should aim for. Every body is different (and some naturally extra-lean bodies conceive and handle pregnancy with ease), but chances are you'll be advised to shoot for a BMI of at least 18.5 but preferably between 20 and 24, the range widely considered optimum for baby making. Not only may a boost in BMI boost your chances of getting pregnant in the first place, but it will allow you to enter pregnancy at an ideal weight—so you'll be able to gain that 9-month standard of 25 to 35 pounds later without worrying about playing weight-gain catch-up first.

"I've always been thin—and definitely underweight for my height—at least according to the charts. But my doctor says I shouldn't be concerned about my fertility. Why's that?"

There's often a thin line between thin and too thin. And that line may be different for different women. The

---

FOR DADS-TO-BE

The Thin Man

If extra pounds weigh on a hopeful father's fertility, do lightweights have the edge in the dad competition? That depends on just how light on weight they are. Being very underweight—with a BMI of less than 20—may be linked to a lower sperm count and decreased sperm function. So if you're on the super-skinny side, you might want to think about adding a few healthy pounds before you and your partner start trying to add to your family.

weight that's right for you may be off the "normal range" charts—especially if it's a weight you've stayed at pretty consistently, without resorting to dieting or overexercising, and if you're otherwise in good health with a healthy lifestyle and eating habits.

That's why weight alone doesn't tell the whole story, particularly when it comes to fertility. You may be thin, but you may have just the right amount of body fat to keep your reproductive health humming along perfectly (regular periods, regular ovulation, and so on) even if your weight and BMI are on the low side. So if your doctor isn't concerned about your weight affecting your chances of becoming pregnant, you don't have to be, either.

Eating Disorders and Fertility

"I've battled with bulimia for years, but lately I've been doing much better. I'm thinking about getting pregnant—will having had an eating disorder affect my fertility?"

Fighting an eating disorder can be a real struggle—as you know all too well. So first of all, congratulations on the hard-earned progress you've made—that makes your pregnancy prognosis very promising. Putting your eating disorder in the past will almost certainly help you put a baby in your future.

Untreated eating disorders are a very different story, however, and a story that's not as likely to have a happy reproductive ending. Fertility can definitely be compromised—sometimes seriously so—by an eating disorder, especially an active one. In fact, as many as 1 in 5 women treated for infertility have either anorexia or bulimia. Not surprising, actually, since such disorders can disrupt the balance of hormones necessary to make conception happen.

Here's how: With anorexia, drastically reduced calorie intake and excessive exercising lead to dramatic weight loss and significant reduction of body fat (usually to levels way below normal). These factors can combine to result in a complete shutdown of a woman's menstrual cycle—no ovulation, no periods—which can obviously make conception virtually impossible. If anorexia continues for years untreated (or treated unsuccessfully), her reproductive system may be permanently damaged, and in some cases, her period may never return. Even if she does manage to get pregnant, extremely low levels of body fat can increase the risk of miscarriage.

Active bulimia can have a devastating effect on a woman's fertility, too—even if she manages to keep her weight relatively normal. In fact, about 50 percent of bulimics don't have regular menstrual cycles (which, again, makes conception less likely). But infertility problems are also possible in bulimics who have regular periods, since the binging and purging can lead to deficiencies in circulating hormone levels.

A nutritionally deprived diet, common for both anorexics and bulimics, can also lead to lowered libido, reduced egg quality, ovarian failure, and poor uterine environment—all of which can make a healthy pregnancy more elusive. Psychological stress from constant anxiety about food and weight monitoring is another potential fertility pitfall for those with eating disorders.

The good news? Taking steps to bring an eating disorder under control—as you've already done and are committed to keep doing—can help you take charge of your fertility and make your healthy-baby dreams a reality. Talk to your practitioner about your plans, and be completely up front about the problems you've had and any you're still grappling with, even if they're minor compared with those you've struggled with in the past. If you still need treatment before you take the pregnancy plunge, now's the time to get that help—from either a program or a therapist who specializes in eating disorders. You may even want to consider continuing the therapy while you're expecting, to make sure that normal pregnancy body changes don't trigger a relapse. Enlisting a dietitian can also help you reshape your eating habits, so you can continue nourishing your body and, hopefully soon, your baby-to-be's. Support groups (you can join one locally or find one online) can help you get your nutritional status back where it should be, as well as help you cope with body image issues that might come up during pregnancy.

The best news of all? Approximately 80 percent of women whose eating disorders are successfully treated will regain their ability to conceive. You can do it, too.

Weight-Loss Surgery and TTC

"My doctor said I need to lose 75 pounds before I start trying to conceive—but dieting isn't getting me anywhere, and I'd really like to get pregnant soon. Should I think about weight-loss surgery?"

When you're seriously overweight—and a lifetime of dieting and exercise haven't helped you melt off the pounds you're desperate to lose—bariatric surgery (gastric bypass, lap-band surgery, or a gastric sleeve, for example) may seem the answer to your weight problems. Especially when baby fever has you sweating the pounds that stand between you and conception. But do weight-loss surgery and baby making mix?

Actually, they can mix—and, with the right post-surgery nutrition, pretty successfully. In fact, such procedures can pave the quickest path to pregnancy for women who are too heavy to conceive. Women who have undergone weight-loss surgery often see a return to regular menstrual cycles within months of the operation, even if they haven't yet come close to their ultimate weight-loss goal. Fertility may return, too, sooner than expected. Some women are able to conceive just months post-op.

But while the surgery may well fast-track your fertility, you may not get the baby green light as quickly as you'd like—even if your cycles are back up and running. Some doctors suggest that women who have had weight-loss surgery put the brakes on their post-op conception plans until their weight has been stabilized for a year—not only so their bodies have time to heal from the surgery and adjust to the new weight, but also so they have time to replenish nutritional reserves that may have been drained by rapid weight loss. Still, regardless of when they conceive, women who become pregnant after weight-loss surgery can have healthy pregnancies and healthy babies—and, in fact, healthier than they would have if they hadn't lost weight at all.

If you're contemplating weight-loss surgery—or you've already had it, and wonder how it might affect your pregnancy plans—talk to your doctor about the best TTC timing for you. Also keep in mind that you'll have to be extra vigilant to make sure your nutritional needs are met during the preconception period and during pregnancy, to prevent shortfalls of vital baby-making nutrients. That's tricky after bariatric surgery, because your food intake will be drastically reduced, but it's definitely possible with some extra focus on the quality of food you eat, the right vitamin supplements, and guidance from your medical team.

Want to get started on TTC sooner? Try the tips starting below to see if you can fast-track your weight loss without surgery.

Reaching Your Ideal Weight

Okay, it's one thing to have a weight-loss—or gain—goal, it's another to actually make that goal a reality. Dieting to lose weight is never easy (and for the super-skinny, eating enough to gain may be tricky, too), but it can be particularly challenging when those pounds need to be shed (or gained) sensibly, as they should be when conception's next up on your agenda. Need a plan to get those numbers where they need to be in the fastest yet most baby-friendly way possible? Read on.

Losing Weight

Losing weight is easier said than done—even if your baby-making plans are making you especially motivated—but it's definitely doable. Your first stop (even before you stop at the market to stock up on yogurt, fresh fruit, and carrot sticks) should be at your practitioner's office. Together, come up with a sensible weight-loss goal and a sensible plan for reaching it—and discuss, too, any health problems that might be contributing to that extra weight, such as a thyroid condition or insulin resistance. It's best to reach your goal about 6 to 8 weeks before you start trying to conceive so your body can get used to its new shape before it starts changing again (pregnancy is definitely a big-time shape changer).

Resist the urge to sign up for a crash diet—even one that's high protein, low carb—because it can too easily deplete your body's stores of vital baby-making nutrients (and after all, it's weight you want to lose now, not nutrients). Steer clear, too, of cleanses, juice diets, diet pills and supplements, or anything that promises a quick fix ("lose 25 pounds in 2 weeks!"). Ditto for many trendy diets (like Paleo and raw food). Weight loss that's too quick can also lead to fertility problems—this time disrupting ovulation—and increase pregnancy risks if you do conceive. Rapid weight loss can also lead to rapid weight gain a few months later, and studies show that yo-yo dieters have a lower rate of fertility than those who lose the weight sensibly. Slow and steady may not have you winning any weight-loss races, but it's definitely the best diet plan when you're planning a baby. A gradual weight loss will give your reproductive hormones ample time to adjust to your new weight reality. Your body needs a steady diet of all kinds of nutrients to be baby ready.

Here's how to lose weight at a steady pace so your body can be in great shape for baby making:

■ Stick to a well-balanced diet that's low in calories and fat but doesn't over-restrict them. For instance, substitute low-fat milk for whole milk, opt for fresh melon or strawberries instead of dried fruit, roast your fish or chicken instead of frying it. Sensible doesn't make many diet headlines, but it's more likely to get the job done.

■ Create an eating plan that focuses on a healthy balance of lean protein, low-fat dairy products, veggies, fruits, and whole grains.

■ Choose foods that fill you up but are low in calories. Think turkey burger instead of fried chicken, frozen yogurt instead of full-fat ice cream.

■ Practice portion control. A serving of meat, poultry, or fish is equivalent to the size of a deck of cards. A serving of fruit is about the size of a lightbulb. A serving of pasta would fill an ice cream scoop. Instead of eating supersize portions (which could add up to 2 to 3 times the recommended daily amount of calories), keep an eye on your portion sizes so you're not eating more than you need to.

■ Get in the habit of grazing on small amounts of food more frequently (a good eating strategy for pregnancy, too).

■ Cut down on sweets, soda, and other junk food—or cut them out if it's easier for you (and it is for some serious junk food fans).

■ Drink lots of water. Lemon slices can add flavor.

■ If you haven't been exercising, start fitting in fitness. Even if it's just a daily 30-minute walk, adding activity will help jump-start your weight loss—and your journey to a healthy pregnancy.

■ Don't forget to take your prenatal vitamin—a standard preconception procedure that will also help fill in any nutritional blanks that dieting may create.

Some women find that a side of camaraderie helps them stay motivated to lose weight (and stick to that side salad, instead of that side of fries). If that's the case with you, check out TTC message boards (you'll find them on WhatToExpect.com) to see if you can team up with other hopeful moms who are eager to lose weight and gain a baby. Or consider joining Weight Watchers or another balanced diet plan that offers support along with those carrot sticks.

If you're feeling discouraged about the weight loss you have ahead of you, here's an encouraging bulletin that's sure to put a smile on your face (and maybe a piece of healthy fruit in your mouth): A loss of just 5 to 10 percent in overall body weight in overweight women (particularly obese women) who haven't been ovulating results in spontaneous ovulation in 60 percent of women. And you know what ovulation can bring you: baby bingo!

Gaining Weight

Gaining weight—like losing weight—is about calories in, calories out. So first, start packing those calories in. If you tend to be a meal skipper, you may also be skimping on your day's quota of calories. Instead, get into the regular-eating habit. Try sitting down for 3 squares a day, but supplement those with healthy, calorie-dense snacks (especially important if a smaller-than-average appetite keeps you from chowing down on too much food at one time). Though the obvious weight-gain formula might be fast food and lots of it (Supersize Me, Mom?), remember that the goal isn't just to gain—but to gain on foods that provide baby-friendly nutrients (fries, not so much). A better way to add those extra calories: Add more "good" fat foods into your diet, such as nuts, seeds, olive oil, and avocados, which can tip the scale in your favor while pumping up your nutritional stores. Focus on complex carbs, too (think whole-grain pasta, whole-wheat bread, and beans). And while you're at it, top them all with some cheese (calcium is your preconception pal, and so are the calories in cheese). Don't skip the fruits and veggies, even though they're low in calories, because they do provide essential baby-making fuel (but do try taking some of your fruits in a healthy higher-calorie smoothie, too). And of course, dig into that ice cream—you'll get a calcium bonus with those calories (add some nuts while you're at it, for extra calories and nutrients).

What about calories out—the ones you're burning through activity? If you're able to gain weight without cutting back on your fitness routine (if you have a fitness routine), great. The exercise may even fuel your appetite for more calories. But if you're taking more calories in yet seeing no results when you step on the scale, take a look at your activity level. If you're exercising strenuously or often, you may just be burning too many calories. Taking your routine down a notch (or maybe two) will still keep you fit, but will allow you to keep more of those calories you've taken in . . . in. And a little extra soft padding on top of that lean frame of yours may be just the ticket to mamahood.

As with hopeful moms and dads who need to lose weight before they step up to the preconception plate, you're wise to make "slow and steady" your motto, too. Gain weight gradually, and be sure to give your body some time to adjust to its new weight before trying to conceive (about 6 to 8 weeks should do the trick).

CHAPTER 3

Eating Well Before You're Expecting

H oping to be eating for two soon? First, you may want to take a look at how you're eating for one. That's because growing scientific evidence suggests that your fertility may be impacted by your diet—possibly improving it or possibly impeding it, depending on what that diet consists of. Which means that getting your eating plan up to baby-making speed may help you close in faster on conception. And there's more to chew on: The right preconception nutrition can even help your soon-to-be embryo get a healthier start in life while helping you enjoy a more comfortable pregnancy. Best of all, it's easier than you might think, and not that different from any sensible eating plan—or from the baby-friendly eating you'll be doing once baby's actually on board (which means you won't have to do much reshuffling of your eating habits later).

Your Preconception Eating Habits

A re you a candy craver? A breakfast skipper? A chip snacker? A soda sipper? Is your idea of a fresh vegetable the slice of tomato on your double bacon cheeseburger—or that side of onion rings? When was the last time you ate something loaded with omega-3s? And are you wondering what exactly an omega-3 is? If you answered "yes" or "huh?" to any (or all) of these questions, it's time to take a close look at your eating habits. That's because your fertility (like the rest of your health) may be impacted by what you eat—and what you don't eat. Plenty of folic acid and the right kind of carbs, for instance, may boost those baby odds. Too much junk food, on the other hand, may trash your conception plans. Bottom line: Filling your stomach with the right foods may help you fill your belly with a baby.

Pretty content with the content of your diet? Good for you—you're ahead of the game. Maybe all you'll have to do is balance your already balanced diet with some especially fertility-focused foods. Never met a vegetable or fruit you liked—or a candy bar or cupcake you didn't? You may have some work cut out for you. Just remember, any nutritional change for the better improves your chances of healthy baby making, even if it's just adding a daily piece of fruit to your lunch, switching from white to whole wheat, or trading in your frosted flakes for bran flakes.

How Well Do You Eat?

So maybe you think you eat really well already. Or maybe you're pretty sure your eating habits are about as bad as they could be. Or maybe you'd rate your diet somewhere in the middle—not too shabby, nothing to brag about. But the truth is, the only way to evaluate your eating habits accurately is to take a good, honest look at them—and the best way to do that is to keep a food journal.

A food journal takes the guesswork out of assessing your diet. It can also be a real eye-opener, particularly if you're a mindless eater—the kind who tends to nibble your way through a bag of chips while watching TV, realizing it only when you find yourself at the bottom. So try keeping track of your diet for a week, writing down (or inputting into

TTC To-Do:

Over the course of 7 days, write down or input into an app everything you eat and drink (including the amount and approximate calorie count, especially if you'll need to be dropping some preconception pounds). Note the number of portions you consume of each food you eat each day. Once your food journal is complete, you'll be able to figure out where your eating habits are—and where they need to be to boost your baby-making profile.

a food journal app) everything you eat, including the handful of M&M's you snagged from your boss's desk and those fries you stole off your hubby's plate at dinner. Be as specific as possible. And be truthful, too: Don't give yourself credit for a side salad you ordered but didn't end up eating. Remember, no one's going to see your food journal but you, so there's no reason to cheat.

Seem like a lot of effort? It is, but it's an effort worth making. What you'll have when you're finished is a complete picture of how you eat, the first step in figuring out how to eat better. You'll see where you're already hitting (or even exceeding) your mark, where you're falling somewhat short, where you're coming up empty—and how changes, either big or small, may be just the ticket you need to help you get that tiny (and cutest) passenger on board.

Making a Change for the Better

So now you know what your eating habits look like (the good, the bad, and the fried) and hopefully, what you'd like them to look like (you'll get the lowdown on what a balanced preconception diet should look like beginning on page 62). Now all you have to do is make a change for the better—which should be easy as pie (or as easy as switching from pie to fresh fruit), right? Maybe, or maybe not. There's no sugarcoating it: Depending on where they stand now and where you'd like them to head, changing your eating habits can be challenging. And even if you're fully up to the challenge, it's not likely you'll be able to transform your diet overnight. Give yourself some time and set realistic goals so you can set yourself up for success. Keeping your eye on the prize—a healthy baby on board—will also help you start making those changes for the better. So will these tips:

Think positive. Unfortunately, the word "diet" doesn't usually stir up positive thoughts—just flavorless flashbacks of rice cakes, celery sticks, and dry boneless chicken breast. Fortunately, eating well for your fertility doesn't have to mean denying yourself eating pleasure. Even if you have serious weight to lose before you conceive, super-restrictive isn't the way to go. Focusing on a wide, well-balanced, and delicious variety of fertility-friendly foods is. And that's a positive change.

Think small. As committed as you are to healthy baby making, thinking too big can be daunting and can make you want to give up before you've really gotten going. So stop thinking that way. Think, instead, of working your way toward your goal (appropriately) in baby steps. Need an example? If your food journal shows that you're not getting any whole grains in your diet, start with small changes: Swap your standard plain bagel for a whole-wheat bagel at breakfast, then start serving your stir-fry over brown rice instead of white. Once you're on a whole-grain roll, drop that midmorning cinnamon roll, adding an oat bran muffin in its place. Before you know it, most of the grains you eat will be whole—and the change will have come so gradually that you'll barely have noticed. Do you have a snack habit at work that propels you to the vending machine? Give the machine 2 weeks' notice, cut back on your visits (once a day instead of twice), and in the meantime try to develop a taste for cheese wedges, fresh fruit, and whole-grain crackers (it's been done!).

Get rid of preconceptions . . . about food. Quick—what do you think of when you think of green vegetables? That they're good for you, but not so good to eat? Whole-wheat bread—something you want to eat, or something you feel you should eat but wouldn't, given the choice? Oatmeal—a chewy, satisfying breakfast (especially when cinnamon and raisins find their way on top), or something Mom made you eat when you would have rather tucked into a Pop-Tart? Maybe it's time to rethink those preconceptions and take a fresh look at food. Instead of serving spinach in the form of your childhood nightmares (that nasty boiled mound that stood between you and dessert at Grandma's house), eat it raw in a sprightly spinach, red onion, and peach salad, lightly sautéed as a bed for grilled salmon, mixed with cheese and stuffed inside rolled chicken breasts, or chopped up in lasagna. With a new perspective and new preparations, you may find the healthy foods you always thought were yucky can actually be yummy, making the change for the better all that much easier.

Plan ahead. The very definition of a habit is that it's something you do all the time, without thinking. Which is why habits can be tough to change—especially when they're long-standing (skipping breakfast since middle school, for instance). So start thinking and planning ahead. Instead of waiting until your stomach is growling in hunger (and that candy bar starts calling you by name), have an eating-well plan in place. Stock up on healthy snacks (think freeze-dried fruit and toasted almonds, crunchy Moon Cheese, individual containers of yogurt, cut-up raw veggies and dip) and keep them within nibbling distance (in your bag, at your desk, in the car, in the office fridge) so you won't be as tempted to make a detour to the drive-through for fries or to the Quickie Mart for a quick bag of chips. Instead of leaving your shopping list up to impulse and the seductive powers of the snack-cake aisle, compose it ahead of time (leaving Little Debbie off), and stick with it—that is, unless a sudden healthy impulse has you reaching for fresh strawberries or a whole-grain cereal you've never seen before. Plan a healthy breakfast the night before so you're not left scrambling in the morning, brown-bag a healthy lunch the

TTC To-Do:

It's never too late to begin making healthy changes to your diet when you're making a baby, but it's never too early, either. So start your diet makeover as soon as you can, and preferably at least 3 months before you plan to get earnest in your TTC efforts. Beefing up your nutritional status and shedding any extra weight will not only help you boost your fertility, but help you provide the baby you hope to make with the healthiest possible start in life. Getting enough of the right nutrients—with the support of a prenatal supplement—may even help you avoid some of pregnancy's most miserable symptoms, too (like morning sickness).

night before so you're not tempted to add pork fried rice to the office takeout order. And have a plan for a nutritious dinner, too—even if it's nothing more ambitious than one of those healthy frozen dinners and ready-made salads you were clever enough to add to your shopping list—so that you won't be tempted to pick up a bucket of extra crispy on the way home.

Keep it real. When you're making your change for the better, take into account the limitations of your lifestyle (and real life)—otherwise, those new habits won't stand a chance. If mornings have you running to catch an early commuter train, a full-on, sit-down breakfast probably isn't in the cards. Instead, blend yourself a strawberry-mango-yogurt smoothie, to be sipped on the train. If you just can't get behind a bowl of oatmeal (or other traditional breakfast foods), break with breakfast tradition and heat up a slice of veggie pizza or toast a grilled cheese and tomato. If you know the chances of your making a sandwich to take to work are slim to none, find a deli that will make it for you, then pick it up on the way. Or get your last licks of sushi (it'll be off the menu once you conceive), picking up a ready-made package of salmon rolls at the market alongside a salad bar selection. If you're certain that willpower won't hold you back from the fast-food fries, visit the healthy wrap place instead of the greasy burger joint.

Don't deny it. If you've ever tried to stick with a diet before, you know that too many restrictions lead to crumbled resolve (and a big slab of cinnamon crumble cake when all you meant to order was a nonfat latte). So don't go there. Craving a bowl of ice cream? Fine, eat it. Just don't eat 3 of them. Longing for a chocolate bar? Munch on a mini instead of a king-size—and savor every morsel. Just keep the balance of healthy foods higher than the unhealthy ones, and find ways to make the less-than-wholesome food a little healthier (add walnuts instead of chocolate chips to your brownies). But recognize your limits, too. If you know you won't be able to stop once the lid's off the half gallon of ice cream, don't open it. Or better still, don't stock it in your freezer—buy single-serve cups or popsicles instead.

A Fertility-Friendly Diet

Since you're not pregnant yet, there's no need to start eating like you are (though if you'd like a preview of expectant eating, check out *What to Expect When You're Expecting* and *Eating Well When You're Expecting*). Still, not surprisingly, the very same kind of balanced diet that best nurtures a baby who's already on board can also best help you get that baby on board. Eating well now, while you're in preconception mode, may increase the likelihood that you'll get pregnant—plus it sets the stage for a healthier pregnancy once egg and sperm meet up.

But a balanced diet—as important as it is not only to fertility, but to general health—is just the beginning when you're eager to conceive. Putting specific foods (and types of foods) on the menu can actually help jump-start a pregnancy by boosting your fertility. Here's what you need to know to make sure your eating plan is fertility-friendly.

Fertility-Friendly Nutrients

Already found balance in your diet? That's definitely a good place to start when you're hoping to eat for two. Want a little more direction to point you toward the baby goal line? Look no further than these fertility-friendly nutrient categories. Each contributes a little something to the baby-making process—but put them together and they pack a powerfully proactive preconception punch.

Full Fat for Full Fertility

Looking for a reason to favor fat? Here's one: Some research suggests that full-fat dairy products (like whole milk, whole-milk yogurt, and whole-milk cheese) offer fertility perks over nonfat and low-fat options, possibly offering protection against ovulation-related infertility. But before you get busy with Ben and Jerry, keep in mind that just 1 daily serving of high-fat dairy—as in 1 glass of whole milk—will net you any potential fertility benefits without the obvious, definite drawbacks (extra pounds, which can actually decrease fertility). Have a lot of preconception pounds to drop? Check with your doctor about whether you should stick with a fat-free approach to dairy.

Bone up on calcium. You already know it's smart to sport a milk mustache when you're pregnant. But upping your calcium intake even before you conceive is smart, too—especially because it might help you conceive a lot sooner. Boning up on calcium will help ensure the proper functioning of your reproductive system, the system you're understandably most focused on right now. Plus, it'll help stock up your stores of this bone-building mineral important not only for your future baby's bone health, but for your future bone health. If your calcium stores and intake fall short during pregnancy, your body will tap into your own bones to build baby's, possibly setting you up for osteoporosis later in life. And if that's not reason enough to raise your glass of milk in a preconception toast, consider that getting enough calcium in your system now will help strengthen your fetus-to-be's developing teeth and bones, as well as help muscle, heart, and nerve development.

The best-known source of calcium is milk (which also comes with a vitamin D bonus), but it's just as easy to find in other dairy-case favorites, including cheese and yogurt. You can mine this mineral from many nondairy sources, too, including calcium-fortified juice, almond milk, soy milk, tofu and other soy products, almonds, sesame seeds, beans, and green leafy veggies. You'll even cash in on calcium when sipping on a smoothie (made with milk or yogurt) and score some when dipping into a bowl of frozen yogurt.

Can't be sure you're hitting your calcium goal? Or just want to give your bones and your fertility every edge? Pop some calcium supplements—aim for 1,500 mg a day—along with your prenatal vitamin. Three Tums, Rolaids, or calcium chews will net you the same total.

TTC To-Do:

How much calcium do you need in your preconception diet? Aim for 3 servings of calcium-rich foods daily. One serving is equivalent to ¼ cup grated or shredded cheese; 1 cup milk, soy milk, almond milk, or calcium-fortified juice; 1 cup yogurt; 1½ cups frozen yogurt; 4 ounces canned salmon with bones; 1 cup cooked collard greens; 1½ cups cooked edamame (soybeans); 3 cups raw kale or arugula; 3 tablespoons sesame seeds.

Power up on protein. Getting ready to build a baby? Then you'll want to put plenty of protein on your plate. Proteins, after all, are considered the body's building blocks—essential for the manufacture of bones, muscles, cartilage, skin, blood, even enzymes and hormones (yours and those of the baby you'll soon be making from scratch).

Does any variety of protein make the baby-making cut? Should you check off the steak or the fish, or maybe the vegetarian option? What about size (of that burger)—does that matter? Maybe. There are 2 general types of protein: animal (meat, chicken, fish) and plant (nuts, seeds, legumes). Either category alone can provide the protein you need to get your body in baby-making mode, as can a balanced combo of both categories. But what some research has shown is that selecting too many high-fat animal proteins—say, that whopper of a burger, those finger-licking ribs, the well-marbled steak—may undercut your chances of getting pregnant, not to mention undermine your general health. Instead, order up lower-fat animal proteins more often—like lean beef and buffalo (aka bison), lean pork (like

TTC To-Do:

Where's the beef? Where it probably shouldn't be is heaped high on your preconception plate, at least if it isn't lean. Current recommendations advise the fertility-focused to get about 2 to 3 servings of protein daily—with at least 1 of those servings preferably being a plant protein, and most animal proteins coming from lean sources. The exception would be higher-fat fish, like salmon, which comes by its fat the healthy omega-3 way. Each protein serving is surprisingly small—equivalent to about the size of your palm. Choose from these (and many other) offerings: 4 ounces (before cooking) poultry, beef, buffalo, or pork; 4 ounces fish or seafood; 3½ ounces canned fish (see page 73 for information on fish safety); 1½ cups cooked beans, lentils, split peas, or chickpeas; 1 cup cooked soybeans (edamame); 3 ounces peanuts. You can also get protein from tofu, nuts, seeds, miso, and high-protein grains such as quinoa and farro.

loin), chicken breast, fish, and shellfish. Just don't over-order. While TTC, it's considered best to limit animal protein—even the lean varieties—to 2 to 3 servings a day, or about 50 to 75 grams (a lot less than you'd net on a Paleo or other high-protein diet). More than 100 grams per day, or 4 servings, can actually compromise fertility (one reason why a high-protein/low-carb diet isn't your best bet; see page 77).

Look to plant proteins, too. Some research finds that swapping out even 1 serving of animal protein (lean or high fat) in your diet for 1 serving of plant protein may help give fertility a boost. Wrap yourself around a black bean enchilada instead of a carne asada. Swap a veggie burger for your usual beef. Stir-fry some tofu instead of some pork. Make your chili full of beans but free of meat.

Pump up with iron. Each month your iron stores are depleted by your period—especially if your flow is heavy (the more blood loss, the more iron loss). Pumping up the iron before you conceive will give your body a chance to replenish those stores before they're needed during pregnancy (it'll take a lot of iron-rich blood cells to nourish and grow that baby-to-be). Pumping up now also makes it less likely that you'll suffer from iron-deficiency anemia during pregnancy (nature takes care of baby's iron needs first, which can leave mom short on her supplies), and after delivery.

But there's even more to the iron-mom story—and in fact, the story begins before sperm meets egg. Researchers have found that women with adequate iron stores have a higher fertility rate than women who are low on iron. Women with iron-deficiency anemia also tend to have irregular periods, which might be the body's way of protecting against further blood loss—and further depletion of iron stores. Messed-up menstrual cycles, not surprisingly, make it more difficult to conceive.

To pump up your iron, turn to leafy greens (collard, kale, spinach), red meat (just keep it lean), dried beans, peas, dried apricots, and oatmeal. To boost absorption, team iron-rich foods with ones rich in vitamin-C (sip some OJ with that oatmeal, or toss in some tomatoes with those beans). You'll also be getting some iron from the prenatal vitamin that you've hopefully started taking already (see page 69). If your preconception blood test reveals that you need more iron than your diet plus a prenatal vitamin with iron can serve up, your practitioner may recommend adding an extra iron supplement. But since far from every woman needs extra iron—and you can get too much of a good thing—don't add a supplement without that go-ahead.

Order up some omega-3s. Never thought fat could be your friend? Well, here's a fat you should definitely get to know . . . and get to love: omega-3 fatty acids. These fabulous fats, most notably DHA, will be essential to your baby-to-be's brain and eye development, so they're definitely a must-have-often during pregnancy, as well as while you're breastfeeding.

But the omega-3 benefits don't just begin once you've conceived your baby. Rewind to the preconception phase (now), when these fatty acids are essential to your overall health, and perhaps to your fertility, too. Omega-3s help regulate hormones—including, possibly, the ones that induce ovulation. They may also increase blood flow to the reproductive organs (for both sexes), always a good thing when baby making's on the agenda. What's more, omega-3s are recognized for their mood-balancing effects, which means that getting your fill may help ease emotional stress (definitely a fertility plus—and absolutely a pregnancy one).

It's easy to get in the omega-3 habit, especially if you're fond of salmon and other higher-fat fish (such as anchovies, sardines, and herring; see page 73 for a safe fish list). Not a fish fan? Grass-fed beef and buffalo are also super sources of omega-3s, as are walnuts and walnut oil, flaxseed and flaxseed oil, chia seeds, DHA (or omega-3) eggs, pasture-raised chicken, and even arugula. Many prenatal vitamins also contain omegas, though dietary sources may deliver the best results.

And while you're feeding yourself these phenomenal fats, don't forget to feed your partner some, too. The preconception perks of an omega-3-rich diet may be even greater for hopeful dads (see the box on page 67).

Consider carbs carefully. A carb is a carb is a carb, and all carbs are bad—right? Wrong. Though carbohydrates have gotten a bad rep (thanks to the popularity of high-protein diets), it's important not to lump all carbs together in the same breadbasket, especially when you're trying to get a bun in your oven. There's a world of nutritional difference between carbs that are complex (whole grains, beans, legumes, fruits, and vegetables) and those that are simple, or easily converted to sugar (such as white bread, white rice, white potatoes, sugary soda, candy bars, and so on). And that difference apparently extends to fertility, too. Researchers have found that women who eat slowly digested complex carbs have higher fertility rates than those whose diets include more of those easily digested simple carbs. What's the connection, and since when is easy digestion a minus? Rapid digestion of noncomplex carbs leads to an increase in blood sugar (as in that sugar high you get after you polish off a red velvet cupcake) and an increase in insulin.

Carbs and PCOS

Opting for complex carbs is an especially important nutritional strategy if you have polycystic ovarian syndrome (PCOS), a hormonal problem that's related to high insulin levels. To keep your insulin from spiking and your reproductive system from derailing, reject those refined carbs and slow down your digestion with whole grains, fresh fruit and vegetables, beans, and legumes. See page 50 and 159 for more on PCOS.

Feed Your Boys

You've probably heard that you are what you eat—but did you know that your sperm are, too? It's true. The healthier your diet, the healthier your sperm—and the more easily you'll likely conceive.

So what foods can give you the fertility edge? A balanced diet, one that includes plenty of fresh fruits and vegetables, whole grains, and lean protein, will almost certainly edge you closer to fertility. Want more specifics? Here are some key sperm-friendly nutrients, as well as the foods you can easily find them in:

- Vitamin A. This A-list vitamin is essential for the production of good swimmers—in fact, vitamin A deficiencies in men have been linked to lowered fertility due to sluggish sperm. You can find plenty of this vital vitamin in leafy greens (dark green lettuce, broccoli, spinach, kale) and orange and yellow vegetables and fruits (carrots, sweet potatoes, red peppers, mangoes, apricots, yellow peaches, cantaloupe), as well as in dairy, fish, and meat, and in oatmeal and other whole grains. Getting your A is as easy as having a V8, tossing back a salad topped with red peppers and carrots, or starting your day with the breakfast of swimming champions: a bowl of oatmeal topped with dried apricots. Really motivated? Earn yourself an A+ by eating all three in the same day.

- Vitamin C. This well-known nutrient will help take your sperm places, increasing motility and viability—and it's easy to find. Start with the obvious sources (grapefruit and OJ), but also look to asparagus, broccoli, cauliflower, kale, red peppers, snow peas, sweet potatoes, tomatoes (they're especially good for you cooked—so pour on that tomato sauce), melon, kiwis, peaches, strawberries, and watermelon—to name a tasty few. You'll find that many C's overlap with A's, giving you extra credit.

- Vitamin D. These days, most people get a D– when it comes to their D intake—making them D-deficient. That's because of less time spent in the sun (the most readily available source of D) and more sunscreen use (sunscreen blocks the absorption of vitamin D through the skin). Fortunately, it takes a severe D deficiency to lead to lowered fertility, in the form of deterioration of testicular tissue. But because you want to give your baby-making effort every edge, try stocking up on the D in your diet. It's actually as simple as pouring yourself a glass of milk or fortified OJ, scrambling up some eggs (it's in the yolks), or chowing down on some sardines (okay, it's an acquired taste). Easier still—score all the D you need by getting a few minutes of sun each day (though if you're dark skinned, you may need 10 times more sun exposure than a light-skinned person). Vitamin D is manufactured in the body from a chemical reaction to the ultraviolet rays in sunlight—but skip the sunscreen during those few minutes. Otherwise you'll be blocking out some of the rays you want to be soaking up.

- Vitamin E. So you've heard a lot about antioxidants, but do you really know what they are, and more importantly, what they do? They're substances found in vitamins that serve to protect cells in your body. When it comes to your fertility, they're busily protecting your boys. Researchers suspect that antioxidants from vitamins A and E (and others) protect sperm DNA from being damaged, ensuring that they stay vital, vigorous, and up to the job of fertilizing an egg. Get your E the easy way, from vegetable oils (choose canola, flaxseed, olive, or sunflower oils), sweet potatoes (yes, the same sweet potatoes that made the A and C lists—so bake a couple tonight for you and your sweetie), mangoes (ditto—share a mango smoothie for dessert), avocados (yes, as in the guacamole you love), spinach, almonds, and sunflower seeds.

- Folic acid. There's plenty of buzz about the importance of folic acid (or folate) for hopeful and expecting moms, but it's a nutrient that's vital for hopeful dads, too. Inadequate amounts of folate in a man's diet can lead to low sperm quality—and may even be linked to birth defects since men with folic acid deficiencies have a higher rate of sperm with chromosomal abnormalities. Plus, prospective fathers appear to need even more folic acid than their partners. Researchers suggest that guys who consume 700 to 1,000 mcg of folic acid daily show the most benefit when it comes to sperm health. Find your folate in leafy green vegetables (time for another salad), most fruits (and another smoothie), avocados (there's that guac again), and beans (you can add even more guac atop that bean burrito). There's also folic aplenty in whole grains, as well as in refined grains (it's added during processing).

- Zinc. As you work your way through the nutrient alphabet, don't forget Z—for zinc. Too little of this virility-vital mineral can lead to low testosterone levels and diminished sperm count. Fortunately, chances are excellent you've already got lots of zinc on your menu—it's found in beef (finally, some good news about burgers!), turkey, yogurt, oatmeal, eggs, seafood, and corn. But if you really want a boatload of zinc (and maybe a really hot night), go overboard on oysters. Apparently what they've always said about these mollusks is true: Oysters are for lovers.

- Omega-3 fatty acids. Fat's gotten a bad name—and, in fact, too much of the wrong fats can mess with both female and male fertility. But here are some fats you can feel good about loving—and eating—in large amounts. DHA and other essential omega-3 fatty acids help improve blood flow to the genitals and increase sexual function. Plus, they also naturally lower blood pressure (which is good for the heart and good for your performance). And here's another reason to reach for these phenomenal fats: Fertile men's sperm contains more of this essential fatty acid than the sperm of infertile men. Find your omega-3s in salmon and other fatty fish, like sardines and anchovies (so order a Caesar salad with your anchovy pizza), grass-fed beef and buffalo, walnuts, omega-3 eggs (you can buy them in any supermarket, and they taste great), arugula, crab, shrimp, flaxseed (look for these nutty-tasting seeds in many whole-grain cereals, crackers, and breads), and even chicken.

- The whole vitamin-mineral gang. Even if you eat well (and especially if you don't), adding a good vitamin-mineral supplement can't hurt. Taking a daily vitamin will act as a nutritional insurance policy, helping you make up any shortfalls in your diet and helping ensure that your health, your fertility, and your sperm are in tip-top shape. Just remember that too much of a good thing can actually be a bad thing. Megadoses of some vitamins and minerals in supplement form can have a negative impact on fertility and sperm production. For example, too much supplementary zinc can be toxic to sperm. The good news for foodie fathers: You can't get too many vitamins and minerals from the food you eat (so go ahead and order that second round of oysters).

TTC To-Do:

What's the plan for complex carbs in your fertility diet? Aim for:

- 6 servings of whole grains. Sound like a lot of dough, or a hill of beans? Keep in mind that whole grains are often stellar sources of plant protein, too, so they perform double nutritional duty. Plus, a serving is a lot smaller than you'd think (a serving of whole-grain pasta, for instance, would only fill an ice cream scoop). Equivalent servings of whole grains include 1 slice whole-wheat bread; 1 serving whole-grain cereal; ½ cup cooked bulgur, whole-wheat couscous, buckwheat, barley, brown rice, farro, or quinoa; 1 ounce (before cooking) whole-grain pasta; and ½ cup cooked beans, lentils, split peas, or edamame.

- 2 to 4 servings of fruit. You'll net a full serving of vitamin C by eating (among many others): ½ grapefruit; ½ orange; ½ mango; ½ cup cubed honeydew; ⅔ cup berries; ½ kiwi; or 2 cups diced watermelon. You'll get a serving of vitamin A (plus a good dose of other essential carotenoids and vitamins) by eating (among others): 1 peach; ½ cup cubed cantaloupe (which also nets you a C serving); ¼ medium papaya; or 6 dried apricot halves. And you'll benefit from the antioxidants, phytochemicals, and minerals in the following fruits, each considered a serving: 1 banana; 2 plums; ½ cup cherries; 1 cup grapes; 1 apple; 1 pear.

- 3 to 5 servings of vegetables. Choose from these vitamin C veggies (among many others): ¼ red, yellow, or orange bell pepper; ½ cup broccoli or cauliflower; 1 tomato; 1 cup raw spinach or green leafy lettuce; ¾ cup red cabbage. Or dip into these veggies, each of which nets a serving of vitamin A: ½ carrot or sweet potato; ¼ cup cooked winter squash; ½ cup cooked spinach; ¼ cup chopped parsley. For servings of veggies that offer other antioxidants, phytochemicals, and minerals, turn to: ½ cup cooked green beans; ½ cup raw mushrooms; ½ cup cooked zucchini, parsnips, or okra; 1 ear corn; ½ cup green peas.

Insulin, besides being a factor in diabetes, also helps regulate ovulatory function. Too much insulin in your body can disrupt the delicate balance of reproductive hormones, throwing your menstrual cycle off kilter and making conception much more elusive. On the other hand, eating complex carbs that take longer to digest (that bowl of shredded wheat and strawberries) doesn't impact insulin levels—and can actually improve your body's ability to ovulate regularly and your ability to get pregnant.

Need another reason to order up your sandwich on whole wheat, reach for the brown rice instead of the white, or toss some beans into your soup instead of noodles, especially when you're trying to conceive? Complex carbs contain an impressive variety of fertility-friendly nutrients—from antioxidants to iron to those baby-boosting B vitamins. Refined carbs have had many of those naturally occurring vitamins and minerals stripped away in processing.

And the reasons to get more complex with your carbs keep on coming. Once that bun is in the oven, opting for whole grains and other complex carbs will, among other perks, provide essential baby-growing nutrients, fiber to help fight constipation (a common pregnancy symptom—stay tuned), B vitamins you'll need to ease any early pregnancy queasiness, and blood sugar regulation to combat fatigue, mood swings, headaches, and more.

Factor in the folic. You've probably already heard how important the B vitamin folic acid (or folate, the naturally occurring form of folic acid) is during pregnancy—it's a vital vitamin in the fight against crippling neural tube defects, such as spina bifida. But studies show that getting enough of this crucial nutrient before you conceive lowers the chances that your baby will develop a neural tube defect (if you take folic acid for 3 months before pregnancy), autism (if you take folic acid for at least 4 weeks before conception), possibly cardiac defects, and perhaps even preterm birth. Relevant in your short-term plans: An adequate intake of folic acid has been linked to increased fertility.

Where can you find folate? Most leafy green vegetables and whole grains are naturally full of it—plus it's added to most refined grain products by law. But since you can't be too careful when it comes to filling your preconception quota, it's recommended that all TTC women take a prenatal supplement containing 400 to 600 mcg of folic acid (yes, even if you're a regular at the salad bar).

Give me an "A" . . . give me a "C" . . . give me a "B₆" . . . What does it spell? A healthier pregnancy—and possibly, a sooner one. You may not be pregnant yet, or even actively trying to conceive, but adding a daily prenatal vitamin to your diet is already a smart move. That's because the same nutrients that will eventually help you grow a baby may also help you conceive a healthier baby—which makes stocking up on them now doubly important.

What makes a prenatal supplement so perfectly suited to the preconception set? It's the carefully selected combination of vitamins and minerals it contains. Here are just a few examples. Many of

Forecast:
Sunny with a Chance of Low Folic Acid

Are you a tanning bed fan? A lover of lying out? Beach babies who aspire to be mamas, take note: Regular unprotected exposure to the sun's ultraviolet rays (or those from a tanning bed) depletes folic acid—a vitamin vital not only during pregnancy but before. Researchers have found that women who regularly spend time outdoors between 10 a.m. and 3 p.m. with little sun protection have a 20 percent decrease in folate levels compared with women who don't spend all that time outdoors. Experts say this drop is enough to make these hopeful moms'

folate levels lower than what doctors consider normal. So if you're going to spend significant time outdoors during the day, be sure to slather on a high-SPF sunscreen. Choose one labeled "broad-spectrum" to screen out both ultraviolet B (UVB) and ultraviolet A (UVA) rays. And stay away from the tanning beds (which you'll be avoiding anyway once baby's on board). Be sure, too, to take that prenatal supplement with 400 to 600 mcg of folic acid every day when you're trying to conceive (and throughout your pregnancy) and to get your fill of folate from your diet.

Should You Curb Your Herbs?

They're sometimes touted for their ability to boost fertility, but could herbs be more of a bust when you're TTC? Check out what's known about herbs and fertility on page 133.

the B vitamins, most notably folic acid, appear to increase fertility. Folic acid, as you've just read, is crucial for the health and wellbeing of your baby and pregnancy, too (see page 69), which is why taking your prenatal supplement for at least 3 months before you start TTC is a smart move. B_{12} is another B vital to healthy reproduction, and in fact a B_{12} deficiency coupled with anemia (both more common among vegetarians) has been linked to ovulation issues and even repeat miscarriages. Vitamin D is hard to come by unless you soak up a lot of sun (exposure that can lead to skin damage, and even skin cancer) or take a supplement, which means many women don't get enough—and some may even be D-deficient. D may also be a fertility friend, particularly for those who have ovulation problems or who are deficient in the vitamin. Iron may give fertility a boost, too, especially if you're low on stores. And the benefits of taking a prenatal continue: from the right amount of A (a baby-friendly antioxidant) to zinc (another notable star in fertility—in fact, a zinc deficiency may slow the maturation of good-quality eggs, something you definitely want to have in your reproductive basket right now). Still another potential perk of popping a prenatal preconception: Take one that's chock-full of B_6, and it's possible

you may experience fewer episodes of nausea and vomiting during your first trimester of pregnancy.

Which prenatal to choose? Check with your practitioner for a recommendation, or look for one that has at least 400 mcg (micrograms) of folic acid, 1,000 mg of calcium, 30 to 40 mg of iron, and 400 IU of vitamin D, plus fertility-boosting nutrients such as zinc, manganese, and even possibly omega-3s. If you find pills hard to swallow (literally, especially when they're horse-size pills), choose one with a slicker coating or one in gel cap form. Powder, gummy, and chewable prenatals are also an option (if not always as tasty as labels promise). Most important, stay with the recommended dosage and don't take extra supplements of any kind unless your doctor recommends them. More isn't better when it comes to vitamins and minerals, unless they're the naturally occurring kind (you can't overdose on the ones you find in food).

It's true you can get plenty of vitamins and minerals from eating a healthy, well-balanced diet—and you should definitely try to do that. But a good

TTC To-Do:

Start taking a prenatal vitamin as soon as you start thinking about getting pregnant—and at least 3 months before you start trying (starting a year before may be even better, if you're planning that far in advance). Not only will it get you into the habit of taking a daily pill (so that it'll become second nature by the time you're actually pregnant), but it could also get you on the expectant express faster. Plus, it'll help ensure a healthier baby and a more comfortable pregnancy. So get popping, hopeful mom!

prenatal supplement serves as a nutritional insurance policy—it not only makes sure that your intake of those vital nutrients is always up to snuff even when your diet isn't, but also acts as a crucial ingredient in the health of your future baby and pregnancy.

Have you recently stopped popping the Pill so you can get busy making a baby? Taking a prenatal may be even more beneficial for you. That's because taking oral contraceptives for an extended period may put some women at a nutritional disadvantage. Make sure all your nutritional stores are fully filled now by popping that prenatal and eating a diet that's chock-full of baby-making vitamins and minerals.

Fertility-Friendly Foods

Though old wives have practically been put out of business by search engines, the tales they told for generations are still making the rounds (more efficiently than ever, thanks to Dr. Google). And one category of tales that seems to have the most legs: foods that make you fertile. You've heard them, you've read them, you've probably told some—and still you're probably wondering, could any of them actually be true? Could there really be foods that enhance fertility? Maybe, and maybe not. So far there really aren't any well-documented studies to back up the claim that putting any one food in your tummy will help put a baby in your belly—but there haven't been any done that rebut them, either. With that in mind, take the following fertile food recommendations (and any others you stumble on during your TTC mission) with a grain of salt—and maybe a side of salad (hey, you can't go wrong with salad). Still, there's definitely no harm in adding these to your balanced diet (they're all healthy foods anyway), and in the case of some there could actually be some pretty substantial fertility perks.

Yams. Since populations that eat wild yams as their staple food seem to have a higher rate of twin pregnancies, some have suggested that yams have fertile properties. Even if yummy yams don't turn out twins, they're definitely a fertile source of nutrients—all the more reason to serve them up.

Nuts and seeds. Walnuts, almonds, and pumpkin seeds (to name a few) are all abundant sources of omega-3 fatty acids, which research shows are vital not only to productive baby making but also to a healthy baby. That's because these fabulous fats (yes, fats can be fabulous!) help regulate hormones—and it's hormones that induce ovulation. Which means that snacking on some trail mix instead of, say, potato chips may help get you on the road to conception. Clearly, this is one fertility food theory that isn't nuts.

Oysters. You've almost certainly heard that oysters can heat things up between the sheets, but did you know that these tasty bivalves can fuel your fertility, too? That's because oysters are off-the-charts rich in zinc, and any food that's rich in zinc can help maintain a healthy menstrual cycle. Zinc deficiency, in fact, has been linked to decreased fertility because it can slow the production of good-quality eggs—something that's obviously essential for conception. Not an oyster lover? No food comes even remotely close to oysters in the zinc competition, but you'll find smaller amounts of this fertility-friendly mineral in other kinds of seafood (such as crab and lobster), as well as in beef, turkey, dairy products, nuts, pumpkin seeds, and legumes.

Fertile Food for Hopeful Fathers?

Hungry for fatherhood? Some evidence suggests that you can feed your fertility by feeding yourself certain foods (and maybe, get yourself a little closer to having that extra little mouth to feed). Though the scientific jury is still out on just how much nutritional input can affect your output (of sperm), there's no downside to adding these healthy foods to your balanced diet, and there could be a significant upside—in more ways than one.

- Oysters. No doubt you've heard that slurping a batch of these bivalves can raise the libido roof, but oysters may also hop up your fertility. That's because they're loaded with zinc, a mineral that helps fuel semen and testosterone production. Can't acquire a taste for oysters? Pumping up your intake of other zinc-rich foods will also help pump up your sperm. Though none can even come close to the oyster's colossal content, you'll find some zinc in beef, turkey, nuts, legumes, dairy products, and in a good vitamin-mineral supplement (which you should consider taking preconception anyway).

- Honey. Put this sweet treat on your "honey-do" list—add it instead of sugar to tea, hot cereal, yogurt, and more. It's packed with boron, a mineral believed to increase the production of testosterone, a hormone that comes in very handy when you're TTC.

- Fruits and veggies. Mom was right about eating your broccoli—except she probably didn't have this benefit in mind: The more fruits and vegetables a man eats, the more energetic his sperm may be. The antioxidants in vibrantly colored produce (such as red peppers, carrots, blueberries, peaches, pink grapefruit, sweet potatoes, tomatoes, and greens of all kinds) give sperm a boost, potentially giving you a fertility edge.

- Pomegranate juice. This juice has made a splash in the nutrition headlines as a powerful antioxidant (its naturally occurring potent purple color can clue you in), but it's also making waves when it comes to male fertility, at least in the lab. Pomegranate juice has been shown to increase sperm count and boost sperm quality in rats—probably because of that high antioxidant content. Researchers are trying to determine if these benefits are reproducible (so to speak) in humans, but so far no published studies have confirmed positive results. Until then, it can't hurt to chug some PJ every now and then—or even to swap it for your morning OJ (they're actually pretty tasty in combo).

- Pumpkin seeds. Naturally high in zinc and essential fatty acids, pumpkin seeds can give your boys a boost as they swim off on their conception quest. So snack on a handful every now and then.

Berries. Berries (think blueberries, raspberries, acai berries, and strawberries) are excellent sources of antioxidants, which can prevent cell damage and aging. How does this relate to fertility? By protecting eggs from damage—especially important for those that have been on the shelf longer (as is true for older moms who are expecting to expect), but helpful for all who want to give their eggs an extra edge. So go berry crazy—toss them on your cereal, in your smoothie, over your ice cream. Try them in crunchy, convenient freeze-dried form, too.

Fertility-Unfriendly Foods

So now you know what foods make the conception cut—and you're likely chowing down on some already. But what about foods—and drinks, and supplements—that are fertility unfriendly? Are there any you should be limiting on your preconception menu? Though scientists are still trying to figure out the science behind fertility-boosting and fertility-busting foods, being sensible about certain foods (cutting back on some, eliminating others) while you're trying to conceive may help get that baby on board faster.

Mercury. This heavy metal is a pretty insidious substance—especially because it can accumulate in your body and linger there, without you even knowing it. What's the connection to fertility? Not only do men and women struggling with infertility tend to have higher mercury levels in their blood than those with normal fertility, but having high mercury levels at the time of conception can be harmful to your baby-to-be's development—even if you're careful to steer clear of this toxic chemical during pregnancy. So it's smart to start cutting back on sources of mercury in your diet, if you haven't already.

Fish is the major dietary source of mercury and probably the only one you need to be mindful of when you're in baby-making mode. If you're pregnant, nursing, trying to conceive, or even thinking about trying to conceive, experts—including the EPA, FDA, and ACOG—suggest avoiding entirely any fish that's typically high in mercury, such as shark, swordfish, king mackerel,

tilefish (especially from the Gulf of Mexico), marlin, and orange roughy, and limiting your intake of recreationally caught freshwater fish to an average of 6 ounces per week. What about tuna? Experts agree that canned light tuna is safe to eat because it's not high in mercury. Solid or chunk white tuna (albacore) contains 3 times the mercury of light varieties, and experts recommend limiting it. Are you a fan of fresh tuna? Skip ahi (bigeye) tuna entirely, since it's especially high in mercury, and limit other varieties of fresh tuna to no more than 6 ounces per week.

But don't take fish off the menu altogether. Fish is packed with lean protein and vitamin D, and loaded with the most fabulous of all fats, omega-3 fatty acids (especially such fatty fish as salmon, herring, and anchovies). So go fish, choosing from salmon (wild caught is best), sole, flounder, haddock, trout, halibut, ocean perch, pollack, cod, light canned tuna, catfish, and other smaller ocean fish. And as you do, here's one fish favorite you may want to go wild

---

FOR DADS-TO-BE

Meaty Men

Is meat a mainstay of your menus (as in bacon for breakfast, bologna for lunch, and burgers for dinner)? Consider this before you order up your next meal: Research shows that men who regularly eat large amounts of beef—especially the processed kinds, like deli and breakfast meats—have a lower sperm count. No need to cut out meat altogether. Just choose healthier forms of it, like lean beef and buffalo (aka bison), and lean pork (like loin), and pile on other proteins like chicken breast, fish, and shellfish.

Tapping Into Safe Water

Tap water: It's the easiest drink in the house—especially when TTC mode has you laying off the diet soda, cutting back on caffeine, and weaning off wine. And happily, most of the nation's water supply is tested frequently and considered safe to drink. But in some communities across the country, the water flowing from the tap doesn't get a clean bill of health—containing contaminants that, at high levels, may pose a risk not only to babies exposed in utero but even to babies not yet conceived. That's because some contaminants can stay in your blood, tissue, and bones for months to years.

What kinds of contaminants could be lurking in your water supply? Most potentially dangerous: lead. Lead can seep into tap water when lead pipes that bring water to your neighborhood or that are in your home corrode. Pipe corrosion is more likely to occur when your water has high acidity or low mineral content, and houses built before 1986 are more likely to have lead pipes. Lead exposure during pregnancy (and possibly exposure before pregnancy as well, since lead can stay in the body for years) has been associated with reduced cognitive function, lower IQ, and increased attention-related behavioral problems in babies.

Other contaminants that can flow from your faucet include infection-causing E. coli, giardia, noroviruses, and other microorganisms and bacteria (from sewage or animal waste contamination), pesticides and industrial chemicals (from agricultural and manufacturing plant runoff) that have been linked to reduced fetal growth and a slightly increased risk of miscarriage, and arsenic (from natural deposits in the earth or from industrial or agricultural pollution) that may increase the risk of miscarriage, birth defects, and preterm birth.

Sometimes, it's obvious that water is contaminated—maybe the taste is off, it smells odd, or it's not running clear. Sometimes, it's not as obvious—the water may look and smell fine. If you have any reason to believe the water flowing from your faucet isn't safe to drink—because of its smell, look, or taste, because you suspect your pipes are deteriorating or your home is too close to a waste disposal area, or because you've heard reports of contaminated water in your community—arrange to have it tested. You can get a list of certified testing laboratories from your state or local drinking water authority. No specific reason to be concerned about your water, but just like to play it extra safe now that you're planning to be drinking that water for two? Since testing doesn't cost much—and can buy you peace of mind—it might make sense to get your water checked out anyway.

What if your family's water comes from a well? It's a good idea to have well water tested every year or so whether

with now: sushi. There are no restrictions on enjoying raw or rare fish or seafood while you're trying to conceive—only after you're pregnant. So belly up to the sushi bar before you've got that belly.

Too much of the wrong kind of fats. Plenty is still not known about the effect of dietary fats on fertility, so stay tuned. In the meantime, some preliminary research has suggested a possible reproductive downside to eating too much saturated fat (say, from greasy bacon or

or not you have concerns about contamination (particularly now that your family will be growing).

If testing reveals your water is safe, drink up. If contaminants are found, figuring out the best way to protect yourself and your future baby will be your next step. Some options for tapping into a safer water supply:

- Install a filter. But not just any filter. The filter you invest in should be designed to remove the specific contaminant or contaminants that were found flowing from your faucets. For example, if your water supply reveals unsafe levels of lead, buy a filtering system (either a whole-house filter or one for each tap) certified to reduce or eliminate lead—then use the filtered water for both drinking and cooking.

- Buy bottled. It's not the easiest or most environmentally friendly option (all that lugging and storage and recycling, unless you're using a water-jug delivery service) and it's definitely not the cheapest, but bottled water can stand in when your water supply isn't safe. Be aware, however, that not all bottled water is free of impurities (some are actually bottled from the tap). Check the purity of the bottled water you're purchasing by looking for the NSF (National Science Foundation) certification on its label, which ensures certain standards of quality.

- Boil before use. If bacteria is contaminating your water, boiling it for at least 1 minute before using for drinking, food preparation, or brushing teeth can kill those microbes. Be sure to use the boiling method only if health officials have told the public that such steps will render water safe. Keep in mind: Boiling will be effective only if the contamination comes from bacteria, not from lead or arsenic.

- Let it stand. If your water smells or tastes like chlorine (which is often used to disinfect water), let it stand uncovered for 24 hours or boil it to allow the chemical to evaporate before using it for drinking or cooking.

- Flush your pipes. If testing reveals that your city's water supply is lead-free but you have lead pipes in your home, you can flush your pipes by running the water until it becomes cold (about 5 to 30 seconds) before using it for drinking or cooking. Remember to tap only into the cold water—the hot-water tap is likely to contain higher levels of lead. If your city's supply is the source of the lead contamination, flushing your pipes won't make it safe—so you'll need to use filtered or bottled water until the city's water gets the all clear from health officials.

---

fried chicken), though the connection isn't clear. One fat more closely implicated as a culprit in decreased fertility is trans fat. According to researchers, the more trans fats you have in your diet (you'll see it listed on food labels as hydrogenated or partially hydrogenated oils), the greater the likelihood you'll have trouble conceiving. Fortunately, avoiding trans fats is pretty easy these days, since most restaurants and food manufacturers have eliminated or reduced the amount of trans fats they add to their foods. In fact, the FDA

A Side of Perspective

Of course you want to get pregnant—that's why you're reading this book. And you're almost certainly in a hurry to get that baby on board (the sooner to snuggle that little bundle!). You'll probably do just about anything—or eat just about anything, or not eat just about anything—to make that baby dream a reality. But speaking of realities, keep this reality check in mind as you fill your plate: Much of the research that's been done on the connection between diet and fertility—and there really hasn't been much yet—is preliminary and not yet fully substantiated. Some may apply more to hopeful moms (and dads) who are already experiencing infertility issues—such as ovulation problems—than to those who are facing no reproductive challenges.

Maybe eating less meat, or switching out the bread on your sandwich from white to whole wheat, or cutting back on the candy in your life will make you a mama faster—or maybe it won't. Either way, all of the potentially (but not necessarily) fertility-friendly dietary changes suggested in this chapter are definitely good for your general health, and absolutely good for the baby you hope to be nurturing soon.

Just remember to order up a little perspective along with your salmon, broccoli, and brown rice. As much good as it can do, a healthy diet doesn't guarantee a healthy reproductive system or fast-tracked conception. Fertility can be affected by many factors—from weight (though that's another compelling reason to eat well) to age to genetics, and much more. There's definitely no downside to eating well before you're expecting—and potentially, there are a lot of benefits. So, if you're experiencing trouble conceiving, eat as well as you can (it can only help), but also speak to your doctor about other steps you can take at the same time to boost your fertility.

---

ruled that beginning in mid-2018, trans fats are not allowed to be in any food products.

Still, while it makes sense to be fat-aware, there's no need to be fat-phobic. Women who eat too little fat can have a harder time conceiving—especially if their own body fat is low. What's more, once you do become pregnant, your baby will need the essential fatty acids in your diet to grow and develop properly (there's a reason why they're called "essential"). Stick to monounsaturated and polyunsaturated fats (olive, canola, avocado, or walnut oil and fats from healthy foods such as nuts and avocados) and omega-3 fatty acids (found in salmon, walnuts, and DHA-rich eggs).

Too much sugar. Before you start trying to imagine life without chocolate—not to worry. You won't have to completely surrender the sweets you're sweet on now that you've got plans to bake that little bun. But limiting your intake of sugar (from cookies, donuts, cake, candy, soda . . . you get the picture) isn't only good for your waistline. It's also good for your chances of expanding that waistline with a baby bump. Why? Because too much sugar can disrupt the balance of hormones vital to making your dreams come true. What's more, overdoing the sugar now (especially in soda form) can raise your risk of developing gestational diabetes during pregnancy.

TTC To-Do:

If you have any reason to believe you may have been exposed to high levels of mercury (for instance, you're a big-time, long-time fish eater or you've had a lot of silver cavity fillings—especially if the fillings have been broken or drilled out in the past), check with your doctor about whether you should be tested for mercury before you try to conceive. If your levels of mercury do test high (and don't try to test yourself, because many at-home tests are inaccurate), discuss ways of bringing those levels down before you start your baby-making engines.

Too many refined grains. How could your bread choice affect your fertility? A diet that's heavy on refined grains (white bread, white rice, white pasta, refined cereal) can come with potential baby-making drawbacks. Carbs that are fast to digest (those refined ones) can raise your blood sugar and insulin levels, in some cases causing a disruption in ovulation. Refined grains are also missing those naturally occurring B vitamins so vital to reproductive function—and the making of a healthy baby and a healthier, more comfortable pregnancy.

Fertile Eating Your Way

Now you know how to eat well before you're expecting, but maybe you're not sure how to apply those general guidelines to your specific eating style. Fortunately, with just a little finessing and fine-tuning, any eating style can become fertility-friendly.

Low-Carb Diet

"I've been on a low-carb diet to lose weight—and it's working, but I have a lot more to lose. Can I stick with it now?"

Going low on carbs may be an effective strategy when you're trying to lose weight, but when you're trying to gain a baby—maybe not. That's because low-carb diets are low not only on carbs (from fruits, vegetables, and grains of all varieties), but on the fertility-friendly nutrients found in carbs—especially the most essential preconception nutrient of all, folic acid. These diets can also send your protein consumption soaring (a girl's got to eat something, right?)—and that's definitely not the best way to give your fertility a boost. In fact, eating more than 100 grams (4 servings) of protein a day—which a high-protein dieter can easily knock back by lunchtime—can result in a fertility dip.

The same goes for any eating plan—or weight-loss plan—that stresses one food group over others or eliminates a food group entirely (unless that food group is "deep fried" or "frosted") such as a juice diet or a raw diet. Good nutrition is a balancing act, especially when you're trying to maintain the complex balance of reproductive hormones that'll help you get that baby on board faster. Not only can nutritionally unbalanced dieting make conception more elusive, but it can also result in a nutritional deficit—definitely not the best way to start your pregnancy. So aim for a daily diet that taps into all the food groups when you're aiming for conception.

Getting your weight to where it should be before you conceive is a smart move, and one that should make conceiving (not to mention pregnancy) a lot less complicated. Definitely keep your weight-loss efforts up, but try to transition to a balanced weight-loss plan to send those numbers down. For more on weight loss, see page 55.

Vegetarian Diet

"I'm vegan. Will that affect my chances of getting pregnant?"

You definitely don't have to eat meat (or chicken, or fish, or even dairy) to make a baby. Vegetarians—including vegans—get pregnant all the time and go on to have healthy pregnancies and healthy (meat-free) babies. That said, as a vegan you'll probably have to be a little more conscious about what you eat while you're on your conception campaign, and also once you've got that baby on board. That's because, though vegan diets are usually loaded with many fertility-friendly and baby-friendly nutrients found in whole grains, legumes, and fresh fruits and vegetables, they're sometimes light on the ones found most plentifully in animal products. Getting enough calories for optimal baby making can be tricky, too, for exclusive plant-eaters.

One key nutrient that you'll have to keep an eye on—especially as a vegan—is zinc. Zinc is found most plentifully in animal products, and if you're skipping those, you may be skimping on zinc. Lacto-ovo vegetarians can get their fill of zinc by dipping into some yogurt or

Can Dads Veg Out, Too?

Is your plate heaped high with brown rice and veggies, instead of meat and potatoes—or granola and fruit instead of bacon and eggs? No reason why you can't veg out while you're trying to make a baby. And in fact, a diet that's full of folate and other baby-friendly nutrients (the kind that are found in the greens and grains vegetarians favor) is a plus when you're in baby-making mode. Just make sure you're getting enough sperm-boosting zinc (most commonly found in animal products, including eggs, but also plentiful in wheat germ, oatmeal, and corn). A multivitamin can fill in the zinc blanks if these foods aren't a regular part of your diet.

cracking open some eggs. If you're a vegan, concentrate on vegetable and grain sources of zinc (black-eyed peas, corn, oatmeal, wheat germ). Either way, a daily prenatal vitamin will fill in any shortfall.

Another nutrient to be mindful of now that you've got baby on the brain is vitamin B_{12}, which occurs naturally only in animal products. If you eat dairy and eggs, you'll be filling your quota, but if you're a strict vegan, you'll need to turn to fortified foods (many cereals have B_{12} in them) to give you what you need. Once again, that prenatal vitamin can fill in any blanks.

Iron can be dicey, too, for vegetarians of all varieties, because red meat is one of the most absorbable sources of this essential nutrient. You'll get some iron if you eat your spinach, dried beans, dried apricots, lentils, and oatmeal, but realistically, probably not enough. That's where an iron-containing prenatal vitamin can step in. If a blood test shows that your iron stores are on the low side, your practitioner may also prescribe an additional iron supplement.

One nutrient you've probably got an edge on is folic acid, found in many leafy greens, whole grains, and other vegetarian-preferred foods. In fact, vegetarians tend to consume more folate-rich foods than meat-eaters, without even trying (and that's a good thing, since there's no such thing as too much folate on your plate). Still, you should take that prenatal vitamin for extra insurance.

Fortified Foods and Prenatal Vitamins

"I eat fortified cereal each morning plus fortified energy bars during the day. I also take a prenatal vitamin. Can getting too many vitamins affect fertility?"

It's hard to avoid fortified foods these days (unless you mill your own flour, bake your own bread, milk your own cows, and make your own cheese). Fortunately, you don't have to. There's absolutely no harm in eating fortified or enriched foods, even if you take a prenatal vitamin—and even if you're totally into Total, or energy dependent on energy bars. In fact, the scientists take into account all the nutrients that likely already find their way into your diet (either naturally or from packaged foods) when they formulate those supplements. You'd have to take megadoses of nutrients (way more than what's in your prenatal vitamin) to mess with your fertility or have any other negative health effects.

All that said, keep in mind that processed foods—the ones that tend to have the most fortification because those extra vitamins and minerals are tossed in to compensate for the ones stripped away on the assembly line—run a very distant second nutrition-wise to whole foods (foods that haven't been processed or refined, and show up at the market as close to their natural state as possible). It's fine to supplement your diet with them—especially when they're made with wholesome ingredients, like whole grains—but smart to balance them with nature's finest. So top that fortified cereal with fresh blueberries, and enjoy that energy bar after you've had a sensible salad for lunch, not instead of it.

Organic Foods

"Will eating organic produce help me get pregnant faster?"

Organic produce isn't necessarily more nutritious than conventional produce (you'll get the same fertility-boosting vitamins and minerals from regular produce), but organically grown fruits, vegetables, and other foods will likely be as close to pesticide-free as possible. Looking ahead, that will be a definite plus during pregnancy, since the pesticides you consume through your diet when you're pregnant will be shared with your baby-to-be. Looking even further ahead, eating fewer pesticides now will mean you'll have fewer stored up in your body later, when they can ultimately make their way into your baby through your breast milk.

Whether the pesticide-free pluses will add up to increased fertility is, so far, unclear. Some research has suggested that women who ingest higher-than-average amounts of pesticides and other chemicals through their food may find their fertility somewhat reduced, but the jury's still out—like it almost always is in the ever-changing fields of fertility and nutrition. It's also hard to separate out whether it's the contaminants in a woman's diet that lead to reduced fertility or the quality of the foods that typically make up such a diet (those that are heavily processed or high in saturated fat, for instance).

So there's no downside—and potentially, a lot of upside—to going organic during your preconception prep period and beyond. Still, it's no secret that organic food is usually more expensive than conventional and sometimes harder to track down, especially out of season. If you have to pick and choose, focus on organic meat and dairy (conventionally raised animal products contain higher concentrations of chemicals that could disrupt your fertility hormones) and the fruits and vegetables you eat most often. Many types of produce—such as bananas, kiwis, mangoes, papayas, pineapples, asparagus, avocados, broccoli, cauliflower, corn, and onions—contain negligible levels of pesticide residue, so there's no need to go organic with them if you can't afford to. Instead, spring for organic when it comes to produce that typically wears the most pesticide residue (the so-called dirty dozen: apples, cherries, grapes, peaches, nectarines, pears, raspberries, strawberries, bell peppers, celery, potatoes, and spinach). For a lower price on organic foods that are also likely to be more nutritious than the ones you'll find in a market, visit the local farmers market if you're lucky enough to have one. The fresher off the farm those fruits and veggies are, the more nutrients they'll have retained, and the more you'll retain when you eat them.

Meal Skipping

"I never eat breakfast, and sometimes I skip lunch. Do I have to eat more regularly while I'm TTC, even though I'm trying to lose weight?"

Not only should you think about switching over to regular eating, but you should think about trading in those 1 or 2 big meals a day for 5 or 6 much smaller ones.

There's no better way for an expectant mom to eat than a little at a time, a lot of times a day—in other words, to graze. The 6-Meal Solution (you'll read all about that once you've graduated to *What to Expect When You're Expecting*) minimizes or eliminates a plethora of pregnancy symptoms, from headaches to heartburn, morning sickness to mood swings. And it's an easy concept to swallow. Instead of sitting down for 3 squares (or 1 or 2, as meal skippers like you do on a regular basis), you simply nibble on 5 or 6 mini-meals or snacks, each containing a source of protein and a source of complex carbs (whole-grain crackers and a cheese wedge; a smoothie made with yogurt and fruit; half a turkey sandwich and a peach).

But how does the graze craze apply to the not-yet-pregnant? How can eating less more frequently boost your fertility? And why would you eat more often if you're trying to lose a few pounds before pregnancy starts packing the pounds on?

Here's the how and why. As far as fertility is concerned, keeping your blood sugar on an even keel can definitely improve your reproductive outlook, especially if you have insulin issues (you have PCOS or you're diabetic, for example). And one of the most efficient ways to regulate blood sugar is—you guessed it—to graze on small amounts of protein and complex carbs throughout the day, instead of chowing down once or twice a day.

And though it sounds counter-intuitive (when has eating more often ever led to weight loss?), grazing can make it easier to drop those preconception pounds, which in turn can help your fertility campaign. Just make sure that the foods you choose to graze on are mainly healthy, low-fat ones and that you don't overdo the calories over those 5 or 6 mini-meals. Otherwise you could end up minimizing your weight loss, or even netting a gain.

PART 2

Getting Pregnant

CHAPTER 4

The Biology of Baby Making

C hances are you already have a pretty good idea of how to go about getting pregnant (insert part A into part B; repeat as needed). But how much do you really know about the science of conception beyond the basics of baby-making biology? If you're like most hopeful moms and dads, probably not a whole lot.

So before you begin your baby-making efforts in earnest, take a moment to marvel at the incredible and improbable process of conception: how 2 tiny cells, 1 from you and 1 from your partner, beat the seemingly insurmountable odds stacked against them to meet, greet, and form a perfect union—a unique human being soon to be your baby. Learning about the science of conception—one of the most amazing biological feats in the body's remarkable repertoire—isn't only fascinating stuff, but practical stuff. It'll arm you with all the biological know-how you'll need to get the job of baby making done, and give you a new appreciation for the miracle that's about to take place in your body.

Anatomy 101

R emember when you were in middle school? When your teachers said you'd be getting "the talk"? The boys got an extra period of gym. And the girls—you got an extra period to learn about your period. And about how each month your ovaries, uterus, fallopian tubes, and cervix (not to mention a bunch of hormones) gear up for baby making—even when there's no baby making on the agenda? Did you pay attention? If you did—great! Go to the head of the class.

If your knowledge of basic anatomy is a little rusty, and if the mysteries of your body are still, well, mysterious, then find a comfortable spot on the sofa and read on. Because knowing what all those reproductive organs inside of you do (and equally important—where they're located) will give you a leg up on understanding how your reproductive cycle works, which in turn can help you get that reproductive process started sooner and get that baby on board faster.

Your Body Basics

Let's get the basics out of the way. As you can see in the illustration on page 86, your internal reproductive organs consist of the ovaries (you've got 2 of them, 1 on each side), the fallopian tubes (ditto), the uterus, the cervix, and the vagina. You probably already know that you have them—and that they come standard issue to the female of the species. But now it's time to learn

a little more about these baby-making must-haves:

- **Your ovaries** are where your eggs (also called ova, or ovum for a single egg) are stored. Each month, one of those eggs matures inside an ovarian follicle and is released from one of your ovaries into a fallopian tube. Most often, your ovaries take turns releasing eggs (left side one month, right side the next). The ovaries also produce the hormones estrogen and progesterone—much more about these later—both of which are essential for conceiving and growing a baby.

- **Your fallopian tubes** are 5-inch-long narrow tubes (you have 1 tube on each side of the uterus) that connect the ovaries and the uterus. It is here, in one of these tubes, that egg and sperm meet up and fertilization takes place. Once conception occurs, the fertilized egg completes its travel through the fallopian tube and arrives at its destination: the uterus.

- **Your uterus** (aka your womb) is the pear-shaped organ where your

---

How Many Eggs in Your Basket?

Ready to count eggs (before they hatch)? Wondering just how many you have in your basket? Consider these fascinating egg facts: When you were a 16- to 20-week-old fetus, your ovaries were housing a mind-boggling 6 to 7 million eggs—way more than one woman could ever use, even if she had her eye on a really big family. From then on, those numbers were all downhill. Not that you would have missed them or used them, but by the time you were born, your egg count was down to about 1 to 2 million, the rest having been weeded out by normal attrition. The gradual attrition continued throughout your childhood, and by the time you reached puberty—and started tapping into those eggs each month through ovulation—you were hosting about 300,000 to 400,000 eggs. By age 37, you're down to approximately 25,000 eggs. Definitely a lot fewer eggs than you started with, but still plenty to go around. After all, it takes only 1 egg to make a baby.

Inside You

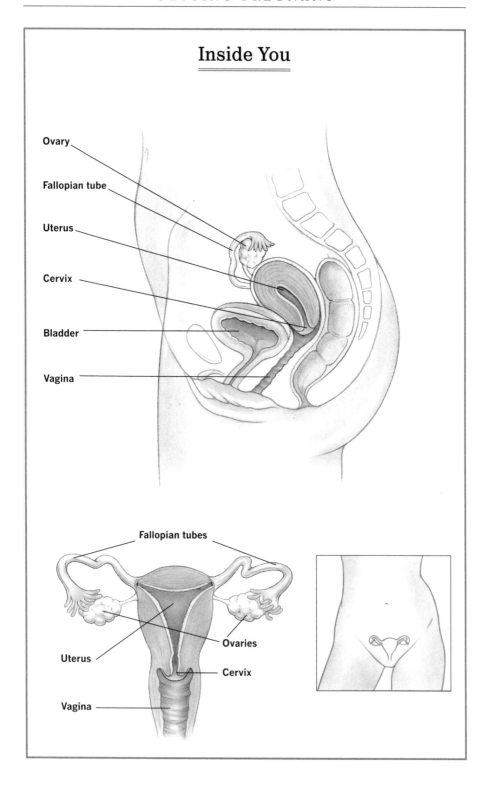

Ovary

Fallopian tube

Uterus

Cervix

Bladder

Vagina

Fallopian tubes

Ovaries

Uterus

Cervix

Vagina

yet-to-be conceived baby will hunker down to grow and develop during pregnancy—essentially, his or her first home. Each month, the lining of the uterus (known as the endometrium) builds up in preparation for a pregnancy—just in case a baby shows up. If a fertilized egg does implant in the endometrium, the cozy uterus incubates the fetus, and eventually, the muscles of this phenomenal organ contract during childbirth to push your baby out. If conception and implantation do not occur—and they don't, of course, most months of your reproductive life—the endometrium will shed in the form of your period.

- **Your cervix** is at the bottom of the uterus and serves as its entrance—essentially connecting the vagina and the uterus. The cervix is shaped like the neck of a soda bottle (the bottle is the uterus) and will stretch up to 10 centimeters (about 4 inches) wide when it's time to give birth. The opening of the cervix (at the top of your vagina) is known in medical-speak as the "os." It's from here that cervical mucus is secreted (more about that super-significant component of fertility later on).

- **Your vagina** is the gateway to the reproductive tract. Here's where reproduction begins (when sperm is

deposited in the vagina during intercourse) and ends (when the baby exits through the vagina during birth—that is, unless you end up with a cesarean delivery). Usually around 4 to 6 inches in length, the vagina is quite elastic, which is why it can feel snug around a slender regular tampon yet can stretch to accommodate the passage of a 7- or 8-pound baby.

His Body Basics

Though females take on the bulk of the reproductive responsibility—actually all of it, once conception takes place—it does take two to make a baby. Without the contribution of sperm, no female human could get pregnant in the first place. Here's the lowdown on what goes on down below on a guy (for a peek inside his reproductive parts, see the illustration on page 88):

- **The testicles.** Unlike his female counterpart who has a lifetime supply of eggs already produced and ready to roll at birth, the male produces fresh sperm each day in his testes (or testicles), the pair of oval-shaped glands that hang below the penis. Ever wonder why the testicles hang—for the most part—outside the body? Sperm can develop only in a place that is 3 to 4 degrees below normal body temperature. The scrotum (the skin that surrounds the testicles) serves as natural climate control, helping the testes stay consistently cooler by thickening and thinning in response to external temperatures (which explains why they hang lower in a hot shower and seem to "shrivel" up after a dip in a cold pool).

- **The epididymis.** The sperm matures and develops the ability to swim—one of its most important skills—in the epididymis, a series of tightly coiled

---

Did You Know?

Did you know that sperm make up only 1 to 3 percent of semen? The rest of that gooey goop consists of fructose and other complex sugars, protein, and trace vitamins and minerals that protect, feed, and fuel the sperm on their journey.

Inside Him

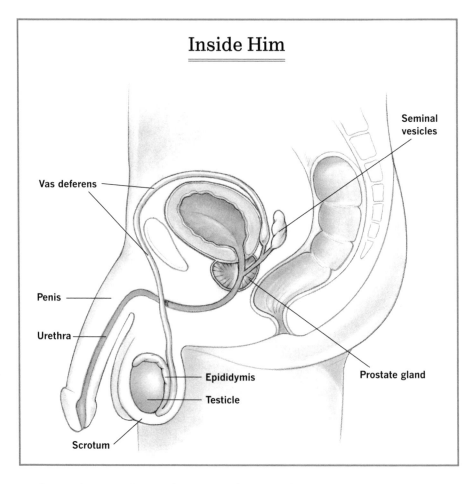

tubes in the scrotal sac right on top of the testicles. It can take 12 to 21 days for sperm to pass through the epididymis in its maturation process. Sperm is stored in the epididymis and the vas deferens until ejaculation.

- **The vas deferens.** During arousal (aka an erection), sperm is pumped from the epididymis to the vas deferens, a pair of 15-inch-long tubes that wind from the top of the epididymis through the scrotum and up into the lower abdomen.

- **The seminal vesicles.** As the sperm travels through the vas deferens, a fructose-filled fluid from the seminal

vesicles—called semen—is pumped into the tubes and mixes with the sperm. This will help push the sperm toward the prostate gland.

- **The prostate gland,** in the lower abdomen under the bladder, adds an alkaline fluid to the semen (to protect it from the acidic environment of the vagina) as the sperm journeys toward ejaculation. From the prostate, the sperm-loaded semen is transported into the urethra (which runs through the penis shaft) and is then released through the tip of the erect penis during ejaculation—with the hopes of meeting its match, in the form of a willing and able egg.

His Olympic Swim Team

Ever stop to think about sperm? With all the fertility focus on your eggs (When will they be ripe? When will they be released? When will they be conception ready?), it's easy to forget about those incredible swimmers of his, who wait on the sidelines, eager to make their vital contribution to Team Baby. Sperm—those tiny tadpole-like cells with whiplashing tails dancing in frantic figure eights—are the smallest cells in the body, but each one potentially packs a powerful punch. A teardrop-shaped sperm head measures only $2/1000$th of an inch (in comparison, the egg—the largest cell in the body—is 30 times the width of a sperm cell).

What sperm lack in size (and who says size matters, anyway?), they certainly make up for in number. Each testicle produces 4 million new sperm per hour (yes, hour)—about 1,200 sperm per heartbeat. Add it all up, and a healthy male can expect to generate 12 trillion (yes, trillion) sperm over his lifetime, compared with the mere million or so eggs a female starts off with. If that number isn't impressive enough, consider this: In each ejaculate,

there are on average 100 to 200 million (yes, million) sperm yearning to become half of a full-fledged human being (though to be fertile, a man needs only a small percentage of those sperm to be capable of fertilizing an egg—the rest are often abnormally shaped, sluggish, or otherwise unserviceable, and that's no problem).

Sperm also make up for their small size with their astonishing athletic ability and mind-boggling speed. The tail propels each sperm forward at the unbelievable pace of $1/12$ of an inch per minute. To put that into perspective, hop onto the treadmill and rev it up to 4 miles per hour. That's the human equivalent of a sperm's speed. Not too shabby for a microscopic cell.

Sperm need all the speed—and strength—they can get to swim from point A (vagina) to point B (waiting egg in the fallopian tube). If that doesn't sound like a big deal, consider that in sperm terms, the distance it needs to travel is equivalent to you swimming 3 (yes, 3) times across the English Channel without stopping. Now, that's some Olympic swim team!

Your Cycle at Work

Ever since you hit puberty, your body has been going through an intricate monthly dance involving brain signals, hormones, and physical changes that ultimately ends with your period— that is, unless it ends with a pregnancy. Whether your periods arrive like clockwork or are a little irregular, your body goes through the same 12-step program during each menstrual cycle:

1. Your period. The first day of your period is considered the first day of your menstrual cycle—though logically, it's more like the end than the beginning (you'll see why when you read on). But forget about logic for now and just remember this: Because a period is the easiest-to-predict, easiest-to-notice, and easiest-to-record reproductive event in the month (unless you count that sudden, uncontrollable craving for all things chocolate), the medical community has taken to calling the first day of your period the first day of your cycle. When you do become pregnant, this day will be crucial to dating your pregnancy—and figuring out your due date.

Over a period (so to speak) of approximately 5 days, the lining of your uterus sheds, causing menstrual blood to flow through the cervix and out your vagina. While you're menstruating, your endocrine system (aka your hormones) starts gearing up for a fresh reproductive start.

2. FSH production. While you're busy bleeding, your pituitary gland (at the base of the brain) is busy, too, secreting increasing amounts of the hormone FSH (follicle stimulating hormone), which stimulates 10 to 20 egg-containing follicles in your ovaries to develop, getting them ready for ovulation (the release of that egg of the month).

3. LH production. By the time your period is ending (around day 5), the pituitary adds another hormone to the mix, releasing increasing amounts of LH (luteinizing hormone). LH works with FSH to stimulate the ovarian follicles and help them mature.

4. Estrogen production. As the follicles in the ovaries are stimulated (thanks to FSH and LH), they in turn begin to stimulate production of the hormone estrogen. Estrogen production stimulates further LH production (talk about positive feedback!), which helps the follicles mature even more.

5. The dominant follicle wins. Sometime around day 8 of your cycle, one of those maturing follicles emerges as the dominant one—the one destined for ovulation. As that alpha follicle establishes its dominant position, the other follicles that had begun to mature in hopes of releasing their eggs now begin to disintegrate instead. (Sometimes, more than 1 follicle continues to mature, resulting in multiple ovulation—and possibly, a multiple pregnancy.)

6. Endometrial cycle. As the dominant follicle continues to mature, it produces more and more estrogen. This increased estrogen production gets the month's reproductive party started in your uterus, and by day 12, the surge in estrogen has caused the endometrium (the uterine lining) to build up anew (remember, that lining was cleaned out after the last period, a week and a half earlier).

Fertility Through the Ages

What are your fertility numbers? That depends, at least partly, on the number of birthdays you've celebrated so far. A woman in her early 20s who isn't using birth control has a 20 to 25 percent chance of conceiving each month. By her late 20s, she has a 15 to 20 percent chance of hitting the baby jackpot each month. That number drops to a 10 to 15 percent chance per month in her early 30s, and an 8 to 10 percent chance each month by her late 30s. By the time the average woman reaches her 40s, that number gets lower still. But notice that, though the numbers decline as you age, they decline relatively gradually—which gives most women plenty of time to clock in their baby making while that biological clock's still ticking strong.

7. Cervical mucus production. Estrogen production has far-reaching reproductive effects, also impacting the glands in your cervix—triggering the production of cervical mucus. As the level of estrogen rises to its highest point midcycle, the quality and quantity of cervical mucus changes, from cloudy and sticky (day 8 or 9) to wet, clear, and slippery (days 10 through 13). Read about this very important fertility sign on page 100.

8. LH surge. The hormone LH now surges to 6 to 10 times its normal value, peaking about 12 to 16 hours before ovulation. Within hours of this LH surge, FSH also surges, but not as dramatically. The surge of these hormones temporarily shuts down the production of estrogen in the now mature dominant follicle.

9. Ovulation. Midway through the menstrual cycle (around day 14 in a 28-day cycle, though it could be anywhere from day 12 to day 18 in a shorter or longer cycle), and courtesy of the LH and FSH surge, the dominant follicle in the ovary begins to swell and then rupture. From the ruptured follicle emerges this month's featured egg, and the force of the rupture propels the egg through the ovarian wall and into the waiting fingers of the fallopian tube. Ovulation has just occurred.

10. The egg's journey. Once the egg leaves the ovary, the fimbriae (the petal-like fingers of the fallopian tube) create a safety net for the egg—catching it and coaxing it into the fallopian tube to begin its voyage toward a possible conception. If sperm has found its way into the fallopian tubes at the same time (and timing is everything when it comes to conception), fertilization might occur. But if there is no sperm around to meet the egg—or if the sperm miss their mark and fertilization doesn't

Give It Time

Of course you're eager to make baby magic happen—and if you had your way, it would happen overnight (or at least, in your first month of trying). But while there's always the chance that you will get that lucky that fast, realistically, the odds are it will take a little longer. In fact, it can take a completely healthy, fully fertile couple 6 to 12 months of active trying before they hit the baby jackpot.

So give it time. Keep an eye on the calendar, but don't obsess over it—and definitely don't stress about it. Instead, relax and enjoy your conception campaign.

occur—the egg will disintegrate within 12 to 24 hours, and this cycle's conception window closes.

11. Progesterone production. Meanwhile, the follicle that was emptied when the egg was released turns into the corpus luteum (translation: "yellow body"), which begins to secrete large amounts of the hormone progesterone and smaller amounts of estrogen. The estrogen continues to build up the uterine lining, and the progesterone acts to mature the uterine lining, readying the uterus for a potential pregnancy. Progesterone also alerts the pituitary gland to limit further production of FSH and LH (since those follicle-stimulating days are over for now).

12. Deterioration of the corpus luteum. If this cycle is destined to end in a period, not a pregnancy, the corpus luteum begins to deteriorate once the residual levels of LH diminish (usually around 12 to 14 days after ovulation). Without the corpus luteum to continue producing progesterone, levels of the hormone drop around day 27, triggering the shedding of the uterine lining—and the beginning of your period, activating the entire cycle all over again. On the other hand, if conception has occurred,

the pregnancy hormone human chorionic gonadotropin (hCG) will signal the corpus luteum to remain viable for a few more months to sustain the pregnancy by secreting progesterone until the placenta gets up and running.

Conception 101

Sure, you know how babies are made, but beyond those basic body mechanics, do you really know what will be going on inside of you after sperm and egg are introduced to each other? Here's the 411 on Conception 101.

Ovulation

Ovulation, as you've just read, is when an egg (smaller than the size of the period at the end of this sentence) is served up from one of your ovaries and caught by the ends of the fallopian

---

Race to Conception

It takes 30 minutes for sperm to reach the fallopian tubes after entering the vaginal canal. It takes another 15 to 20 minutes for the sperm to find the egg and start attempting penetration (of the egg, that is). And it takes a good 20 minutes for the winning sperm to drill its head through the tough shell surrounding the egg and officially get lucky—while officially kicking off conception. Add it up and you'll see that this incredibly intricate process—from sex to fertilized egg—can take as little as an hour. How's that for a game of beat the clock?

---

tube. The key to planning conception: knowing when the big O occurs. Why? Because to make a baby, you need to make sure sperm and egg meet up during a very tight window of opportunity—right around ovulation. And that window is even slimmer for an egg than it is for the sperm. Though sperm can hang around and get their job done (assuming they're in the right place) for 72 hours after ejaculation or even longer, eggs are viable for only 12 to 24 hours after ovulation. Once a released egg has expired without meeting its sperm match, the conception window closes for the month. For more about predicting when ovulation will occur so you can time your conception efforts right, flip ahead to page 96.

Fertilization

The journey to fertilization starts with sex. You're probably familiar with this part of the drill: With his climax, your partner's sperm shoot their way from his penis into your vagina in a sea of semen. What you might not know is what lies ahead for the sperm. Semen provides the perfect travel environment for the sperm as they set out on the long trip ahead, keeping them well fed and protected on their journey while helping deliver them safely to Destination Egg. Semen coagulates in the vagina

Conception Close-Up

You've heard about sperm meeting egg, but have you ever wondered how the miracle of conception actually plays out—start to amazing finish? Take a look at this conception close-up.

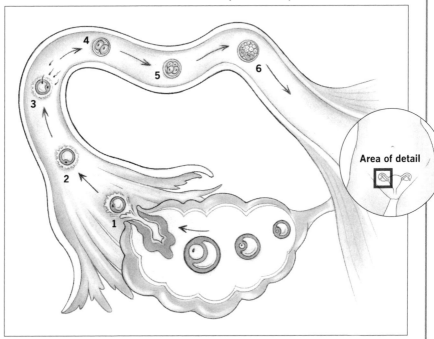

Area of detail

1. An egg is released from its follicle and propelled out of the ovary into the fallopian tube.

2. The egg, viable for only 12 to 24 hours, begins its journey down the fallopian tube.

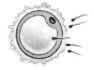

3. Sperm reach the egg and fight for their chance to fertilize it. Only 1 sperm—the first to achieve penetration—succeeds.

4. The fertilized egg divides into 2 cells and starts making its way to its new home, the uterus.

5. The egg, called a zygote, floats down the fallopian tube for 5 days, dividing into more and more cells.

6. Now called a blastocyst—and made up of 100 cells—this soon-to-be baby is ready for implantation in the uterus.

Phase Facts

And now, more cycle facts that can come in handy when you're trying to make a baby. The first part of the menstrual cycle (from the start of your period through ovulation) is called the follicular phase, and its length varies considerably from woman to woman, depending on the length of her cycle. The second part of the menstrual cycle (beginning at ovulation) is called the luteal phase and usually lasts 12 to 14 days. This second phase is more consistent from woman to woman, no matter how long or short her cycle is, making it easier to look to for fertility clues.

How can these phase facts help you in your quest for conception? By helping you pinpoint that all-important monthly event essential to baby making: the release of that egg of yours. If you have longer cycles (say, 33 days or even 40 days), it's likely to be because your follicular phase is longer than average—not because your luteal phase is. Chances are you'll still be ovulating approximately 12 to 14 days before your next period. Likewise, if your cycles are on the short side, that's a sign that your follicular phase is shorter than average. Even if your periods arrive 24 days apart, figuring out your ovulation date is often as easy as counting back 12 to 14 days from the beginning of your period (most of the time; read on to learn when that's not the case). If your cycles are irregular, you'll have to focus on other tools to help you pinpoint ovulation (such as those starting on page 100).

Have you noticed that your luteal phase is sometimes (or consistently) shorter than the predictable average of 12 to 14 days? When the time from ovulation to the next period lasts 10 days or fewer, a diagnosis of luteal phase deficiency (LPD) is made. What does this diagnosis mean? As far as your fertility goes, probably nothing at all. Experts believe that a short luteal phase has no clinical significance—that is, it doesn't affect fertility and doesn't need to be treated. See page 165 for more.

---

right after ejaculation to prevent the sperm from getting off track and wandering too far in the wrong direction, such as right back out of the vagina (and that's a good thing—you know how few guys are willing to stop for directions). About a half hour after ejaculation, the semen reliquifies (and usually ends up dribbling out of you, sometimes in a post-sex gush). But don't worry about any loss of semen at this stage of the game. Any sperm that haven't made it up through the cervix by then are clearly not worth saving. What's more, any sperm stragglers who find themselves left behind in the vagina for more than a few minutes don't have much of a chance of surviving anyway, thanks (or no thanks) to the vagina's sperm-unfriendly acidic pH.

The sperm quickly pass through the inhospitable vagina toward the more welcoming cervical canal that is awash in cervical mucus (the thin, clear mucus associated with ovulation is specially designed to transport sperm more efficiently). The cervical mucus separates the sperm from the semen, which includes bacteria, white blood cells, and assorted substances that could be toxic to your waiting egg. Cervical mucus also helps the sperm undergo an important biochemical change, releasing enzymes (in a process called capacitation) and allowing them to transform from sluggish slackers into tail-thrashing dynamos, ready to jump the starting gate and propel through the uterus and fallopian tubes toward their target—the egg. Without the capacitation process, the sperm would be unable to burrow into an egg and fertilize it.

But those boys are not home free yet. For starters, sperm have to get their timing just right. If they reach the fallopian tube too early, they risk dying before the egg shows up. Too late, and the egg will be long gone—and the sperm will have missed their once-in-a-lifetime opportunity to fertilize. They also need to pick a tube—and not just any tube. An egg is usually present in only 1 of the 2 fallopian tubes in any given month. Pick the wrong tube, and the sperm come up empty.

Even the sperm that are resourceful enough to reach the egg still have their work cut out for them. Hundreds of sperm will fight for the chance to fertilize the same egg, swarming around it and attempting to plow headfirst through its hard outer layer. The best man wins—as long as he's the first man to break into the egg's inner sanctum. As soon as the one lucky sperm cell succeeds in penetrating the egg, the egg immediately forms a barrier to keep the other sperm from getting through. Then, without so much as a celebratory toast, the victorious sperm plunges into the egg's nucleus, releases its own genetic contribution, and the egg is officially fertilized, combining equal shares (50 percent each) of dad's genetic makeup with mom's genetic makeup. Within a matter of hours, the microscopic fertilized egg (called a zygote) divides, then splits again and again. It continues to divide and float down the fallopian tube toward the uterus—a journey that takes around 5 days—and by the time the cluster of cells (now called a blastocyst) reaches your uterus, it numbers around 100 cells strong.

So You Think You're a Stud?

Get ready for a reality check, courtesy of the animal kingdom. Consider this: A male pig ejaculates 1 pint (yes, pint) of semen each time he mates, while the average human male ejaculates only ½ to 1 teaspoon of semen. Here's another stat that may leave you a little, well, deflated. The average bull ejaculate contains 10 billion sperm. In comparison, the average healthy man's ejaculate contains 100 to 200 million sperm. But before you start feeling sorry for yourself—or a little envious of those other male animals—remember that pigs and bulls don't get nearly as many opportunities to get lucky as humans do. So who's the stud now?

Implantation

When the blastocyst reaches its residence for the next 8½ months (your uterus), it wastes no time in making itself at home. First, it begins to burrow deep into the uterine lining (the endometrium) that was built up in anticipation of the tiny occupant's arrival, attaching itself firmly. Once snug and secure, the ball of cells differentiates into 2 groups. Half (now called the embryo) will become your baby; the other half will become the placenta, the amazing lifeline that channels nutrients to the fetus and carries waste away. As soon as the fertilized egg implants, it starts to release hCG—the just-for-pregnancy hormone that will turn your home pregnancy test positively positive. Score!

Predicting Ovulation

....

O f all the complex processes involved in the making of a baby—and, as you've read, there are plenty—there's no more important one than ovulation. Sure, knowing precisely when that egg will be ripe, released, and ready for fertilization definitely isn't necessary for conception. Many a baby has been made without any ovulation heads-up (typically it's just a matter of time before an egg and a sperm find themselves together in the right place at the right time), but it does takes a lot of the guesswork out of getting pregnant. Whether you're just looking for some general guidelines to direct your TTC efforts or you're looking to micromanage Project Conception by employing every ovulation prediction tool known to reproductive science, this chapter will point you in the right direction.

How to Pinpoint Ovulation

During each monthly cycle, a released egg is open for the business of fertilization for only about 12 to 24 hours—after which your reproductive shop shuts down until next month. But before you get discouraged by what seems like an impossibly short fertilization time frame, remember that sperm have a much longer shelf life than eggs do—and can live to fertilize for 72 hours or even longer. Though it's ideal to have sex the day you ovulate—giving sperm and egg the best chance of hooking up successfully—you may score a fertilized egg even if you have sex a couple of days before ovulation. After all, there may be plenty of viable sperm still hanging around in your fallopian tube waiting patiently for the egg when it finally emerges. And it takes only one Mr. Right to make a baby.

Even with that encouraging news from the sperm front, the goal of fertilization becomes a little more challenging when you factor in the very limited use-by date of each egg. Which is why pinpointing when ovulation occurs—and when that egg will be ready for the taking—is key to making a baby.

How can you pin down the big O, so you can pin each other down for some baby-making action? For one, by tuning in to changes in your body—changes you may have largely ignored up until now. Mother Nature wisely drops clues each month that signal the imminent arrival of ovulation. Knowing how to read those clues will help you better predict when that monthly egg will be released so you'll know to time sex and up the odds that your conception quest will end in success.

Cycle Length

As with everything reproduction related, there's a wide range of normal when it comes to menstrual cycles. Some women have short cycles lasting a mere 23 days or so, and others have a long reprieve between periods—say, 35 days. Most women find that their cycles fall somewhere in between.

The variations in length typically happen in the first half of the cycle, called the follicular phase. On the other hand, the second half, or luteal phase, of the monthly menstrual cycle (the time span between ovulation and the onset of your next period) is typically pretty predictable, usually lasting 14 days (though it may be as short as 12). Which means that if your period usually starts 30 days after the previous one started, it's likely that you ovulated on about

TTC To-Do:

Looking to schedule in baby making? Keeping an eye on your calendar (or your fertility app) now can help you pencil in that bundle of joy sooner. A few months before you plan to begin TTC, and after you've shelved any hormonal birth control you've been using (you'll need to pause at least 6 months if you've been on Depo-Provera shots), start tracking the first day of each period. After a few months, you'll be able to determine your natural cycle length. Count back about 14 days each month to get an idea of when you ovulated during the previous cycle. This will help narrow down when you'll likely be ovulating in the next cycle (and more important, during the cycle when you're going to begin giving conception a try).

day 16 (though it could have happened as late as day 18). And if you have a fairly regular cycle and keep track of cycle lengths, you'll be able to estimate when you'll likely ovulate during your next cycle. If you get your period every 24 days, for instance, ovulation most likely occurs on about day 10 (though it could happen as late as day 12). If your period comes every 35 days, ovulation probably takes place on about day 21 (but could occur as late as day 23). If your periods are irregular and there's no discernible pattern you can count on (one month you have a 27-day cycle, the next a 49-day cycle, the next a 33-day cycle, and so on), you won't be able to look to your cycle for fertility bulletins. Instead, you'll need to be more alert for other signs of ovulation.

Basal Body Temperature

You know all those hormones that make you feel, well, hormonal during your cycle? For most women, the ups and downs of those trademark female hormones—most notably estrogen and progesterone—cause plenty of typically unwelcome emotional and physical changes (from crankiness to cravings, bloating to breakouts). But one by-product of those hormonal fluctuations that isn't as noticeable, unless you're really paying attention, is the subtle changes in your body temperature. More precisely, your basal body temperature (BBT)—the baseline reading you get first thing in the morning, after at least 3 to 5 hours of sleep and before you get out of bed, talk, or even sit up (and definitely before you indulge

The Art of the Chart

To make a baby, consider starting in bed—and not for the obvious reason. Taking your BBT with a digital basal thermometer each morning before you get out of bed (yes, even before you pee or take a sip from that bedside water bottle) or using one of the BBT temperature wearables can help you figure out when during your cycle you ovulate—so you'll know when during your cycle you're most likely to succeed in conceiving. You can keep track old-school-style by marking each daily reading on a graph and connecting the dots—but it's a lot easier to let the fertility app on your smartphone do the calculating. You can find a sample fertility chart and empty ones to fill in beginning on page 258.

You should see evidence of ovulation a day or two after it has occurred by noticing a half-degree jump in temperature. Over the course of a few months, you should be able to detect patterns of highs and lows, and you'll be able to pinpoint the dramatic increase in temperature, giving you a clue for the next month about when ovulation typically takes place—about a day or two before that jump—and giving you a heads-up on when to hop back into bed for baby making. As an example, if your BBT jump occurs on day 16 each month, you're probably ovulating a day or 2 before that—on day 14 or 15, which means you should be having sex on days 13 to 16 (since sperm can hang around for a few days waiting for the egg to show up).

One thing to keep in mind when it comes to BBT: Keeping track of it, at least once the novelty wears off, can be a major drag—especially on those mornings when you don't have time for lounging in bed (though the thermometers and wearable monitors that seamlessly sync to your smartphone do make the charting a little less tedious). A meticulously kept fertility chart or app can definitely provide some clues to better help plan the best time for conception, but remember that it can issue that ovulation bulletin only after the fact—at which point, it may be too late to put that just-released egg to good use. To make it a more effective conception-planning tool, you'll probably need to keep at the charting for at least 2 cycles so you'll know when to anticipate ovulation in the next cycle based on your ovulation history.

Sick of taking your temperature after the second day—and can't imagine keeping it up for 2 months? Skip this preconception step altogether, and move on to other, less time-consuming ovulation clues.

A Confusing BBT Chart

Wouldn't it be great if BBT readings were reliably consistent from month to month, with clear, predictable patterns of highs and lows—and without any outlying (and confusing) temperature numbers? Unfortunately, rare is the BBT chart that is neat and tidy. Real life often gets in the way, making your real-life charts a little more mysterious than you might have thought—at least some of the time.

So what if you've been getting reassuringly regular-looking charts, but then one month you get a temperature reading that's much higher than it should've been, throwing off the pattern you've come to expect? Not to stress. Just remember that your BBT measures your temperature at total rest, and it's extremely sensitive to any change (which is why it's recommended that you take the reading immediately after waking and around the same time each morning). Perhaps the day you noticed that elevated temperature reading was a Saturday and you'd slept in, taking your temperature at 10 a.m. instead of your usual 6 a.m. Since temperatures rise as the day goes on, that might account for your bumped-up reading. Or maybe that soup-bowl-size margarita you sipped with your enchilada plate last night caused a spike in your waking temp. Or maybe your body was busy fighting an infection that day (and fighting so effectively, you never got sick—but your temperature was temporarily elevated). Or your 5 a.m. trip to the bathroom (it was dark, so you thought it was still nighttime) caused the higher reading at 6 a.m. when your alarm woke you for real. Or you tossed and turned for hours before you actually got up. For best results from your BBT chart efforts, remember that you're looking for an overall pattern, rather than analyzing individual daily readings—which may occasionally stray from your "norm."

in any early-morning loving). If you ever needed an excuse not to jump out of bed at the first sounding of the alarm, this is it (hey—you just bought yourself a few extra minutes under the covers).

During the first part of your cycle—before ovulation—estrogen dominates. Once ovulation occurs, there is a significant surge in progesterone—the "pro" gestation (pregnancy) hormone—which helps ready your uterus for a fertilized egg. With that bump in progesterone comes a rise in your body temperature—an increase of about half a degree (think of it as nature's way of getting your body warmed up for baby making). In other words, your temperature will be lower before ovulation than it is during the second part of your cycle—after ovulation. If you're charting your BBT, you'll notice the bump in temperature a day or two after ovulation day.

Keeping track of your BBT can help you pinpoint ovulation—at least after the fact. You'll need a special basal body thermometer, which measures temperature in increments of $\frac{1}{10}$ of a degree instead of the standard $\frac{2}{10}$ of a degree—a regular thermometer won't get the job done. Also available are BBT wearable monitors, sensors, patches, armbands, and in-ear thermometers—as well as vaginal rings and sensors—that automatically and continuously collect temperature measurements and transmit the data to your smartphone and fertility app. This eliminates the need for tedious temp taking and charting. Keeping track of your BBT over a few months will help you see a pattern to your cycles (once again, assuming your cycles are pretty consistent), enabling you to predict when ovulation will occur—and baby-making conditions are ripe—in future months.

Cervical Mucus

It's time to get up close and personal with your underwear—really. Because it's here that you'll discover the next fertility clues.

Ever notice that sometimes the crotch of your underwear is really wet and sticky, but other times you're quite dry down there? Ever wondered why, or even wondered if that occasional discharge was a sign that an infection was brewing?

Actually, it's your cervical mucus (CM) at work—and it's one bodily substance you'll definitely want to get to know as you go about the business of baby making. That's because it reflects the normal hormonal ups and downs of your cycle, which you can use to help you pinpoint ovulation day.

Did You Know?

Did you know that fertile CM tends to form a circle on your underwear, while CM during the nonfertile parts of your cycle is more likely to appear as a rectangle or line on your panties? So circle those circle days on your calendar!

Taking a closer look at your underwear (or the toilet paper you wipe with after you pee)—and keeping an eye on the cervical mucus you find down there—may not be the most appealing activity, but it's really a pretty effective way of tracking your fertility. Here's what to look for as your cycle progresses (there's a cervical mucus change for every phase!):

- Dry. Right after your period ends, don't expect to notice any cervical mucus. This dry spell—when your underwear will stay nice and fresh—usually lasts about 6 days to a week on average.

Getting in Touch with Your Cervical Mucus

Wonder exactly how you're going to obtain a sample of your CM so you can properly assess it? For some women, the CM faucet is always flowing—all they have to do to secure a CM sample is touch their vaginal opening (in fact, when they're fertile, these women might feel like they're swimming in egg whites). For those who produce CM on the scantier side, it may be necessary to insert a finger into the vagina and touch the cervix to cop a feel

of CM. But if you're like most women, paying attention when you wipe after peeing will tell you much of what you need to know about your CM. When you're fertile, the toilet paper will glide easily. During the unfertile times of the month, it'll feel drier when you wipe the toilet paper across. And of course, one of the easiest ways to keep track of your CM is to keep an eye on your underwear. When you're at your most fertile, your panties will likely spill the beans.

- Sticky. As your dry spell ends, things may start getting pretty sticky in your vaginal area (and your underwear)—and generally stay sticky for a day or two. The texture and consistency of your CM during the sticky phase may be crumbly, tacky, rubbery, pasty, springy, or similar to drying rubber cement (see how personal you're getting with it?). The color of CM during this phase can be yellow or white.

- Creamy. For the next several days (beginning, on average, around day 8) your CM will take a turn for the creamy. It may have a lotion-like consistency or a milkier one, but it'll most likely be white or pale yellow. This is where things can start getting pretty damp, too, or even pretty wet—often noticeably, and sometimes uncomfortably, so. In fact, you may be reaching for the panty liners at this point, to keep this creamy mess out of your underwear. If you try to stretch this CM between your fingers (how's that for fun in the bathroom?), it'll break apart.

- Slippery. Bingo! This is the sign you're looking for if you're TTC—CM that's slippery, stretchy (in fact, if you stretch it between 2 fingers, fertile CM may stretch up to a few inches), clear in color, with the consistency of egg white. This is the most fertile CM, and it indicates that ovulation is occurring (and that it's definitely time to schedule in sex, if you're already actively trying). There is usually more CM present during your most fertile time than there is during other parts of the cycle, but keep in mind that quality is more important than quantity when you're looking for the most fertile CM.

- Mostly dry. Right after ovulation, the CM forecast is mainly dry—and it's

TTC To-Do:

Now that you know everything you ever wanted to know about CM—or actually, probably a whole lot more than you ever wanted to know—it's time to start paying attention to it daily. Each day, take a look at your CM and note on a chart or app the consistency of CM you accumulate. Over the course of several months, you'll see a pattern, and you'll be able to pinpoint when your CM is at its most fertile (egg white slippery consistency, and most likely lots of it), so that you and your partner can hit the baby dance floor.

likely to stay dry until your period arrives. Some women, though, notice a thicker, cloudier discharge during this time, and others feel a little wet-and-watery a day or two before their period begins (a result of the normal drop in progesterone that precedes menstruation).

Don't confuse fertile CM with that wet (and wild) slippery sensation you get when you're turned on. CM is something that you'll be able to detect throughout the whole day—while arousal fluid (feeling "wet" when you're sexually aroused) is noticeable only when you're turned on, something you're not likely to be around-the-clock. Arousal fluid is also thinner and will dry on your fingers, while CM remains on your finger until you wipe it off.

If you're diligently checking CM each day to get to know your cycles, you'll also want to avoid confusing it with the semen that often dribbles out of your vagina after sex. To stay out of that sticky situation, try to remember to do your CM check before you have sex—not after.

Cervical Position

You're not done with your cervix yet. This tiny body part that you've probably never given a first thought to plays a pivotal role not only in pregnancy, but also in figuring out how to get pregnant. You've already explored the fertility clues your cervix leaves on your underwear or toilet paper, and now it's time to explore the cervix itself—that is, if you're game to. Feeling the shape and position of your cervix at different points in your cycle will fill in even more fertility blanks—and you don't have to be a gynecologist to do it.

During most of your cycle, your cervix is firm (it's often described as feeling like the tip of your nose—go figure), closed, and low in your vagina. As ovulation draws near, your cervix rises, opens slightly (thanks to the increase in estrogen), and becomes soft (described as feeling like your lips, which seems a little more like it). The reason for these changes? A soft, open cervix allows the sperm to pass through more easily on their quest for the egg.

Other Fertility Signs

Not all women notice the following other fertility signs, but if you experience any or all of them (many are easy to miss if you're not paying attention), you've got extra TTC know-how to go on:

Crampy ache. Some women notice some sort of mild pain in their lower abdominal area around the time of ovulation. This pain, known in medical-speak as mittleschmertz ("middle pain" in English), can be felt near the ovaries (on one side or the other—likely the side that's about to release an egg) or in the lower abdominal area as a dull achiness, a cramp, or a sharp pain. Experts hypothesize that the pain might be caused by the swelling of the maturing follicle or the bursting of the follicle at the actual moment of ovulation. Or the

TTC To-Do:

Ready to get to know your cervix? It's easier than you'd think. No stirrups or speculums necessary—all you need is a very clean finger with a short, smooth nail so you don't inadvertently scratch something sensitive. To check the position and feel of your cervix, insert that finger into your vagina each day or every other day of your cycle, after your period ends. You may find it easier to locate your target when you're checking in the squatting position, though you can also check while you're sitting on the toilet or with one foot up on the toilet seat. Relaxing your body will also help (if you clench those muscles, you'll have to fight your way in). For consistency's sake, assume the same position (sitting, squatting) each time you check. Once your CM kicks into high gear, it'll be even easier to check because you'll be lubricated. It may take a few cycles for you to get used to your cervical position differences (practice makes perfect), but once you start making sense of them, you can chart your findings on your fertility chart or app.

If you've already had a vaginal delivery, your cervix will always feel slightly opened (no matter what time of month) and more oval than that of a woman who's never delivered a baby before, but you'll still be able to notice the subtle changes if you're consistent about checking.

TTC for You and Me

In the market for some TTC friends to share your baby-making adventure with? Someone who can really relate? Someone who you can describe your cervical mucus to without hearing, "Ewwww . . . gross!"? Who you can swap baby dance tips with? Pass the time with while you're waiting for testing day to come (again!)? Someone to pump you up when a negative pregnancy test result deflates you, or to share your excitement with when you finally see the readout of your dreams (and who won't think it's weird when you post that pee stick for all to see)? Check out the TTC boards at WhatToExpect.com. You'll make friends, find support, gain insights, and tap into an amazing community of hopeful, expecting, and new moms.

pain might be the result of contractions of the fallopian tubes around ovulation. The pain can last anywhere from a few minutes to a few hours.

Swollen vaginal lips. Just before ovulation, some women feel a fullness in their vulva and vaginal lips, often on the side they're ovulating from.

Spotting. A few women notice light spotting midcycle, right around ovulation day. This so-called ovulatory spotting is thought to be caused by the sudden drop in estrogen right before ovulation and the lack of sufficient progesterone at that moment to maintain the uterine lining. If that occurs, a little blood leaks out until progesterone kicks into higher gear and continues to build up the endometrium.

Ovulation Predictors

Don't want to mess around with mucus or get close and personal with your cervix? You don't have to. Visit the fertility aisle in your pharmacy (or shop online) and stock up on any or all of the following (though be prepared to cough up a good chunk of change—technology doesn't come cheap). And keep in mind that no ovulation predictor tests can promise an accurate fertility forecast (or guarantee conception)—they can only indicate when ovulation may be occurring.

Ovulation predictor kits (OPKs) can help pinpoint your day of ovulation 12 to 36 hours in advance by looking at levels of LH, which is the last of the hormones to hit its peak before ovulation actually occurs. All you have to do is pee on a stick (or into a cup and dip the stick or strip into the pee) and wait for the indicator to tell you whether you're about to ovulate. (You'll be an expert at peeing on a stick by the time you're ready for your pregnancy tests.) Unlike pregnancy tests—where any line (faint or dark) indicates you're pregnant—the test line on an OPK has to appear the same or darker than the control line. Since there are always low levels of LH in your body, a sensitive OPK can detect it and show a faint line, but what you're looking for is the LH surge (higher amounts of LH)—and a test line that reads bright and clear. You can bypass this confusing line-reading detection by choosing those OPKs that have digital readouts—no squinting required.

When You're Not Ovulating

What happens if you've been charting your BBT and checking for CM and even using OPKs, but for some reason, it seems that you're not ovulating every month—or maybe, not ovulating at all? You're not alone. About 6 to 15 percent of women have anovulatory cycles—in other words, they get their period but don't release an egg (and without that egg, conception can't occur). The most common reasons why otherwise healthy women may not ovulate in a particular month include illness, traveling, strenuous exercise, weight gain or weight loss, or extreme stress. Being chronically underweight or overweight or having a medical condition, such as PCOS or a thyroid problem, may also cause anovulatory cycles. If you think you might not be ovulating, check with your gynecologist. He or she can turn to a host of low- and high-tech methods to help induce ovulation—and help you get closer to that baby of your dreams. See page 159 for more information.

Some OPKs ask you to insert your daily test stick into a digital reader, which will then compare your hormone levels with the levels you've had on previous days, helping you detect that all-important LH surge.

It's best to use an OPK between noon and 8 p.m. because most women experience their LH surge in the morning and LH won't be detected in the urine until at least 4 hours later. To make sure your urine is concentrated enough, don't pee for an hour or two before you plan on testing. If you miss the LH surge when it actually happens and detect it only on the way down, you may think you're ovulating a day after you truly are—throwing your baby-making sex schedule off and possibly missing your monthly window of opportunity altogether. If you really want to make sure you catch your LH surge, consider testing twice a day (once between 11 a.m. and 3 p.m. and a second time between 5 p.m. and 10 p.m.). Whether you test once or twice a day, be consistent and test at the same time (or times) each day.

It's best to start using the OPK tests a little before midway through your cycle (about 3 to 4 days earlier than your cycle midpoint). For a 28-day cycle, start using them on days 10 to 11. For a 31-day cycle, start on days 12 to 13. If your cycles are irregular, use the length of your shortest cycle in the last 6 months as a guide and begin testing 3 to 4 days sooner than the midpoint of your shortest cycle. The more irregular your cycles are, the more OPKs you'll likely use up, so figure that into your cost estimation. Most kits come with 5 to 10 test sticks.

As soon as your LH surge is detected, begin having sex on that day and for 2 to 3 days after.

Some caveats about OPKs: First, these kits work best for women whose cycles are relatively regular. Women who have very irregular periods (and therefore have a hard time figuring out when they're due to start ovulating) may start using the tests too early or too late, and they might miss the ovulation window altogether because they ran out of test sticks. Second, the kits are not accurate for all women. For example, a woman with PCOS (see page 159) might experience multiple LH surges during a particular month, rendering the results of an OPK unreliable, since those surges don't necessarily mean ovulation is about to occur. Third, the kits look for the LH surge, but can't detect ovulation itself—which means that there's no way of knowing for sure that you've definitely ovulated in a particular cycle, even if you've had a positive LH surge. While most women do ovulate each month, some women don't (see box, facing page), even with an LH surge. Finally, OPKs won't always be accurate if you're taking certain medications, like some types of fertility drugs, hormones, or even antibiotics.

Fertility monitors take ovulation detection one step further. Instead of testing only for the LH surge, a fertility monitor will test for both LH and estrogen in the urine, giving you a 6-day window of fertility opportunity. You use the monitor each day, beginning on day 1 of your cycle (the first day of your period), by turning on the device with the press of a button. The monitor keeps track of your cycle days, and the digital indicator reminds you when to start using the urine test strips that come in the package. When you get the heads-up signal from the monitor, you'll pee on the test strip, insert it into the monitor, and wait for the monitor to indicate whether your fertility status that day is low, high, or at its peak. When you see a high or peak readout, you're at your most fertile—which means it's time to get busy.

A saliva test allows you to monitor levels of estrogen in your system. Estrogen rises before ovulation—and before the LH surge—so by tracking estrogen, you can get an even earlier indication of when you'll be ovulating. What does estrogen have to do with saliva? When estrogen increases, so do the electrolytes (salt content) in your saliva. Testing your saliva for electrolytes can indicate when estrogen is on the rise and when your fertile time is approaching (and you thought you were done with the bodily substance samples).

Each morning before brushing your teeth, eating, or drinking, put a dab of saliva onto the tip of a clean finger and gently smear it onto the lens of the saliva test. Some test brands suggest you put the saliva on the lens directly from your tongue. Wait about 5 minutes until the saliva is dry and then take a look under the test's eyepiece. When you're about to ovulate, a look at your saliva will reveal a microscopic pattern that resembles the leaves of a fern plant or frost on a windowpane (the rest of the time, you'll just see random dots). Once you see your fern, get ready for baby-making sex. Ovulation will likely occur within 24 to 72 hours.

The downside to this type of test is that not all women get a good "fern," and it can be very hard to interpret the test results.

A fertility "watch" is a biosensor worn on your wrist each day (or at night, if it's not your preferred fashion statement).

TTC To-Do:

Now that you know when ovulation is happening, you know when you should time sex for the best chance of conception. But don't wait too long. Remember that your actual fertile window consists of the day of ovulation plus the 5 cycle days *before* ovulation. Wait until the day after you've ovulated to have sex, and you've missed your monthly shot at conception.

The watch can detect the numerous salts (chloride, sodium, potassium) in yet another bodily substance, sweat—because the salt amounts change during different times of the month. Before ovulation (and even before the estrogen and the LH surge), there is a surge in ion levels, called the chloride ion surge. Once the watch detects this surge, you've got a 4- to 6-day heads-up that ovulation is approaching, giving you plenty of time to schedule in some baby-making sex.

A fertility tracker bracelet—think of it as a fertility Fitbit—is a wearable fertility monitoring device that syncs with your smartphone to give you a window into your fertility. You wear the fertility bracelet at night, and while you're sleeping, the bracelet monitors your pulse, breathing, sleep quality, heart rate variability, skin temperature, and other metrics, each of which is affected by the monthly surge in reproductive hormones estrogen and progesterone. When you wake up, you sync the bracelet with its companion app, and your smartphone will show you which cycle phase you're in and whether it's time to TTC.

CHAPTER 6

Figuring Out Your Fertility

Wondering how your fertility stacks up on paper before you put it to the test in bed? If you're the curious type, you'll probably want to dig into this chapter for clues about your fertility—how your cycles, your genetics, and your age (and your partner's age) might influence your reproductive profile. Keep in mind as you read, however, that no fertility forecast is a sure thing. Every woman's fertility is different, which means that certain fertility factors may never factor into your baby-making experience. It also means that you may end up getting pregnant a lot faster in bed than you would on paper.

Rather just plunge into baby making without any fertility forecast? Skip this chapter and get right to the action.

Am I Fertile?

Inquiring (and hopeful) minds want to know: Am I fertile? How easily will I conceive once we start trying? There's no telling for sure how your fertility stacks up until you actually take it for a test-ride. Even if it's been tested in the past (and passed the test in the form of a previous pregnancy), fertility can keep you guessing. Still, there's no need to be completely clueless about your fertility—especially when there are so many clues that can reveal at least part of the baby-making picture.

Your Cycle and Your Fertility

"We're about to start TTC. Is there any way to tell whether I'll be able to conceive or not, or how long it will take?"

There's really no way to know right out of the gate whether you can expect a smooth ride or a bumpy one to the baby finish line. It can take a healthy couple 6 to 12 months of active trying to successfully make a baby. And short of either getting pregnant or undergoing a fertility screening (which you certainly don't need yet—and might never need), there is no way to find out definitively what your fertility prospects are at this early stage of the baby-making game.

Still, you can look to an old familiar friend—your period—for some hints about what might lie ahead in your TTC future. In fact, tracking your monthly periods is one of the best ways to gauge your fertility and clue yourself in on the state of your reproductive health. So as you embark on your fledgling campaign to fill your nest, asking yourself some questions about your cycle can be a great place to start. Keep in mind that you won't be able to get a good read on your cycle if you've been on oral contraceptives or another hormonal birth control method, because such cycles are "artificial" and don't reflect what's normal for you. That's why it's a good idea to get back to cycling naturally, after quitting hormonal birth control, before you start trying to conceive.

How long are my cycles? A "normal" cycle can last anywhere from 21 to 35 days between periods, with 28 to 30 days the average. If your cycles are much shorter or longer than what is considered "normal," it may be a clue to some fertility issues (though it may not be, too). Are your cycles all over the place? Occasional cycle-length irregularities aren't cause for concern. They're usually just the result of stress, travel, weight loss or gain, too much partying, or another temporary blip in your normal routine, and as long as they reregulate, they won't keep you from reaching your baby goal. But consistently irregular cycles can make conception slightly more elusive. If there's an underlying condition (like a thyroid problem) contributing to your irregular cycle, treating it can help you get regular—and pregnant.

How much bleeding do I have? A normal period begins with light bleeding, builds to heavier bleeding, and then slowly tapers off, ending with light staining. Excessive bleeding (extremely heavy blood flow, blood clots, or large volumes of blood loss) or a flow that's watery or exceptionally light in color could (but doesn't always) signal a reproductive problem.

It's Not Just Your Period, Period.

Your period can tell you a lot when it comes to the state of your fertility, but it can't tell you the whole story. For the rest of the scoop, you'll need to keep an eye on ovulation—the most important component of fertility. If you don't ovulate, you can't get pregnant (without a little help from medical science, that is). And sometimes, even women who have seemingly "normal" periods may not be ovulating (this is called an anovulatory cycle). How can you tell if you're ovulating each month? See Chapter 5.

Another Clue to Your Fertility

Interestingly, some women who do not ovulate regularly and/or have other fertility issues have a slightly increased amount of male hormones (and that's probably what's contributing to the irregular ovulation). How can you tell if that's the case with you? One sign is hirsutism: You're hairier than average on areas of the body normally not associated with hair on a woman, such as on the nipples, lower abdomen, face, even the big toe. Another clue? Acne that persists beyond the midteens can indicate increased male hormones. Check in with your doctor if you've noticed these symptoms.

How long do I bleed? Most women have their period for 5 to 7 days, though bleeding is usually heavy for 2 to 3 days. Bleeding typically lessens by day 4 and continues with only light staining up to day 7. Heavy bleeding that lingers longer than 6 days or periods that last longer than 8 to 9 days may possibly (but by no means necessarily) be a sign that something is off the mark reproductively. Ditto for periods that have very light blood flow for longer than 8 or 9 days or ones that end abruptly after 1 or 2 days.

Do I have pain or cramping? Some aches, pains, and cramps come with the time-of-the-month territory, though a few lucky women don't feel a thing. What's not normal is extremely severe cramping, nausea, vomiting, acute backache, dizziness, or headaches right before or during your period. Any of these could signal a reproductive problem (though not necessarily).

Are my cycles erratic? If you go months without a period, then have a few periods in a row, and then go months again without bleeding, it could signal fertility challenges ahead (unless it's a sign of stress on your body—in which case the erratic cycles and the potential for fertility challenges should disappear when the stress does).

If there are any red flags in your period assessment—or if you have any other reason to believe you may be facing a fertility issue—talk over your concerns with your gynecologist. Chances are, you'll get the reassurance you're looking for—and marching orders right onto the baby dance floor. If it turns out that your menstrual irregularities may signal a fertility problem, now's the time to have it checked out, diagnosed, and treated, so you can get back on the track to parenthood as quickly as possible.

Genetics and Fertility

"My mother had trouble conceiving me. Does that mean I'm going to have trouble conceiving, too?"

Like mother, like daughter? While it's not necessarily true that your mother's reproductive difficulties will be passed on to you, there are genetic components to some fertility-related disorders, and it's worth exploring your female family tree to see what may—or may not—be lurking beneath the leaves. If family dynamics allow you to comfortably have such a conversation, ask your mother, maternal grandmother, any sisters or maternal aunts, and even female cousins on your mother's side about their TTC experiences and whether they had or have endometriosis, ovarian cysts, fibroids, thyroid disorders, celiac disease, or other potential fertility stumbling blocks. It may also be helpful to know (if you're comfortable asking and they're comfortable sharing) how long it took each of them to conceive and at what age they went through menopause (if early menopause runs in your family, that may impact the timing of your family planning). Take all this information with you on your baby-making journey—and be sure to let your practitioner know about it, too.

Getting Pregnant After 35

"I'm 37 years old. Should I expect a harder time conceiving?"

Thirty-five may be the new 25, and 40 the new 30—but the question is, have your reproductive parts gotten the message? Can baby making be on your calendar no matter how many calendars you've gone through?

Absolutely. Birth rates are on the rise for women (and men) well into their 30s and 40s—proof positive that babies can come to those who wait (even if they sometimes come with a little help from a fertility specialist). If it's true that a woman's life begins at 30 (or even 40), it's also true that, more and more often these days, so does her active reproductive life. Fewer women are jumping on

How Fresh Are Your Eggs?

Since a woman is born with all the eggs she'll ever have—and they're gradually used up or break down as the months (and years) pass—she's left with fewer and fewer fertilizable eggs in reserve as she moves later into her reproductive life. But how do you know how many eggs you've still got left in your basket—and whether they're still functioning and healthy enough to make a baby?

When women over 35 are trying to conceive for 3 to 6 months or more without success, doctors use a blood screening test to determine "ovarian reserve." (There are other times when a doctor may suggest ovarian reserve screening; see page 175). This is done by measuring a few hormones that can give a picture (though not with 100 percent accuracy) of a woman's fertility potential.

The first hormone tested is follicle stimulating hormone (or FSH)—the all-important hormone that signals the ovary to release an egg. When lots of young and eager eggs are ready to burst out and get busy, a little FSH goes a

long way—and less is needed to get the ovulation job done. But as the number of eggs dwindles, the brain senses that getting them ready to ovulate won't be as easy as it used to be—and that it will take a little extra stimulating in the form of a lot of extra FSH. So the brain issues a signal to the pituitary gland to release more FSH. The fewer good eggs (and good follicles) left, the more FSH is released—the body's way of getting a productive egg up and running, and of compensating for the less-fertile conditions that come with aging. In fact, sometimes the body overcompensates by producing too much FSH, which explains why older women are more likely to drop 2 eggs at a time, upping their chances of conceiving twins (those follicles can get a little overstimulated from the flood of FSH). What's more, the body—never a quitter—keeps up its follicle-stimulating campaign long after there are no eggs or follicles left to stimulate. In fact, FSH levels are permanently elevated in menopausal women—a souvenir of their reproductive years.

the baby train in their 20s, with a full 1 in 5 opting to wait until they're well into their 30s and 40s to start a family.

Many of these moms are able to conceive within just a few months of trying (and have healthy pregnancies and healthy babies to show for it soon after). But some "older" hopeful moms find that it takes longer to conceive or that they need some help—sometimes a little, sometimes a lot—from fertility treatments to make their baby dreams a cuddly reality. That's because women are at their most fertile in their very early 20s, well before most are ready to tap into that fertility. By their early 30s, fertility has started to wane—the chances of getting pregnant gradually go down from 25 percent per cycle for women age 25 and under to about 15 percent per cycle for women in your age bracket, 35 to 39. Average chances of conceiving naturally at age 40: about 5 percent per cycle. Still potentially doable, but clearly not as easy to do.

What causes this drop in fertility? Fewer eggs (by age 30, only 12 percent of the eggs you started out in life with are left) and less frequent ovulation, for one thing. For another, your eggs have been sitting on the shelf longer. As a woman ages, so do her eggs—and

By measuring a baseline FSH on day 3 of a woman's cycle through a simple blood test, doctors can get an indication of how close a woman is to menopause—and how close she is to having fewer and less viable eggs. The higher the baseline FSH, the lower her egg supply, or ovarian reserve. And most of the time, the lower the egg supply, the lower the quality of the remaining eggs will be, too. A normal FSH level is usually under 10. Measurements between 10 and 15 are borderline, and anything above 20 to 25 is considered low ovarian reserve.

Estradiol hormone levels are also measured along with FSH. Estradiol (a type of estrogen) is released from the ovary during follicular development, and an elevated level on day 3 can indicate low ovarian reserve (because the eggs are developing too quickly). Another hormone—AMH (antimullerian hormone), detected via a blood test—can also be used to determine ovarian reserve, and in some cases can be more accurate than FSH because there are no monthly fluctuations in AMH levels as there can be with FSH levels. What's more, the test isn't dependent on a woman's menstrual cycle, meaning the test can be given at any time. AMH is secreted by the small follicles (called preantral and early antral follicles) found in the ovaries at the start of a menstrual cycle. AMH levels reflect the number of follicles present in the ovaries and can estimate how close a woman is to menopause. A higher AMH level would indicate a large number of preantral and early antral follicles and therefore an adequate ovarian reserve, while a lower value would indicate a lower ovarian reserve. A high AMH level could also be a marker for polycystic ovarian syndrome (PCOS; see page 159).

Your physician might also perform a transvaginal ultrasound to view the ovaries and count the number of antral follicles. A high antral follicle count not only indicates a better ovarian reserve, but can also help predict whether the ovaries would respond well to ovarian-stimulating drugs (see page 190) in the case of fertility treatments. A lower antral follicle count (along with other indications of lower ovarian reserve) might encourage a woman to fast-track her TTC efforts, as well as expedite any necessary fertility treatments. She might also want to consider freezing some of her eggs for future use.

Fertility and the Older Man

It's long been documented that a woman's biological clock eventually runs out, limiting her baby-making years. But what about men? Is your reproductive life also on a timer?

Actually, it might be, at least to some extent. Guys can—and do—continue their baby-making careers long after they've passed retirement age (and decades after a woman's fertility expires). And more and more are waiting longer to father that first child (about 25 percent of first-time fathers are over age 35). But researchers have found that fertility does decline in men, too, albeit more gradually than it does in women—beginning at about age 30, and dropping more rapidly after age 45. In fact, it may take up to 5 times longer for a man to get a woman pregnant once he's 45 than it would have when he was 25.

And though a guy can continue producing viable sperm well into his AARP years, his age can affect the quantity of sperm (there may be fewer sperm in each ejaculate), the quality of sperm (aging sperm are more likely to be genetically damaged, and that's linked to a higher rate of miscarriage, possibly Down syndrome, and other chromosomal defects–even if the mom is much younger), the motility of the sperm (if they can't move fast enough to reach the egg, conception can't happen), and the strength of the sperm (weak sperm will not be able to penetrate the egg's membrane to fertilize it).

Other facts of older life for guys: decreased potency (the force of a younger man's ejaculation is often more powerful than that of an older man, enabling the sperm to be ejected farther into the vaginal canal) and problems with erectile dysfunction (which can definitely make fertility more challenging). And even those lucky older guys who notice no reduction in sexual function do experience a fertility drop-off. (By the way, taking Viagra or Cialis to make the mechanics of baby-making sex easier to accomplish hasn't been linked to decreased fertility, but since research has been limited so far, check with your doctor before popping that pill.)

That's not to say that your baby-making days are ever over when you're a guy. Far from it—only that there is a point of somewhat diminishing fertility returns for men as well as women. Though it's possible that you may have to wait a little longer to make that miracle happen, babies are always worth waiting for.

older eggs are less easily fertilized. Still another challenge: Older women don't make cervical mucus like they used to—the quantity and quality of this fertility-friendly fluid also tends to lessen as a woman ages. A woman in her 20s can expect 2 to 4 days of fertile (clear, thin, slippery, stretchy, egg-white-like) cervical mucus per cycle, while a woman in her late 30s often has only 1 or 2 days of fertile CM. Less CM may spell more challenging swimming conditions for egg-seeking sperm. Gynecological problems that can interfere with fertility—such as endometriosis or fibroids—are also more common as women get older, as are general health issues such as high blood pressure or type 2 diabetes that can make it harder to conceive. Those who do conceive have a somewhat higher rate of miscarriage, in large part because of those aging eggs.

Feeling daunted? Don't. The majority of women your age—50 to 70 percent—conceive naturally and without a hitch. Even women who've passed their 40th birthday have about a 40 percent chance of conceiving naturally. So don't bog yourself down with the numbers now. Instead, relax and go about your baby-making business. Just a couple of things to keep in mind as you do. First, you'll probably want to pay some extra attention to your cycles, so you can give yourself every fertility edge (see Chapter 5 for tips). Second, you'll probably want to seek help sooner than a younger mom. If you're 35 to 38 and haven't conceived within 3 to 6 months of active efforts, check in with your practitioner to see if it's time for a little help in the fertility department. Check in sooner (after 3 months) if you're over 38, and check in before you start trying if you're over 40.

And here's something else you may want to keep in mind. Being over 35 means conception can be a little trickier, but it can also make it more fruitful—meaning that when it rains babies, it can pour. Older moms have a greater chance of conceiving twins, even if they conceive naturally, without the benefit of fertility treatments. That's because

TTC To-Do:

If you're over 35, you might want to put in a call to your doctor after 3 to 6 months of TTC with no luck. If you're over 38, consider making that call after 3 months of active efforts. If you're 40 or over, there's no reason to wait—check in right from the very beginning of your conception campaign. Why the earlier medical input for older moms? Not because you're definitely going to need help in the form of assisted reproduction (and in fact, you may conceive naturally—and much sooner than you'd think). It's just that taking a more time-sensitive approach to TTC makes sense when you're trying to conceive later in your reproductive years. If you do end up needing some help, it's a good idea to start the ball rolling sooner, so you're more likely to have time on your side.

older moms tend to ovulate irregularly, and because they produce more follicle-stimulating hormone (FSH), their ovaries are more likely to be stimulated into dropping 2 eggs at a time. Two fertilized eggs—and bingo, you've got 2 babies.

CHAPTER 7

Getting Busy Getting Pregnant

....

So, say you've done your preconception prep. Your diet's on track, your weight's on target, and you've downsized from a 5-cup-a-day coffee habit to a 2-cupper. Your nest egg is busy solidifying, and you've paid a visit to your doctor and dentist. You've gotten to know your cycle and your cervix, and you're an ovulation prediction pro. Or maybe you've opted to skip the prep phase altogether and cut straight to the good part—getting pregnant. Either way, all reproductive systems are go and it's time to make a baby. But how, exactly, do you go about doing that?

No doubt, you're pretty clear on the logistics of sex—but how do you put that knowledge to its best baby-making use? Are there do's and don'ts to doing "it," now that your goal is conception? Should you let nature take its course or give nature a helpful nudge? And what if nature takes her sweet time—how much doing it will you have to do? Are there ways to do it that speed conception or might make your pink or blue daydreams more likely to come true? Should you tap into the complementary and alternative medicine (CAM) camp for a fertility boost? Read on for the answers to all your baby-making questions.

Making Love to Make a Baby

Before jumping into bed, you might want to give sex a second look. Sure, you've probably been doing it for years—and chances are you're pretty good at it by now. But will sex for procreation have to be different from sex for pleasure? In most cases, not at all—after all, egg and sperm often end up meeting spontaneously, without special scheduling or preparations. Still, a few minor adjustments here and there might be just the ticket you need to hop onto the baby express.

Stopping Birth Control

"We're ready to TTC. Do I just stop my pills and get started?"

Ready to take the plunge into unprotected sex? Baby making might seem as easy as tossing the pills, pulling off the patch, or letting the condoms gather dust in your bedside drawer. But you'll need to look before you leap into the sack without that prophylactic protection, and give your birth control method a preconception assessment first. Here's the lowdown on how your pregnancy protection can affect your pregnancy planning:

Pills, patches, and rings. These contraceptives prevent pregnancy by stopping your body from ovulating (no ovulation, no pregnancy). How do they accomplish this neat birth-controlling trick? By turning off hormone signals from your brain and your pituitary gland to your ovaries—effectively flipping off the ovulation switch. Quit the Pill, the patch, or the ring, and your ovaries will begin receiving those brain and pituitary signals again—picking up the ovulation process where you left off. To avoid breakthrough (midcycle) bleeding, finish up the month's pack before calling it quits.

Most women start to ovulate within a couple of weeks of shelving their hormonal contraceptives, but that first egg may drop sooner or later than that (it could take a few months in some

Hot to Trot

Feeling frisky? Most women report feeling their sexiest—and most in the mood for loving—right around the time they're ovulating. Convenient for baby making—and not surprising, given Mother Nature's master plan to keep all species reproducing. Just as female animals go into heat when they're primed for procreation, females of the human race, too, have developed a heat of their own—biological responses to increase the odds that mating will occur when the chances for pregnancy are highest (at ovulation).

Both testosterone and estrogen peak midcycle, just about the time you ovulate. Testosterone sends your libido into action (bringing out the sexual aggressor in you), and estrogen hones your senses (which come in very handy when it comes to sex). What's more, these hormonally triggered friskiness factors (nature's answer to scented candles and mood music?) seem to increase as LH rises, peaking right before ovulation occurs—just in time for sperm to get in line for the egg's release. And leaving you wondering: Is it hot in here, or am I ovulating?

women). There's no risk to getting right down to baby-making business as soon as you're off the hormones, but to make dating a pregnancy easier, it's a good idea to hold off TTC efforts (using a barrier method in the meantime) until you've had a full natural cycle (including a period) after stopping the Pill, ring, or patch. If you do get pregnant before your first period and consequently don't have a starting date for the pregnancy—early ultrasound can

Your Voice Says It All

You may not hear it, but believe it: Your voice sounds sexier when you're most fertile. Think of it as a mating call, researchers say—a subliminal signal to your mate that you're ready to conceive. Even if he's not aware of the voice change, his reproductive parts apparently are—and they respond accordingly. All of this seems less random and more ingenious when you consider this fascinating fertility fact: The hormonal changes that result in egg release also change the shape and size of your larynx. These findings add fuel to the theory that women give off subtle signs (from scents to style) about their fertility—signs that can help put that fertility to good use. Now you're talking.

step in and solve the dating mystery. Also good to know: There's no added risk to the baby or the pregnancy if you conceive inadvertently while on hormonal birth control or if you conceive before your cycle is up and running again. In fact, there is some evidence of a decreased risk of miscarriage for women over 30 who have used the Pill in the past.

Barrier methods (diaphragms, sponges, caps, condoms). No need to plan way ahead with these types of contraception, so they're perfect for the spontaneous set. Just ditch the diaphragm or condom anytime (how happy are you about that?) and you're ready to get busy baby making. And while you're ditching your diaphragm, you might as well toss it out, too. You'll need to be fitted for a new one after delivery, since

pregnancy and childbirth change the shape of your cervix (and diaphragms that don't fit don't do their job).

Spermicides. Like barrier methods, spermicides don't need to be stopped until you're ready to roll. Don't worry if you accidentally conceive while using a spermicide—it won't hurt your baby.

Intrauterine device (IUD). Stop anytime by having your doctor remove the device. Once it's out, you may be able to start your conception efforts pronto (check with your doctor). Typically, your fertility will be the same as it was before the device was put in, with little or no downtime. Even an IUD that releases hormones shouldn't delay your TTC campaign, since the level of hormones is much lower than that in the Pill and other hormonal forms of birth control.

Depo-Provera. There's plenty of advance planning required here, because it can take 6 months to a year for ovulation to resume after you stop getting these progesterone shots. Talk to your ob-gyn about the best timing for you. And plan on using another method of nonhormonal birth control (condom, spermicides, or diaphragm) while you wait for your cycles to return to normal. Not to worry if you do become pregnant as soon as ovulation returns and even before your cycles regulate. An ultrasound will help date the pregnancy, and there's no added risk for the baby.

Implant. Within 48 hours of having the implant removed, the hormones it releases to switch off ovulation are no longer circulating in your system—which means you'll probably resume reproductive business as usual within a few weeks (though it can be sooner or longer). Still, it's a good idea to wait a cycle before you start TTC (use a barrier method in the meantime) so that you can more easily date a pregnancy. If you conceive inadvertently before then, there's no increased risk, and early ultrasound will determine your due date.

Fertility awareness method (FAM). As a practitioner of this method, you're ahead of the baby-making game, since you're likely an expert on your own fertility. Now that you're ready for a baby, just reverse your efforts. Instead of avoiding sex during fertile times, bring it on!

Sex Positions

"Is it true that some sex positions are better than others when it comes to conception?"

Is there a better way to do "it" (get pregnant, that is)? Or will any way do? Will just getting it on get that baby on board—or will you have to get creative, too? Or even technical?

Though there's no need to pull out the old *Kama Sutra* (unless you're in the mood for some spicy gymnastics), you also don't have to go back to on-your-back basics (as in the missionary position) either. The bottom (or top) line is that as long as sperm from your partner is deposited close to your cervix, you're in business. That's because healthy sperm are pretty good swimmers—even when they're swimming upstream without the help of gravity—and they normally don't need any extra nudging along. Plus, though baby-making sex serves a brand new purpose, its other purpose still applies: having fun in bed (or wherever you choose to do it). After all, you're going to be doing it a lot while you're TTC, so you might as well relax and enjoy it. And don't get bent out of shape, literally, if you're happier in your same-old, same-old position. Medical studies haven't yet supported the theory that some positions are more effective for getting pregnant than others.

Of course, there's no harm in doing a little research of your own and trying a few of the positions often touted for optimum fertility success. After all, it can't hurt to head the little guys in

Do Headstands Give Sperm a Head Start?

Wondering how to spend your post-sex time for best baby-making results? You've probably heard it all: Lie down for 20 to 30 minutes after sex to fast-track those sperm to your cervix. Or put your knees or legs up to enlist gravity. Or stand on your head—or twist yourself into some other kind of sperm-preserving pretzel position. And whatever you do, don't get up and pee.

But is there any truth to these tips? While they can't hurt—and potentially might help a little—don't get too hung up on hanging out upside down after sex. Lingering in bed with your sweetie is always sweet—and if it helps make a baby, all the better. But advanced yoga moves aren't called for. And neither is enforcing after-sex bed rest for yourself if you haven't got the time (you have to get to work after that early morning loving or back to work after that lunchtime quickie). Remember, healthy sperm are little men on a mission—and many of them will accomplish that mission without any help from you or gravity. After all, that's why a man's ejaculation is so forceful—to send those boys flying to their target.

Take Your Sperm to a Movie

Did you know that watching a sexy movie with your mate right before you have TTC sex may actually help you conceive faster? Researchers (who apparently research everything) have found that when men watch a scene with sexual content (and it doesn't have to be X-rated) right before making love, the sperm they produce is of higher quality. Why's that? You can chalk it up to good old-fashioned evolutionary male rivalry. When you see someone else getting it on, your innate sense of male competitiveness kicks in ("Hey, I can do that, too, and I can do it better!") and your body revs up to produce superior sperm ("I'll show him!").

the right direction, especially if your partner has a low sperm count. It might even give sluggish sperm the mojo (or gravitational pull) they need to get the job done, or help them access that cervix of yours more easily. Because your vagina naturally tilts toward your back, lying on your back (with man on top)—and with a small pillow under your hips, if you'd like—can allow the sperm to pool right at the cervix. Too big a pillow, though, and you risk directing the sperm behind your cervix instead of up through it, so elevate your hips only slightly to give gravity an edge (as opposed to a steep slope). If you have a tipped uterus (if your uterus tips toward the front—ask your practitioner if you're not sure), doggie-style (hands-and-knees position with penetration from behind) may give sperm that full-access pass to your cervix.

For now, you may want to avoid positions that allow the sperm to leak out (though it takes only 1, there is strength in numbers when it comes to fertility odds), including any position in which you straddle your partner—sitting, standing, woman on top, and so on—though again, such a change isn't necessary for conception, and it could actually work against you if you find it doesn't float your love boat (if you're not having fun, you're going to start dreading TTC sessions—and that's not going to get you anywhere). Whichever position you choose, make sure your mate ejaculates deep within your vagina—and that he lingers in there as long as possible (you want to get every last drop of sperm).

Lubricants

"Now that we're timing sex so we can get pregnant, the sexiness is gone—and I'm finding that I'm not as wet as I used to be. Is it okay for me to use lubrication?"

It's always easier (and much more comfortable) to get wild when you're wet—and vice versa, too. But when you're trying to conceive, you're better off sticking with nature's lube—your own vaginal secretions. Most experts agree that many commonly used lubricants—particularly oil-based ones such as Vaseline or massage oils, but even some water- and silicone-based lubes—can not only mess with your cervical mucus, preventing it from doing its job optimally, but also alter the pH in your vaginal tract, causing it to be extra inhospitable to sperm. Some types of lubricants (ones that contain glycerin, for instance) can even be toxic for sperm, killing them off before they can get started (and believe it or not, another natural lubricant—saliva—falls into the sperm-killer category). Also off the bedside table: slippery stuff

Winter, Spring, Summer, or Fall

Flipping through the calendar, trying to figure out when to start penciling in baby making? According to researchers, conception may be more seasonal than you'd think. With birth rates peaking in the summer and fall (and counting 9 months back), they speculate that the best time to conceive is from October through March—slow season on the beach, high season in bed. And there is more seasonal data you may want to factor in if you're thinking blue: More boys are conceived in October, researchers say, when there are 12 hours of daylight and the average outdoor temperature is 54°F. The possible explanation? An October conception results in an early summer birth instead of a harsh winter one—a good thing for boys, who tend to be less hardy at birth. Pining for pink? Girls are most often conceived in April and born in the winter (the girls, it seems, can handle the chill better than the guys can).

The season when conception is less likely, according to these studies? Early fall. Just don't tell that to all the people whose birthdays are in late spring.

---

you might find in your pantry or fridge (such as olive oil or egg whites). In other words, it's best to lay off your usual K-Y until baby's on board—at which point you might not need any help in the lubrication department, since pregnancy hormones typically step up secretions.

There are a number of sperm-friendly lubricants specifically marketed as TTC compatible (such as Astroglide TTC and PreSeed). These lubricants are designed to mimic cervical mucus,

possibly aiding sperm motility, and have the same pH as sperm, helping them feel at home in the vagina. If you do opt to use one of these lubricants, be sure it's FDA-approved.

If TTC has made sex feel like a chore, try putting some pleasure back into the work of procreation. Spending more time (or at least some time) on foreplay before getting the deed done can pay off big time and get your juices flowing again naturally. For tips on heating things up while trying to conceive, see page 127.

see page 127.

FOR DADS-TO-BE

Like What You See?

Is your mate looking extra, well, mate-able to you lately? Strange as it sounds, a woman's facial features are at their most attractive just as her ovary gets ready to drop its egg delivery. This monthly makeover (which is pretty subtle, yet scientifically identified by researchers) makes her more desirable to her partner—so that the couple is more likely to partner up for baby making.

Orgasm

"Does my having an orgasm increase our changes of conception?"

It's no secret that for conception to have a shot (so to speak), the male partner has to reach orgasm—ejaculating, so that sperm-loaded semen can be released and sent on its merry baby-making way. No male orgasm, no baby. But female orgasm, apparently, is optional. In other words, you don't have to climax to conceive.

The Smell of Love

Smell something? Smell everything? A baby—or at least an opportunity to make a baby—may be in the air. Your sense of smell, like your other senses, becomes heightened when you're in egg-release mode—thanks to stepped-up hormone production, particularly of estrogen. You'll wake up and smell the coffee more keenly, the aftershave of a guy passing you on the street, the flowers in your boss's office, the hamburgers grilling down the block. But what your nose knows also apparently allows you to sniff out a smell that no one else can: the musky pheromones of your male partner. This sensory response is instinctual and isn't something you're conscious of (so you won't be literally sniffing around your spouse's armpits, which could be embarrassing in public). But before you know what hit you (the pheromones), your nose will lead you and your mate into the bedroom for a little baby making.

Still, some experts speculate there may be more to female orgasm than a good time. Here's why: When you have an orgasm, your uterus contracts, and these contractions may allow the cervix to dip into the semen pool to "suck up" more sperm. And once those sperm are in the uterus, the small contractions from a female orgasm can help move sperm toward the fallopian tubes. All these theoretical benefits are, of course, contingent on both of you climaxing at the same time (or relatively close in time)—a nice goal to work toward as a couple anyway.

So if you enjoy a good climax (and who doesn't?), go for it—that's at least half the fun of baby making. But don't get yourself all worked up trying to get all worked up in the name of conception. And don't sweat it if you don't get it. Though sperm always appreciate a helping hand—or a little push from those uterine contractions—they can also swim exceptionally well on their own.

Frequency of Sex

"I've heard conflicting advice on how often to have sex when I'm ovulating. Every day? Every other day? Twice a day? Which is it?"

Is Underwater Sex All Wet?

You already know that hanging around in hot tubs can land a guy in hot water, at least as far as his fertility is concerned. But did you know that underwater romance can also undermine your chances of conceiving—no matter what the water temperature? If you're fooling around in a pool, the chlorine can alter the pH in the vagina, making it extra inhospitable to sperm. But even plain water, the kind you'll be splashing in if you're doing it in the bathtub, can water down the cervical mucus that your partner's sperm count on as they try to hitch that ride to your waiting egg. For best results, save the water play for foreplay—and do your actual baby dancing on dry ground.

For men with a normal sperm count, the latest evidence seems to indicate that more is more. Which means that once-a-day sex during your fertile period is optimal for conception. For men with a low or marginal sperm count, however, sex every other day is probably best because it allows the troops to build up again between deployments.

As for even more, that seems to be less. Making love more than once a day will not only wear out your man (and you, too, most likely), but might actually decrease your chances of getting pregnant. That's because a guy needs time to regenerate his boys, and if he ejaculates more than once a day, he'll be doing so with a depleted number of sperm—which means those encore performances won't be packed, and they could be wasted. Any ejaculation (from masturbation or oral sex, too) has the same effect.

Time of Day

"What's the best time of day to have sex if we're trying to conceive?"

Simply put: There's no better way to start the day than by making love—especially when baby making's on the schedule. Some research has shown that sperm levels are higher in the morning than later in the day. It could be related to your man's cooler testicles (body temperature is at its lowest after sleep, which explains why you take your BBT immediately upon waking), and you already know that cooler testicles make for happier—and more plentiful—sperm. What's more, a guy's hormones peak in the morning—probably why he often wakes up with an erection. So putting that early morning erection to good use may be a smart baby-making move.

Not a morning person—or just can't fit sex into the stressful get-to-work

Hands Off

You've already heard that having sex more than once a day is probably too much of a good thing when you're trying to make a baby. That's because each ejaculation temporarily depletes your sperm count—and those depleted troops need a chance to build up again to give them the best shot at success during Operation Conception. Same applies to taking matters into your own hands (ahem) between TTC sex sessions. Masturbation may never seem like a waste of time, but it is a waste of sperm—at least on days of the month when baby dancing is scheduled. So try making every drop count—stick to once-a-day sex and a hands-off approach until you've hit the baby jackpot.

rush? Don't let the clock stop you from scheduling TTC sex at a more convenient—or appealing—time. Sperm concentration may be higher in the a.m.—but there are still plenty of sperm hanging around after hours, and definitely enough to get the job done 24/7. In fact, other evidence suggests sperm count might be higher in the p.m., specifically during the 3 p.m. to 7 p.m. block. Besides, the best time to make a baby is when you're relaxed, ready to roll, and thoroughly in the mood—not when researchers say it's time to do it.

Oral Sex

"I heard saliva kills sperm. Is oral sex okay while TTC?"

You'd think bodily fluids would all just get along—but it's true, saliva is a sperm killer. Which means you'll probably want to limit the amount of saliva deposited in or near the vagina when you're trying to conceive, and that you'll definitely want to skip the saliva when you're looking for lubrication. Happily, this saliva stipulation doesn't mean oral sex is off the table (or the bed) for now. If you enjoy it, go for it— or tell your partner to go for it. Just keep the slobbering to a minimum. And don't worry about saliva you deposit on his penis when you offer him oral— there probably won't be enough left by the time he ejaculates inside you to harm any sperm.

Vibrators

"Can using a vibrator hurt the chances of conception?"

Your good vibrations can continue even when you're trying for a baby. Having a good time with sex toys of any kind won't keep you from getting pregnant—and in fact, if a session with a vibrator puts you in the mood for the real thing, it can actually help you get pregnant, at least indirectly. As always, just practice proper sex toy hygiene (clean them with soap and water after use, don't share them with others, and so on).

More good news on the vibrator front: While a guy's recreational self-pleasuring may sabotage procreational efforts during fertile days, there are no such restrictions on the number of orgasms you can enjoy while you're TTC.

Douching

"Is it okay to keep douching while I'm trying to get pregnant?"

In trying to tidy up down there, you can actually mess up your fertility plans. The truth is, your body knows how to clean itself naturally, and douching can upset the balance of good bacteria in your vagina, possibly setting you up for infections (and that goes for all the time—whether you're in the market for a baby or not). But that's not the only downside to douching when you're trying to conceive. The drawback conception-wise is that douching can wash away that very important (and fertility-aiding) cervical mucus—something the sperm will miss, even if you don't know it's gone. Douching can also change the

---

Dressing for Fertility Success

Looking for another sign that you're fertile? Take a look in the mirror. Researchers have found that women tend to dress (and primp) to impress when they're ovulating. This is probably nature's way of making sure you— like all the other females in the animal kingdom—attract your mate's attention and are more likely to mate (and make a baby). So next time you find yourself unexpectedly reaching for the clingy sweater with the plunging V-neck or the stilettos that make your man weak in the knees—or suddenly taking more pains with the blow dryer and painting on that pouty red lip and those smoky eyes—consider that it might be just the time of the month to rip those clothes off, rumple your hair, and smudge your makeup.

Gee, You Smell Nice

The smell of love works both ways, it seems. Just as a woman can sniff out her mate's natural sexual scent, pheromones, when ovulation perks up her sense of smell—guys are more likely to respond sexually to a woman who smells like she's about to ovulate. Though you won't be aware that your partner smells different or conscious of this animal-like response to her scent (you'll just know that you feel more like an animal) any more than she'll be aware of the pheromones that are attracting her to you, these subtle signals are among the many that nature transmits when the Egg Train is getting ready to pull out of the station (so your sperm can get ready to hop on board).

---

pH in the vagina, making it even less hospitable to sperm. What's more, if you douche after sex, you can be washing away the sperm—and washing away your odds of conceiving. And if that's not enough reason, women who douche regularly are at a higher risk of developing pelvic inflammatory disease (PID), a leading cause of infertility.

The same drawbacks may apply to homemade douches designed for sex selection (they haven't been proven to work anyway) or so-called natural douches. So bag the douching—and keep it bagged for good while you're at it.

Love that fresh feeling? Take a shower or bath but skip the feminine hygiene sprays and wipes. Not only do you not need them to stay clean, but they, too, can compromise your conception chances.

TTC To-Do:

So what's the plan when you're looking for TTC action? Here's a recap: Sex every day, man on top, on dry land, in the morning, stay put for 20 minutes, no lubricants allowed, simultaneous climaxes. Got it? Good. Now feel free to forget it. Though all those game plans may boost your chances of scoring that baby, they don't make it a slam dunk. You can do everything according to plan and not get pregnant. Or you can break all the TTC baby rules (you have sex when you feel like it, how you feel like it) and still end up making a baby. So bottom line: Go for your bottom lines. Follow the how-tos if you want, skip them if you don't. Approach procreational sex any which way that feels right for you, both physically and emotionally.

Staying Connected While You're TTC

Trying for a baby can be fun, and it can be exciting—but it can also be trying . . . and take a lot of trying. Though all those baby-making efforts may bring you and your partner together physically more often than ever, the emotional connection can sometimes take a hit in the process. But you can nurture your twosome even as you strive to become a threesome—and even fire up some of the romance that charts, ovulation predictor kits, and sex-on-demand may have left out in the cold. Just add a little TLC to your TTC.

Your Relationship

"We're so focused on trying to conceive that I'm afraid our relationship isn't what it used to be."

When you're baby making on all cylinders, it's understandable that you've both got less energy and time to put into romance. And though you're almost certainly having a lot of sex while you're trying to conceive, it's easy to lose sight of the other kind of intimacy that's needed to maintain a healthy twosome—the emotional kind.

But now, when you're striving to form that most perfect union (of sperm and egg), it's more important than ever to pay attention to the other significant union in your life: the one with your partner. These tips will keep your relationship on track even when you're tracking your monthly cycle, tracking your BBT, tracking your cervical mucus, and tracking your sex life.

Stay connected. Sure, your bodies may be connected now (as when the OPK says all systems go), but how about your minds? With all the sex you're having, don't forget about the other kind of intercourse—the talking kind. Stick around for some pillow talk after sex.

TTC Stress Cycle

Have you gotten yourself stuck in the TTC stress cycle? You chart, you have sex, you wait, you test, and you stress. And you stress a little more each month your baby-making efforts end in a period instead of a positive pregnancy test. And then, if that's not stressful enough, you start stressing about whether all the stress over conceiving is making it even harder to conceive.

Many TTC moms who've been at it a while find themselves caught in the same stress cycle, and it's not surprising. After all, deciding to make a baby is exciting, but actually getting that baby on board, especially if the boarding process takes more than a few months, can be, well, stressful.

Though normal amounts of stress don't typically affect fertility, it makes sense to try to break the stress cycle before it starts spinning out of control (and increasing your stress to the kinds of excessive levels that may be implicated in lowered conception rates). For relaxation tips, see page 28.

Date Your Wife

Thought your dating days were over? You may want to think again. Dating your partner regularly is one of the best ways to make sure you stay partners for life—plus, it can help strengthen your twosome as it weathers the emotional and physical challenges of trying to become a threesome. A little rusty on the whole courtship thing? Here's a refresher course on romance:

Surprise her. Most women find surprises pleasing—and romantic. And if your partner has come not to expect any surprises, she'll be even more pleasantly surprised when you spring one on her—whether it's a bouquet of flowers, a reservation at her favorite restaurant, or just a sappy, sweet text or hand-drawn love note taped on the bathroom mirror (or tucked into her handbag, for her to discover later). An occasional surprise will keep her guessing—and keep her loving you more than ever. A little spontaneity will also be a welcome change of pace from all the scheduling you two have likely been doing lately that can quickly make even the most passionate relationship feel routine.

Notice her. When sex becomes procreational instead of recreational, it's easy for the mechanics to become the focus, for romance to leave the building (and the bedroom)—and for both of you to start taking each other for granted. So stop and smell her perfume. Grab her hand just because it's there. Tell her how much you appreciate the view when she bends over to retrieve the keys she dropped. When you're having another session of scheduled sex, let her know how much you love her as your lover and not just as the woman you're trying

to make a mother and who's trying to make you a father.

Date her. Recreate those early days of courtship. Meet her for a latte at the coffee bar you two always hung out at after the movies. Make a reservation at the restaurant where you lingered over your first dinner—and impress her by remembering what she ordered (and if your memory's really good, what she was wearing). Take a drive to see the changing leaves, like you did that first fall—and don't forget the picnic lunch. Hold hands at the movies, when you're at the mall, on the sofa—and whenever her hand is handy. Just because you've moved on to bigger and better things doesn't mean you can't go back to basics (which, by rekindling the romance in your relationship, may actually help heat up those bigger and better things).

Treat her. You already have her love, so you don't have to buy it. But that doesn't mean you can't occasionally do a little relationship reinvestment. Celebrate your baby-making adventure with a commemorative bracelet or necklace, one that you can add charms to as you fill your nest. Or with a scrapbook that you can fill together with the memories you'll be making as you make a baby (ending, soon, with that positive pregnancy test!). Buy her a teddy bear that can one day reside in baby's room. And don't forget that some of the best treats don't cost a thing besides a little effort: Bring her breakfast in bed or a bowl of ice cream with 2 spoons for an after-sex snack. Offer her a foot massage, complete with scented lotions. Or a neck rub while you watch TV.

Is Her Stress Stressing You Out?

Planning a baby is exciting stuff—especially if it's a life event that you've looked forward to your whole lives. But it can also be stressful, particularly when it starts becoming too much like hard work. Between the temperature taking, kits, and apps—and the monthly sex marathon that can make one of your favorite activities feel like a drag—it's no wonder if anxiety is in the air. Though both of you are equally invested in baby making, it's often the woman who becomes a little (or sometimes a lot) more hyper about it. Females tend to excel at micromanaging, as you might have noticed, and sometimes to a fault. If your partner is driving you both a tad crazy these days—and is running Operation Conceive with more flowcharts than

you've ever seen in a conference room and more precision than a military mission—maybe it's time for an intervention. Try explaining that though you both want this baby very much and are both giving this team effort your best efforts, the stress isn't good for either of you or for your fertility chances. And while all of those tools of the modern conception age may help you achieve your most adorable of goals, making them the focus of your daily lives can step up the stress unnecessarily (which can actually get in the way of that goal). For best results, suggest you both jump off the baby-planning roller coaster every now and again and take a moment (or 2 or 3) to appreciate each other—and the amazing ride that's about to begin.

Snuggle on the sofa when TTC sex isn't scheduled (and your phones are off), and share what's on your minds. Take a walk for the workout, but also for the chance to talk, without interruptions. Your mate is the one person in the world who not only knows you best, but knows best what you're going through—because you're going through it together. And don't always stick with the baby talk. Healthy relationships are multidimensional, just like both of you are.

Get out of the bedroom. Maybe you haven't spent this much time in the bedroom since your honeymoon—but even back then you probably took a break in the action every once in a while and ventured out for a swim or a bike ride or a meal. So for a change of pace, schedule something else to do together besides sex, and rediscover the other

side of romance. Splurge on a couples massage. Head out for a romantic dinner—or cook one together, and enjoy it with a side of mood music and minus the phones. Take a nightly stroll around the neighborhood at dusk. Plan a weekly movie night, complete with popcorn. Make a date for a game of miniature golf or bowling—or something else you can't help but have fun doing together.

Get out of town. Treat yourselves to a preconception vacation (once your conception mission is accomplished, traveling won't be quite as carefree). A week at a beach isn't feasible or financially possible? A night in a local hotel (with room service) can also take you away from all that conception stress—even if you'll be baby making during your stay—and remind you both why you're a couple in the first place. That's not in the (credit) cards, either? Improvise economically by staging a romantic stay-cation weekend.

Have a laugh. Making a baby is serious business—sometimes too serious. So loosen up a little. Stream that comedy that was too dumb to pay to see in a movie theater—but is just dumb enough to keep you both rolling off the sofa at home. Play a silly board game that's sure to get you giggling. Challenge each other to a round of bad jokes—or watch some crazy YouTube videos together. And whenever you can, see the humor in the TTC process (there's plenty if you look objectively—like those comical mad dashes to the bedroom) and get a good laugh over it. Laughter isn't only the best medicine for your relationship, but also one of the best ways to relax, which means it may help you with your conception efforts, too.

Making that love connection stronger isn't just important as you try to make a baby. It'll be important once that baby has arrived, too—and maybe more so. Remember, even when you're a couple of parents, you'll still be a couple—and that's ultimately the most important relationship in your life.

Sex-on-Demand

"Sex seems like so much of a chore these days. How can we make it more fun?"

Take this little quiz: Which scenario best describes your love life these days?

A. Candlelight, back rubs, whispers of sweet nothings, leisurely foreplay, satisfying mutual climax.

B. Pee on a stick, shrieks of "it's time," missionary position with shirts still on, wham, bam, thank you, ma'am, drive-thru deposit made in under 3 minutes.

Say Goodbye to Your Tighty Whities

Looking for another way to enhance your fertility? Take a look inside your underwear drawer. Though scientists have yet to rule definitively on the boxers versus briefs debate (at least on the fertility front), the facts so far seem to favor boxers. And it doesn't really take a scientist to figure out why: Boxers allow your testicles to have breathing room, as well as a cooler, sperm-friendly environment to hang out in. Briefs (or boxer briefs, or bikini briefs) keep the scrotum pushed up against your body, where your boys can become overheated, potentially lowering sperm count and quality. Same goes, too, for those spandex shorts you may wear to work out or bike in.

How much of a difference does your underwear choice make on your fertility chances? Probably not that much. For a guy with a normal sperm count, wearing briefs won't push fertility over a cliff, or even over the edge—though if you're open to pulling a switch, it definitely couldn't hurt. If you're a brief-wearer with a sperm count on the lower side, converting to boxers is probably a smart move, experts say. Worried your briefs history might have already taken its fertility toll? The good news is that any potential harm your sperm count may have experienced in those tight white quarters will resolve after just a couple of months of breathing freely in boxers.

If you answered "B," chances are you've stumbled—or fallen headfirst—into the sex-on-demand rut that many hopeful parents-to-be find themselves stuck in when sex becomes a means toward an end (a baby) instead of a means toward a "happy ending." All work and no play makes any sexual relationship—even one that used to be all fun, all the time—dull. So it's not surprising that sex these days is more about getting it done than getting it on. After all, how sexy is temperature charting? How mood making is a beeping ovulation monitor? And who can get worked up over watching a fertility watch?

The good news is that trying to score (a baby) doesn't have to feel like a chore—even when OPKs line the bathroom counter and you're stretching cervical mucus between your fingertips. Here's how to keep the sparks flying even as you try to put a bun in the oven:

Get him thinking (of you). Leave love notes on his pillow or hide them in places where he'll find them throughout the day—in his car, with his laptop, in his underwear drawer. Write him suggestive text messages or Snapchat him alluring pictures to whet his appetite for tonight's special (you). Tell him what you'll be wearing, and what you won't be wearing. Tell him what you'll be doing to him, and what you'll want him to do to you. Anticipation always adds sexual tension (the good kind of tension) to a lovemaking session—even if it's a fully scheduled one. And if you've never tried naughty on for size, don't knock it until you've tried it.

Rev up the romance. You know the drill, but it's probably been a while since you practiced those romantic moves that used to be lovemaking business as usual. Take a bath together, light scented candles, bring out the massage oil, play some soft music, dip some strawberries in chocolate (oh heck, just dip each other in chocolate) . . . you get the picture.

Turn up the heat. Debut a new piece of sexy lingerie each month. Play strip poker or nude Twister or an R-rated board game. Press play on an erotic movie or unveil a sex toy. Bring on the whipped cream for a different kind of dessert. Get kinky to your comfort level, of course, but if there was ever a time to push the sexual envelope, now would be it.

Don't just do it. Yes, you're goal oriented these days. But you can reach that goal and still have fun along the way. So don't just do it—take your time doing it. Serve up some foreplay appetizers before you dive into the main course. Try for a slow build to increase tension and make the ultimate climax more explosive. Mind you, sometimes a quickie can be just as explosive—especially if plenty of groping under clothes is involved—and on a particularly busy day, it may be the only way to get the job done (you have 15 minutes to do it, change, and get to a client dinner). Just try, as you go about reaching that all-important goal you're so understandably focused on, not to forget the other goal in all this: mutually satisfying sex and intimacy.

Change the scenery. You've likely been spending a whole lot of time in bed these days. But guess what—babies can be made in other locations, too. In a car. On the kitchen table. Even in the laundry room (talk about a spin cycle). And don't just assume your positions, either, without some thought to the pleasure component. Nothing says rut like the same-old, same-old—so spice things up with a brand new *Cosmo*-worthy move or two.

Talk him up. At times you may be feeling like a sperm receptacle, which is understandable. But keep in mind that he may be feeling like nothing more

TTC: To Tell or Not to Tell

Hoping to start a family soon, or add to it—but not quite sure when (or whether) to alert the social media (as well as the mother and mother-in-law)? Do you tell as soon as you begin making the plans? Wait until your efforts are fully under way? Or keep your mission a secret until it's a mission accomplished?

If you're already being bombarded with questions about that baby-making barometer at each and every family gathering, not to mention on each and every call from the folks (and your sister, and your great-aunt, and your friends), then you may be tempted to tell all about your plans, just to get everyone (and your mother) off your back. You may be inclined to share the news, also, if you're feeling like you need a little TTC support or cheerleading—or if you're just too excited to stay mum about your plans to become a mom (and a dad).

You might want to think it through before you spill the TTC beans too soon. That cheerleading squad may be nice—as can having Mom's number on your favorites list when you need a preconception pep talk—but will you really want to deal with that monthly deluge of questions from friends and family? And all that advice? Those comments you could definitely do without ("You're just trying too hard" or "You're not getting any younger!")? The added pressure of offering up pregnancy test results to a long list of well-wishers eager to hear the monthly update?

Don't feel obligated to tell if you're afraid that spilling those beans will open up too many cans of worms. In the meantime, try to field those inevitable questions about your future plans to start your family with a sense of humor. "You'll be the first to know" is sure to get you off the hook (who can argue with that?).

On the other hand, if you decide you're happy to make the whole gang part of your pregnancy planning, go right ahead—after all, you know yourself and your family and your social media network better than anyone. And if the barrage of unsolicited advice you'll inevitably receive on how to become pregnant makes you second-guess your decision, you may want to arm yourself with this one-size-fits-all comeback: "Thanks, but we actually know how to get pregnant."

than a sperm provider, which is equally understandable. Remember, too, that he's the one who's under all that performance pressure, to rise to the occasion at the beep of a fertility monitor. So make sure you let him know how much you love him and appreciate him (and find him stud-like when he's not performing those services), even as you're asking him to hop into bed for yet another round of fertilize-my-egg.

Get physical. Even when it's not ovulation time, stay in tune by touching each other often, swooping down for unexpected kisses, catching each other for hugs, cuddling whenever you can, and yes—making love at other times of the month, too . . . just for the fun of it.

Take a break. Not from the pleasures of lovemaking, but from the stress of baby making. Remember that sex isn't only about getting pregnant (though it may seem that way these days). There's

You're Up ... Again

Feeling a little like a performing chimp lately (or maybe like a performing Chippendale)? That's not surprising if you've been TTC. After all, while the logistics of planning those baby-making sex sessions to coordinate with ovulation may be your partner's department, the sole responsibility for getting the deed done falls on your shoulders (or on, let's just say, another part of your body). Even if you're performing your favorite activity ever, being asked to perform it at a moment's notice, at inconvenient times (half an hour before you have to be at work, or after an extra-long day), and when you're not even remotely in the mood—can be a drag, and sometimes a stressful drag, one that can even make performance elusive.

You're not alone. Just about every guy who's in the thick of TTC experiences performance anxiety—or performance dread—at some point, and that's nothing if not understandable.

You're only human (as opposed to the studs in the rest of the animal kingdom, who don't give performance a second thought). But that doesn't mean you have to keep your feelings to yourself—and in fact, you shouldn't. Let your spouse know that the sex scheduling is getting you down—and maybe, keeping you down when you'd rather not be. Suggest that you try adding a little spice to the sex-on-demand schedule, even if spontaneity isn't practical. You'll see plenty of tips on how to keep TTC sex exciting—and fun—on these pages. Thinking of giving that little blue pill a try, to give you a little extra boost on those down days? Ask your doctor for the lowdown on using Viagra or Cialis when you're TTC.

Not having a hard time, so to speak, with all the sexual demands being placed on you these days (and nights)? Having the time of your life, actually? That's normal, too. So just sit back—or lie back—and enjoy the show.

also an important emotional connection that's involved, one that often gets neglected when the mechanics of conception get in the way. If you're finding that the CM stretching and BBT charting is taking its toll on your relationship and on your quality of life, ditch it and let nature take its course. Not only can taking a break from all those gadgets and charts help you reconnect as a couple, but it can help you relax about conceiving (and remember, the more relaxed you are about it, the more likely it is to happen). Consider this: Studies show that the average unstressed couple has sex 2 to 3 times per week. If you're on that type of schedule, chances are nature will work pretty well on its own and you'll likely get pregnant within 6 to 12 months (and maybe a whole lot sooner) even without "working" at it. So take a break from TTC, and who knows—you might find you've conceived without even trying!

Getting Pregnant with CAM

There's nothing more natural than making a baby—so what could be a more natural way to boost your fertility than tapping into the CAM camp? Complementary and alternative therapies—from acupuncture to hypnosis to herbal medicine—are being used more and more often to give Mother Nature (and sometimes medical science) a nudge. Whether that nudge works hasn't been demonstrated consistently through research, and a lot more research will have to be done before any conclusions can be drawn. Still, here's what's known so far about so-called natural fertility boosters.

CAM for Fertility

"My friend says using acupuncture helped her conceive when she was undergoing IVF. Is there any truth to that?"

Can a little bit of CAM go a long way in your fertility quest? It's possible. Though the modern study of these therapies—which are rooted in ancient practices—is still in its infancy, more and more research seems to be showing that they do have applications to successful baby making. In fact, some studies suggest that adding acupuncture and/or other mind-body techniques to infertility treatments may increase your chances of getting pregnant (though other studies don't show a benefit). By extension, proponents say, the therapies may also help speed the conception process in a woman without known fertility issues.

Long respected in Eastern medicine, alternative treatments have gained increasing popularity in the West for a variety of illnesses and conditions. More and more often, these treatments are being integrated into traditional medical care, in the form of CAM.

East is meeting West, as well, when it comes to fertility—and some preliminary feedback has been promising. A few published studies have shown that acupuncture may help a variety of fertility issues at almost every age and promotes reproductive health in general (though technically, there's no scientific consensus on how much, or even if, acupuncture really helps). Acupuncturists contend that the technique increases nerve stimulation and blood flow to the ovaries and uterus, improving reproductive function. What's more, acupuncture may increase the production of feel-good endorphins that also play a role in regulating your menstrual cycle and, therefore, your fertility. Acupuncture may ease fertility-busting stress, too.

Some evidence indicates that chiropractic techniques can also help the fertility cause in certain women. Chiropractors hold that if the nerves going to your reproductive organs are impaired, fertility can be impaired as well. Manipulation of the spinal column and nerves in those areas may restore balance and, possibly with it, fertility.

Hypnosis and hypnotherapy may also boost fertility, particularly in cases when the mind (often a stressed one) is interfering with the body's normal reproductive functions. Some CAM practitioners say that the reduction in stress and the relaxing benefit of hypnosis can even aid in embryo implantation, resulting in an increased rate of pregnancies among women who practiced hypnosis while undergoing fertility treatments.

A few less obvious examples of mind-body techniques are proving

Cough It Up to Some Medicine

Could cough syrup actually be good medicine for fertility? While no scientific studies have backed up the anecdotal evidence, some women aren't sneezing at it. Here's how an expectorant, theoretically, can help you expect:

The active ingredient in cough medicines (like Robitussin and Mucinex) is guaifenesin, a substance that helps thin the mucus in your lungs—helping to decrease coughing. But it doesn't differentiate between the mucus in one part of your body (in your lungs) and the mucus in another. Which means that guaifenesin also thins cervical mucus, possibly allowing sperm to move through it faster and better, and potentially making it easier to hit their target on time.

Willing to do your own clinical trial? Take 1 to 2 teaspoons of Robitussin or the equivalent dose of Mucinex Expectorant tablets once a day beginning a few days before ovulation. One major caveat: Read labels carefully before purchasing your cough syrup or before pulling it out of your medicine cabinet, and make sure the only active ingredient is guaifenesin. Not all cough medicines are alike—and some contain antihistamines, which can actually have an anti-fertility effect by drying up that sperm-friendly mucus.

to be effective as well. For example, emotionally connecting with others is a powerful component when it comes to getting pregnant, and researchers have found an increase in pregnancy rates for infertile women who take part in support groups (another reason to check out those WhatToExpect.com TTC message boards). Other mind-body strategies include diet changes, movement, meditation, relaxation, yoga, and visualization.

It's still unclear if these documented fertility improvements are the result of the actual CAM technique being used or a placebo effect (and if they work, does it really matter why?). Still, most experts agree that as long as the CAM techniques do no harm, there's no harm in trying them—and there could be many benefits, especially if the therapies make you feel less stressed and more empowered. If you do decide to incorporate these and other alternative techniques in your baby-making mission, take the safe route. First, make sure any CAM practitioner you engage is qualified and experienced and specializes in women's health and fertility. You can visit the American Association of Acupuncture and Oriental Medicine (aaaomonline.org) to find an acupuncturist in your area. Other resources include the American Physical Therapy Association (apta.org), the National Center for Complementary and Integrative Health (nccih.nih.gov), the Center for Mind/Body Medicine (cmbm.org), and the Academy of Integrative Health & Medicine (aihm.org).

Second, be sure to remember the "C" in CAM: complementary. For CAM to be a valuable part of any medical care, it needs to be integrated into your traditional care. So let your traditional doctor know about any CAM techniques you might be using or considering, because some therapies could interact with each other negatively,

CAM for Men

CAM isn't just for women looking to get a leg up on fertility. Acupuncture practitioners say that CAM treatment reduces the number of abnormal sperm and increases the number of healthy sperm in men with a low sperm count. It can also be used to pump up blood flow, which may definitely help pump up something else. Mind-body strategies, including hypnosis, massage, relaxation, yoga, and visualization, can reduce stress and promote healthy blood flow—important components of a healthy libido, which in turn is an important component of making a baby.

making your goal of conception more elusive. And if you're having fertility issues, don't rely on CAM alone to find your way out of them—also seek the help of a doctor who can diagnose and treat any reproductive problem.

Thinking Positive

"I've heard that it's possible to boost fertility just by thinking positive. Is there any truth to that?"

The power of positive thinking may be more powerful than you think when it comes to scoring that positive pregnancy test. Really—your ability to conceive could actually be impacted by your thoughts and feelings. Not directly, of course (as in "If I just wish it hard enough, I'll get pregnant"), but indirectly. It is becoming more recognized that physical health, including reproductive health, is related to emotional health. A negative state of mind (as is common with excessive stress, depression, or even just being really pessimistic) can have a negative effect on hormone levels and fertility. Experts well versed in this mind-body theory suggest that you can boost your fertility by boosting your emotional wellbeing. You may even benefit from an emotional boost if you learn that your fertility challenges have a clearly physical cause—in fact, it may make other forms of treatment more effective. Managing stress, depression, anxiety, and other emotional challenges through yoga, meditation, acupuncture, visualization, and relaxation exercises, according to these researchers, may indeed help give your fertility a boost—and bring you one step closer to the baby you're hoping for.

Will trading in a Debbie Downer attitude for a Pollyanna approach definitely make your baby dreams come true? As powerful as positive thinking can be, it's also important to be mindful of the mind's limitations. If stress is interfering with your fertility, thinking happy baby thoughts may be just what the doctor ordered—without the doctor. But if it's another fertility issue that's standing between you and conception, seeking medical help—while continuing to think those happy baby thoughts—is always a smart strategy. For more on the stress-conception connection and stress relief, see page 28.

Herbs and Fertility

"I take herbals daily, just for overall health. Are any unsafe now that I'm trying to conceive? And are there any herbs I can take to increase my chances of getting pregnant?"

That depends who you listen to. According to some holistic practitioners, certain herbs can give your

Supplementing Fertility

It seems as if everyone's hopping on the supplement bandwagon these days, including guys who are hoping that hopping will help make them a pop. But what can herbals and other supplements really do for your fertility? The scientific jury is still out on that. A small study showed that Pycnogenol can boost male fertility. L-carnitine and arginine are said to promote good sperm motility and sperm count. Ginseng is a classic Chinese aphrodisiac and, according to classic Chinese medicine practitioners, also a fertility booster, upping testosterone levels and increasing sperm count. Astragalus may increase sperm motility, and lycopene may increase sperm count.

On the fertility flip side, however, large amounts of St. John's wort can negatively affect the genetic makeup of sperm, echinacea can change the composition of the sperm head (making it less able to penetrate an egg), and ginkgo biloba can have a detrimental effect on sperm health. Ditto, possibly, for other herbs. Which means that before you pop a supplement, ask your doctor (one who knows you and your partner are trying to conceive) whether it's safe and what the risks may be. That goes even for supplements you've been taking forever. One exception: omega-3 fatty acids. Since an omega-3 deficiency could be linked to lowered sperm production, getting your fair share of this fabulous fat—whether from food or in supplement form—can possibly boost your fertility.

reproductive efforts an edge. For example, black cohosh is touted as a way to establish regular ovulation and thicken the uterine lining. Siberian ginseng and dong quai are said to help regulate the menstrual cycle. Chaste tree berry is said to stimulate the release of LH and regulate the levels of progesterone and estrogen. Red clover blossom is rich in estrogen-like isoflavones and might be helpful in regulating hormones and readying the uterine lining for a pregnancy. Stinging nettle tea is supposed to nourish and tone your uterus.

Sounds promising, huh? The only problem is, when it comes to most herbal supplements, it's hard to know how effective, or how safe, they are—especially when it comes to fertility. Here's why: First, the FDA does not evaluate herbal supplements the way it does prescription and over-the-counter medications, so the safety and risks associated with them aren't scientifically established. Neither is effectiveness, which means a promising claim on the supplement bottle is just that—a promising claim (one that hasn't been proven). Second, there's still a significant shortage of clinical studies on these supplements—especially when it comes to reproductive matters. So it's not clear whether they help fertility, have no effect on fertility, or may even compromise fertility. Another reason to proceed with care: regulations in the United States don't govern the manufacturing and selling of herbal products, so there's no way of knowing whether you're actually getting what you think you're getting—or what you're paying top dollar for (though products from Germany, Poland, Austria, and the United Kingdom are regulated and therefore may be more reliable). Further complicating the supplement equation: Some herbals (including some of those purported to promote fertility) are considered unsafe during pregnancy—which means that taking them while you're TTC could put your baby at risk if you do end up conceiving.

The bottom line when you're trying to create that very cute bottom line: Though herbs are natural, natural doesn't always mean safe. As with any medicine, herbs should be taken only under the supervision of your doctor and/or an alternative-medicine practitioner who knows you're trying to become pregnant. Not only to find out if they're safe, but also because some herbals may interfere with other medications, fertility boosters, or treatments you're already using. Also keep in mind that different people can react very differently to herbs, so even though your sister-in-law swears her herbal concoction put a baby bun in her oven practically overnight, that same potion might not work for you (and besides, she might have gotten pregnant even without taking the herbs—that's what makes anecdotal evidence so unreliable). So ask before you pop. And until more is known, you'll probably want to be cautious with supplements in general—just to stay on the safe side.

One CAM supplement—albeit not technically an herbal—you can feel good about taking: omega-3s. Whether these phenomenal fatty acids can boost your fertility is still open to debate (and further scientific investigation), but

Baby Help from a Box?

Been trying for a few months to hit baby bingo without success? No need to panic. Remember that the average couple conceives within 6 to 12 months of trying, so you probably need to give baby making a little more time. Not a patient waiter? You may find the help you're looking for in a box. Couples eager to conceive ASAP can turn to conception kits (some needing a doctor's prescription) that aim to bring you one step closer to a baby without going that extra mile to the fertility specialist's office.

The product premise is pretty basic: By concentrating your partner's sperm as close as possible to your cervix, you'll boost the chances of conceiving. Here's how it works: The kits contain nonlatex condoms that don't contain spermicide (for obvious reasons) that are used during intercourse to collect semen from an ejaculation. There is also a cervical cap into which the collected semen is transferred (though some conception kits don't require the transfer step since the condom itself is attached to the cap). The cervical cap is then placed (either by hand or with the special tampon-like applicator, depending on the kit you're using) into the vagina and onto the cervix for 6 to 8 hours—allowing the sperm to bypass the vagina and head right into the cervix sooner and in a more concentrated form.

These kits aren't cheap, and though there's no harm in using them, they're definitely not necessary for most fertile couples, who can conceive the time-honored (and arguably more fun) way. They also aren't helpful for couples who have more complex fertility challenges. Those with the most potential to gain from spoon-feeding sperm into the cervix could be those who are dealing with a diagnosed low sperm count, since the cervical cap can get the boys closer to where they need to go.

there is evidence they may help lift your mood—a lift that could give your fertility a leg up. Plus, they offer plenty of other potential health benefits—particularly once you're pregnant (they're super baby friendly).

Wondering about the supplements you take for general wellness (without ever giving them a second thought)? Like that echinacea you pop to ward off a winter cold, the ginkgo biloba you swallow to give your brain a boost, or that St. John's wort you take to turn your frown upside down? These, among many others, may interfere with conception in both hopeful moms and hopeful dads. Another good reason to think twice (once for yourself, once for the baby you're hoping to make) before taking any supplement—and to review all medications with your practitioner before you TTC.

Making a Baby Boy—or a Baby Girl

Pink or blue? Of course, either will do—as long as that baby of your dreams is healthy. But what if you could choose your baby's sex even before you've conceived that sweet bundle of (girl or boy) joy? The concept of sex selection may be extra tempting if you're hoping to add a blue member to your predominantly pink team or a pink member to your gang of blue—or if you've always had your heart set on starting your family with a baby of one gender or the other.

But do do-it-yourself sex selection methods you've read about and heard about really work? Can they influence those time-honored 50-50 odds in favor of a preferred gender? Maybe . . . but probably not. Still, in most cases there's no harm in giving them a shot—as long as you don't count on the results, and just have fun trying.

Choosing the Baby's Gender

"Is it possible to choose the sex of my baby? We already have 2 boys, and we'd love a baby girl."

Thinking pink? Eat lots of veggies and pile on the chocolate (and perhaps the pounds?). Make sure the moon is full when you conceive, and take the sexual lead. Have sex only on a certain day of the month based on calculations involving the calendar and your birthday. Rooting for the blue team? Have sex lying on your right side, be sure there's a quarter moon, and eat lots of red meat.

There's no shortage of far-fetched methods promising to deliver you the baby of your gender dreams—and you can access dozens without consulting a single old wife (your favorite search engine is loaded with them). The only thing is, they work just 50 percent of the time—giving you the same 50-50 odds of having a girl (or a boy) that you'd have if you left the selection of your baby's sex up to nature (and your partner's sperm).

Not thrilled with those odds? Hoping to give sex selection an edge, even if it's just a slight nudge in the direction of your choice? Old wives' tales and internet legends aside, a number of low-tech techniques claim to up the odds of conceiving one or the other

Pick Your Food, Pick Your Baby's Sex?

Can the food you eat affect the sex of your soon-to-be-conceived baby? There's plenty of conjecture (and message board rumors) to answer that question. You may have heard, for instance, that eating a diet rich in calcium and magnesium and cutting back on red meat and salty food will increase the odds of conceiving a girl. Or that eating foods rich in sodium and potassium will up your chances of making a boy. Some salt with that banana?

But is there any grain of truth to these theories? That's still unclear. Some research has pointed to a possible link between a baby's sex and a mom's diet around the time of conception—with one controversial study even suggesting that eating your Wheaties (or your Cheerios, or any other cereal) may increase your chances of conceiving a boy. Ditto for a diet high in energy foods (aka high-calorie foods) and in such nutrients as potassium, calcium, and vitamins C, E, and B$_{12}$.

Does that mean you should switch from yogurt to Special K if you'd especially like a boy—or quit cold cereal cold turkey if it's a girl you're hoping for? Should you increase your calorie consumption around conception time if your heart's set on a baby boy, or cut back if sugar and spice would be nice? Not so fast. First, it's not smart to increase or decrease your caloric intake when you're trying to conceive unless your practitioner has specifically advised you to do so (to gain or lose weight preconception)—or to restrict nutrients by eating only certain foods and avoiding others. Second, this research is definitely not conclusive—and in no way promises that a change in diet can help you choose your baby's sex. In fact, the boy-to-girl proportion of babies born in the overall sample studied by these researchers was about 50-50—pretty much the same as would be expected without any diet modifications. Food for thought, but not necessarily for breakfast.

gender, but have no scientific evidence to back up their claims. A few high-tech (and expensive) sex-selection methods are more likely to work but involve assisted reproduction, and are consequently not available to every couple.

First, the do-it-yourself techniques. Try these at home, if you're so inclined, keeping in mind that all 3 recommend completely different approaches, often conflicting—and none has been proved to work the way it claims:

The Shettles Method. This theory holds that the Y-sperm (boys) are faster swimmers yet don't live as long and are not as strong as the X-sperm (girls). Because of the resiliency of X-sperm, female babies are more often conceived in less

ideal conditions, such as when there is a lower sperm count or when the sperm are kept waiting a long time for the egg to be released (and only the fittest—and most resilient—are still surviving when the egg finally shows up). On the other hand, males are more often conceived when conditions for fertilization are ideal because, as the faster swimmers, they will win the race to the finish.

To up the odds you'll conceive a girl, according to the Shettles method:

- Have lots of sex starting 3 days before ovulation (more frequent ejaculations mean fewer Y-sperm, and the longer sperm wait for the egg, the better the odds that the stronger X-sperm will be the last women standing).

And They Say Girls Keep You Waiting

Laugh all you want at this twist—but interestingly, the longer it takes you to conceive, the greater your chances that a baby boy will show up. How do researchers explain these late-breaking boys? First a basic fact: Y-sperm (male) sperm swim faster in thick cervical mucus, while X-sperm (female) swim faster in thinner mucus. Another fact: Women with thick cervical mucus have a harder time conceiving in general, so it takes them longer to get pregnant. Put these 2 factors together, and it makes sense that women who take a while to conceive because of their thicker cervical mucus are also somewhat more likely to end up playing on Team Blue.

- Use the missionary position.

- Avoid female orgasm, which will only help the weaker male sperm along. (Clearly, this involves some sacrifice on the part of the female partner—how's that for a touch of irony?)

If you're trying for a boy, take the opposite approach:

- Avoid intercourse until the day of ovulation (this way the faster-swimming boy sperm won't be kept waiting for the egg—and will, hopefully, race their way to the finish line faster).

- Achieve female orgasm (to help propel those less hardy boys to the egg and to improve the alkalinity of the vagina).

- Use the rear-entry position.

- Have the male partner drink something caffeinated an hour before sex (to speed up his boy-making boys).

The Whelan Method. This method contradicts the Shettles Method completely (go figure). According to this theory, the closer to ovulation you have sex, the more likely you are to conceive a girl. That's because of certain biochemical changes that could favor Y-sperm the earlier you are in your cycle. Therefore, if you want a boy, have sex 4 to 6 days before ovulation, and if you want a girl, have sex only when you're ovulating.

The O + 12 Method. This method claims to up the chances for conceiving a girl by having sex 12 hours after ovulation (hence the name of the method: ovulation plus 12 hours). Contrary to the Shettles technique, this method requires waiting to have sex until 8 to 12 hours after ovulation—and then to have sex only once.

Getting a lot more high tech, pricey (very, in some cases), and invasive (and leaving it up to the pros) are these options:

The Ericsson Method. This in-the-lab technique separates the faster-swimming boy sperm from the slower-swimming girl sperm. The method relies on the theory that the faster Y-sperm will be able to swim through a solution and reach the bottom of a test tube faster than the X-sperm, allowing the 2 types of sperm to be separated. Once the X- and Y- sperm are separated, the desired gender is introduced via intrauterine insemination (IUI). There is no guarantee of success (the odds of conceiving the gender of choice using this method range from 50 to 80 percent), and many say this technique has not been shown to work reliably at all.

The Microsort Method. This high-tech (and costly) method also separates the X- and Y-sperm in the lab. Though not foolproof, the technique seems to work because Y-sperm contain less DNA than X-sperm, making them a bit smaller and lighter, and allowing the male-producers and female-producers to be sorted. It appears to be more successful in producing a girl than a boy.

Preimplantation Genetic Diagnosis (PGD) or Screening (PGS). This procedure, which is also used to screen embryos for genetic defects, is an effective sex-selection method—but one that's typically reserved for couples who have a medical reason to choose their baby's sex (when there's a genetic condition that's X-linked recessive, for instance, such as hemophilia or fragile X syndrome, that is inherited by sons, but not daughters). Using embryos conceived via IVF, doctors determine the sex of each, implanting only the embryos with the gender of choice. While some centers do offer PGD/PGS to any couple who chooses it, especially if a couple is already using IVF for infertility issues, it sometimes comes with parameters, such as only if the couple already has at least one child of the opposite sex they're trying for. However, most experts maintain that using it for nonmedical reasons is ethically problematic and should be discouraged.

Sex-Selection Kits

"I already have a girl and would really like a boy. A friend of mine mentioned something about sex-selection kits. What's the deal with them?"

You've seen them advertised, you've heard other TTC couples chatting them up, and you've probably wondered: Do these do-it-yourself sex-selection kits really work? Do those gender vendors have any scientific leg to stand on—or are they just peddling false hope at inflated prices to those thinking pink or blue?

Sex-selection kits claim to improve your odds of conceiving the gender of your choice by using nutritional supplements and herbal extracts that allegedly alter the conditions around the egg and sperm, vaginal pH testing, and douches that supposedly make the vaginal tract receptive to one or the other sex-specific sperm. Most experts consider these claims to be scientifically suspect, especially since there's a 50 percent chance that you'll get the gender of your choice without doing anything at all. In other words, buyer beware—or at least be aware. (Also, wise to be aware of the potential risks of douching; see page 122 for more.)

CHAPTER 8

Are You Pregnant?

You've charted, you've checked your cervical mucus, you've had sex at all the appropriate times and in all the recommended ways. And now you're wondering: Were those TTC efforts successful? Has our conception mission been accomplished? Did we score that fertilized egg? Hit the baby jackpot? Could I be pregnant? Sure, you can just wait until you expect your period to take a home pregnancy test and find out for certain. But what if you're not the waiting type? Read on for the very early pregnancy scoop.

Early Pregnancy Signs—or Are They?

Is this month *the* month? Or is it just that time of the month—again? Are those early pregnancy signs—or early PMS signs? Or just your imagination gone baby wild? Unless you've produced that positive pregnancy test, you won't have proof positive. But it doesn't hurt to wonder . . . does it?

Tender Breasts

"My breasts feel achy on the sides. It's sort of what I feel right before I get my period. Could I be pregnant—or is it just PMS?"

Breasts are often the first body part to get the message when sperm meets egg, at least the first part noticeable to you. Their response to the big news varies from woman to woman, but newly pregnant breasts can be tender, full, achy, swollen, tingly, sensitive, and even painful to the touch. Sometimes these signs show up within a few days of conception, sometimes they hold off until weeks later. Sometimes the changes are over the top (and have you quickly coming out of your tops), and sometimes they're more subtle (especially if they come on gradually instead of seemingly overnight).

There's just one little catch. As you're already figuring out, early pregnancy breasts are not all that different from PMS breasts—except that breast changes caused by pregnancy hormones stick around instead of disappearing with the arrival of your period. Problem for you—and lots of other hopeful TTC moms—is that until your period begins (or doesn't), it's really tough to tell these 2 types of breast changes apart. The puzzle is even harder still to solve in women whose breasts normally change a lot premenstrually, since these same women are more likely to experience pronounced breast changes with pregnancy.

Confused? Frustrated? Eager for a sign that you can actually take to the baby bank? Well, here's one to look out for: changes in your areolas (the circles around your nipples). Early pregnancy hormones can cause the areola to darken in color and increase in diameter somewhat in the weeks after conception—though, again, that timetable can vary a great deal. You may also notice, as those hormones kick in, an increase and enlargement in the tiny bumps on the areola (they'll resemble goose bumps). Those bumps are actually glands that produce oils to lubricate your nipples and areolas in preparation for lactation (talk about planning ahead!). These areola alterations will appear only if you're pregnant, not if you're PMS-ing. However, because every mom-to-be experiences these changes to a different extent and also at different times (some will notice obvious changes almost immediately, others won't notice any at all until much later), not seeing these differences in your areolas now doesn't mean baby isn't already on board—just that you might have to wait until that passenger list is officially confirmed by a pregnancy test.

Implantation Spotting

"I'm TTC, and though it's a week before I'm due to get my period, I'm noticing some pinkish discharge when I wipe. Is my cycle messed up?"

The spotting you're noticing could actually be the positive sign you're looking for—or, at least, a prelude to the positive sign you're hoping to see on that as yet unopened pregnancy test. A significant minority of newly expectant moms (around 20 to 30 percent) notice scant spotting when an embryo burrows its way into the uterine wall. Such so-called implantation bleeding will likely arrive earlier than your expected monthly flow—usually around 6 to 12 days after conception. Much lighter than your period (it'll be spotty, not continuous bleeding) and lasting anywhere from a few hours to a few days, implantation bleeding is usually pale to medium pink or light brown in color—sometimes merely pink-tinged mucus. It's rarely red, like a period.

Don't have any spotting at all? Remember, implantation bleeding is the exception, rather than the rule. The majority of moms-to-be (70 to 80 percent) do not have any spotting when an embryo implants, which means you definitely don't have to spot to be expecting.

On the other hand, not all preperiod spotting is related to implantation or a sign that you're expecting—and this can lead to frustration. Women with irregular cycles (or cycles that are disrupted in a particular month for whatever reason) may assume that the pink they're seeing on their panties or on the toilet paper is implantation bleeding, only to find later that it's a midcycle blip or a harbinger of that monthly visitor coming a little earlier than expected. Adding to the frustration is the fact that home pregnancy tests (HPTs) may not be able to produce a reliable result this early (though if the result is positive, you can be positive, too—if it's negative, you can't consider it definitive yet). If your spotting does end up being implantation bleeding and a pregnancy test confirms your happy news—congratulations. If the spotting turns to bleeding, and ultimately ends up being your period, don't be discouraged. Next month might be the one that's marked for success—so try, try again.

Urinary Frequency

"All of a sudden, I feel like I have to pee all the time. Could it mean I'm pregnant?"

Feel like you're peeing for two? It's possible you are. The need to pee with annoying frequency can appear on the pregnancy scene fairly early—usually about 2 to 3 weeks after conception. That's because pregnant kidneys must work overtime (keeping moms-to-be on the toilet overtime) to filter waste from the blood once there's an extra waste producer on board. What's more, even a just-pregnant uterus has begun to grow, and because it's still low in the pelvic cavity, it presses squarely on the bladder, triggering that gotta-go feeling. Also sending an expectant mom to the bathroom more often: those pregnancy hormones, most predominantly, progesterone.

The best way to find out if all this peeing is a sign of pregnancy is to pee—on a home pregnancy test. Since this symptom typically appears right about the same time reliable results can be expected on an HPT, this purposeful peeing should give you your answer. And weren't you on the way to the bathroom again anyway?

If it turns out you aren't pregnant—and retesting confirms this—the need to pee frequently could be a sign that either you've been increasing your fluid intake (which is fine) or that you may have a urinary tract infection (which isn't so fine, and needs to be treated). Check in with your practitioner to find out for sure, especially if it burns or hurts when you're urinating.

Not peeing up a storm? That doesn't mean there isn't a baby brewing. It could just mean this particular symptom hasn't kicked in yet or won't be kicking in at all. After all, the first rule of pregnancy is that every pregnant woman is different—so no pregnancy symptom is experienced universally or at the same time by all pregnant women. Test when the time is right to find out for sure.

Elevated BBT

"I've been tracking my BBT and noticed the expected temperature rise right after ovulation (luckily we had sex the day before)—but it hasn't come down, like it usually does. What's going on?"

If you've been tracking your first morning temperature for a few months, you're probably pretty familiar with your BBT ups and downs. As you've noticed, your BBT shifts upward right after ovulation, thanks to the increase in progesterone. Your temps will drop back down again when you get your period, thanks to the dropping levels of progesterone. But if you've conceived, there is no drop in progesterone (in fact, elevated progesterone is what keeps a new pregnancy going)—and that means there is no drop in your BBT. So if you notice 18 or more consecutive days of elevated BBT, there's a pretty good chance you're already hosting a baby. And if for some reason you were to continue taking your BBT each morning during your pregnancy (though there's definitely no need to do that, unless you've become really attached to that thermometer), you'd see those increased progesterone levels keeping your temperature up throughout your pregnancy.

Does a persistently elevated temperature provide proof positive that you're expecting? Not exactly—you'll also need a positive pregnancy test to positively confirm your happy news. There are other, far less common explanations for a continued elevated temperature (such as an ovarian cyst), so if you don't see a drop in your temps, and if you don't get your period, yet all your pregnancy tests come out negative, put in a call to your practitioner to find out what's going on. It's definitely still possible that you're pregnant. Sometimes it's just too early to call on an HPT, especially if you've been testing before your period was expected, but it's always a good idea to check out the situation.

Other Pregnancy Symptoms

"I'm TTC and wondering if I'm pregnant, but it's too early to take a pregnancy test. Are there any other symptoms—besides breast and temperature changes—I can look for to know for sure?"

The only way to be positively sure that you're positively pregnant this early on is to get a positive result on a pregnancy test—and that may be impossible to secure just yet, depending on how early you're testing and how sensitive the test is. While you're waiting for testing day to dawn—and that waiting can be tough—you can be on the lookout for any early pregnancy clues your body may be sending (such as those tender breasts or that perpetual peeing). Unfortunately, those clues

(plus the ones listed here) can also point to unrelated conditions (most notably PMS, but stress or a stomach bug are among the other possibilities). Still, experiencing any of these symptoms may be just the excuse you need to run to the store for an HPT:

Fatigue. Too pooped to pop? You may be on your way to becoming a mom. Early pregnancy—actually the first 4 months—is typically exhausting, leaving you feeling sluggish, sleepy, and sofa loving. That's because your body is beginning to crank up its baby-making machine (particularly the placenta manufacturing), and that takes a lot of energy—just about all the energy you have on hand. Those newbie hormones surging through your body also do a number on your energy levels—and your ability to keep your eyes open (would you believe all that extra progesterone can actually put you to sleep?). Lower blood sugar, lower blood pressure, and increasing metabolism can also zap you of energy. Does an attack of the sleepies guarantee that you're providing bed and board for a baby? No—it can also indicate that you're PMS-ing, fighting off an infection, working (or playing) too hard, stressing too much, or not sleeping enough.

Nausea. Here's a symptom that can sign on early—in some cases, just days after conception, though it's more likely to show up 4 weeks later, at about 6 weeks of pregnancy—and that, hopefully, will check out by the end of the first trimester. Though pregnancy hormones are responsible for so-called morning sickness, not every mom-to-be gets the queasies, and far from all experience vomiting, since hormones affect every woman differently. Not feeling green? That morning sickness could be just around the corner, or you may dodge it altogether. Still, nausea—or even a bout of vomiting—isn't a definite sign of pregnancy. It can also be caused by PMS, by a stomach bug or food poisoning, or even by mind games (it's possible to talk yourself into feeling queasy if you're really eager to be expecting).

Smell sensitivity. Does your nose know something you don't know (but are hoping for)? Some newly pregnant women report a heightened sense of smell early on—and that could be owing to the increasing amount of estrogen in your system during early pregnancy. If your sniffer's suddenly more sensitive and easily offended, pregnancy might be in the air. But (and there is a but), some women also experience this smell surge during PMS.

Bloating. That bloated feeling can creep up (and out) on you very early in a pregnancy—though it may be difficult to differentiate between a pre-period bloat and a pregnancy bloat. While it's too soon to attribute bloating to your baby's growth (remember, your baby's

not much bigger than the size of the period at the end of this sentence), it's likely due to early pregnancy hormones, particularly progesterone. These hormones slow down your digestive tract (to better allow what you eat to feed baby), allowing gas to hang out in your intestines. Of course, as every woman knows from many months of experience, bloat doesn't always spell baby— it can also spell P-M-S.

Cervical mucus. If you've become a student of your CM (maybe a grad student if you've been at it awhile), then take this test: Check your CM. If it becomes creamy and stays creamy after ovulation, that's a good sign that you'll pass the pregnancy test.

Missed period. In the stating-the-obvious department, if your 2-week wait doesn't end with a period (especially if your periods generally run like clockwork), it may be time to celebrate. Break out the pregnancy test, and hopefully the sparkling cider!

Diagnosing Pregnancy

Maybe boxes of pregnancy tests are stacked up in your bathroom waiting for the right moment to be ripped open and peed on. Or maybe you're waiting until the last minute (as in the day you miss your period) for a mad dash to the drugstore to pick one up. Either way, you're sure to have questions about taking that pregnancy test (when? how? how often?). Keep in mind that even though pregnancy tests may answer one question, they often leave you with lots more.

Pregnancy Tests

"How soon can I use a home pregnancy test to find out if I'm pregnant?"

Soon . . . but definitely not soon enough for most hopeful moms.

Though it would be nice (note to Mother Nature and manufacturers of home pregnancy tests) to get the heads-up—or thumbs-down—as soon as the last baby dance of the month is over, that's not the way it works, at least not yet. There's an average of 2 weeks of waiting from the time you ovulate until

Who Needs a Blood Test?

With HPTs as easy as 1-2-3-pee, why bother with a doctor's office blood test anymore, especially if you're not fond of needles? Actually, a blood test offers more information than those pee-on-a-stick tests can. Since it measures the exact amount of hCG (an at-home test lets you know only whether it's there), and those values change as pregnancy progresses, a blood test can help confirm that the pregnancy is proceeding normally. That's why some practitioners will follow up with a blood test even if you've had a positive HPT, and also if your HPT was negative but your period hasn't shown up or if you're not sure when you conceived.

Blood tests are routine if you've been undergoing fertility treatments (so the pregnancy can be detected as early and as accurately as possible).

the time you have (or miss) your period. And that's a lot of waiting, especially if you already feel like you've been waiting forever for that hopefully happy news.

Luckily, HPTs are quick, accurate, and reliable—and most important of all, they can keep the waiting to a minimum. You can start using many of them even before your period is scheduled to arrive, though the closer to P-day, the more reliable your results.

So how exactly can peeing on a stick give you the pregnancy scoop, and what's the earliest it can issue that baby bulletin? It's actually pretty simple. All those HPTs lined up on the shelves of the pharmacy work by measuring the levels of human chorionic gonadotropin (hCG) in your urine. HCG, a developing-placenta-produced hormone of pregnancy, finds its way into your bloodstream and urine almost immediately after an embryo begins implanting in your uterus, between 6 and 12 days after fertilization. As soon as hCG can be detected in your urine, you can get the positive result you're looking for—theoretically, that is. But HPTs aren't always sensitive to hCG until levels begin building up, which they do as the days pass. Though some hCG is in your urine a week after conception, it's not likely to be enough to register on the HPT—which means that if you test 7 days before you expect your period, you're likely to get a negative result even if you're pregnant. That's a good reason to hold off breaking open that HPT until your period's expected.

Waiting's not your thing? Some tests promise 60 to 75 percent accuracy 4 to 5 days before you expect your period. Not crazy about those odds? You'll have a 90 percent chance of netting the correct result if you sit tight until your expected period. Test a week later, and the accuracy rate jumps to 99 percent (so if at first you don't succeed, or get your period, try that test again). Whether you test early or late, the good news is that false positives are far less common than false negatives—which means if your test is positive, you can be positive, too. The exception to this rule: if you've been undergoing fertility treatments (see page 148 for the reason why).

HPTs offer a very accurate diagnosis very early in pregnancy, all in the privacy of your own bathroom. Still, you'll

HPTs, Circa 1350 BCE

So you thought peeing on a stick to find out if you're pregnant was an invention of the modern era? Well, the stick may be—but the peeing, apparently not. An Egyptian papyrus from 1350 BCE describes a home pregnancy test that definitely predates EPT. To test for pregnancy—and her future baby's sex—a woman would urinate on a pile of wheat and barley seeds. If barley grew, it meant she was pregnant with a boy. If wheat grew, it meant she was expecting a girl. No sprouts at all? Then there was no little sprout growing in her, either.

Were those ancients on to something? Believe it or not, there's some grain of truth (both barley and wheat) to this wisdom from the ages. When replicated in our times, it's been found that this test is 70 percent accurate for predicting pregnancy (not a baby's sex), probably because the elevated levels of estrogen in a pregnant woman's urine cause those seeds to sprout. Farmers, take note.

have to leave the bathroom and follow up with a professional. If the result is positive, you should schedule a prenatal checkup, where your practitioner may confirm the HPT result with a blood test. If repeated tests are negative, but your period still doesn't show up, check in with your practitioner to see if there's another reason why you're so late.

Can't test on the day your period's expected because you never know for sure when that day will come? Your best testing strategy if your periods are irregular is to wait the number of days equal to the longest cycle you've had in the last 6 months—and then test. If the result is negative and you still haven't gotten your period, repeat the test after a week, or after a few days if you're not the patient type.

Best Way to Test

"I heard it's better to take a pregnancy test in the morning. Is that right?"

Any time is a good time for a home pregnancy test, and with today's extra-sensitive tests, there's no need to stick with your first morning's urine.

As for other test prep tips, start by reading the package directions thoroughly and then following them. No, it's not rocket science, but since different pregnancy tests may have slightly different protocols, it pays to look before you pee. Depending on the brand, you'll either hold the test stick in your stream of urine for a few seconds or collect your urine in a cup and then dip the stick into it. Midstream urine is usually preferred for any urine test because it serves up the cleanest sample. (And you might as well master the midstream now, if you haven't already: If your test is positive, you'll be spending

TTC To-Do:

Though you might not want to hear it, the truth is, it's best to wait until the day you expect your period (or a few days before, depending on the brand of test) to break out the HPT. The results will be more accurate and you'll save yourself a lot of uncertainty—not to mention all the money you'd be spending on retests.

Stress Tests

Is it that time of month again—testing time? If you've been TTC for a while, you know the drill, and maybe you've come to look forward to it—and at the same time, dread it a little bit. That's understandable. All those efforts you're both putting in to your baby-making mission each month, all the anticipation, all the excitement, all the hopes and dreams—all come down to a trickle of urine, a stick, and a knot-in-the-stomach wait for a sign (or a line, or a readout).

If the monthly testing—and monthly second-guessing of her symptoms—is stressing you both out, hang in there. Getting pregnant can take longer than you'd think (ironic, considering how much effort you may have made over the years trying *not* to get your partner pregnant), but most often, it does happen—and it's always worth waiting for. In the meantime, try taking some of the stress out of the monthly testing by planning a little something special each month: a dinner out, a bouquet of her favorite flowers, a cupcake from her favorite bakery, even a card that lets her know how happy you are to be working on making a baby with her. Whether you end up celebrating a baby-to-be or toasting next month's efforts, it'll remind you both not only how lucky you are to be starting a family together, but how lucky you are to have each other.

a lot of time providing these samples to your practitioner at your prenatal appointments.) To perform a perfect midstream, pee for a second or two, stop, hold the flow, and then put either the stick or the cup in position to catch the rest of the stream.

Once you have a properly peed-on stick, take a deep breath and get ready to read the result. Make sure you follow the recommended waiting period; not waiting long enough, or waiting too long, can affect that result. In fact, it's possible for a test that originally came out negative (using the timing indicated on the packaging and directions) to turn into a positive result hours or days after it was done, even if you're not really pregnant. The test result that's accurate—and the one you should count on—is the one that appears after the recommended waiting time. If you see a different result hours later, take another test before jumping to any conclusions.

Faintly Positive

"When I took a home pregnancy test, it showed a really faint line. Am I pregnant?"

Get ready to faint—from excitement. Any positive line (or readout) is a positive sign—and a sign that you're positively pregnant. That's because the only way an HPT can produce that positive result is if there's hCG circulating in your system and making an appearance in your urine. And the only way that hCG can show up is if you're pregnant (only pregnant bodies can manufacture this pregnancy-centric hormone)—or you've been undergoing certain fertility treatments (see box, page 148). Bottom line on that line (or that digital readout), no matter how faint: It means you're officially expecting.

Not the dark, emphatic, no-doubt-about-it line you were looking for—the one you were going to snap a picture of and post on social media? That's

Pregnancy Testing and Fertility Treatments

If you've been undergoing certain fertility treatments, you've likely been told to skip the HPT and wait until a blood test can be done (which, depending on your fertility clinic, may be a week to 2 weeks after conception or embryo transfer). Why can't you turn to the pee-on-a-stick method to find out if you're expecting? Since hCG, the hormone tested for in an HPT, is often used in fertility treatments to trigger ovulation, and because it may remain in your system (and therefore show up in your urine) even if you're not pregnant, HPTs can provide unreliable results for fertility patients. By measuring hCG in the blood (you'll probably have several blood tests), your doctor will be able to see not only that there's hCG in your system, but also that the level of hCG is increasing, indicating that you've got a bun in the oven and all is going well so far.

probably because the type of test you used wasn't supersensitive, or because you're testing so early that there isn't enough hCG to generate that loud-and-clear baby bulletin you hoped to see (those levels rise each day, so if you test early, there's only a little hCG to tap into).

If you feel you need a more definitive result before you start celebrating (or if you're just determined to get that photo op), wait until at least the first day of your missed period and test again. Chances are you'll see the line that will delete your doubts and convince you that you've conceived after all.

Positive Result . . . Then Negative

"My first pregnancy test was positive, but a few days later I took 2 more and they were both negative. And then I got my period. What's going on?"

Early testing does come with a downside, and unfortunately, it sounds like you may have experienced it: the diagnosis of a chemical pregnancy. Because an HPT can diagnose a pregnancy so very early in the process, it can sometimes also diagnose one that isn't meant to continue—one that isn't capable of developing or surviving, and ends practically before it begins. In a chemical pregnancy, the egg is fertilized and starts to implant in the uterus, but for some reason it never completes implantation. Instead of turning into a viable pregnancy, it ends very quickly in a period. Though experts estimate that up to 70 percent of all conceptions are chemical, the vast majority end before a woman even realizes that she's conceived (certainly in the days before home pregnancy tests, women didn't know they were pregnant until much later, so chemical pregnancies weren't diagnosed at all). Often a very early positive pregnancy test, followed by negative testing and then a late period (a few days to a week late) are the only signs of a chemical pregnancy. Unless you tested early, you never would have known about it.

Technically, a chemical pregnancy is more like a cycle in which a pregnancy never actually occurred than it is a true miscarriage—it's a random event that requires no medical treatment or

I'm Pregnant, Now What?

Maybe it was your first time at the baby-making plate, or maybe you've been swinging away for months. Either way, sperm and egg have made contact—and you and your partner have conceived. Congrats on a job well done! But guess what? Your work is just beginning. If you thought making a baby was demanding, wait until you start growing that baby. That's why you're going to need all the help you can get, not just from the daddy-to-be in your life, but from the prenatal practitioner of your choice. Haven't made the choice yet? Now's the time to get busy on your search for Dr. (or Midwife) Right. Don't know where to begin with that important assignment—or where to begin on anything pregnancy related (what to do, what not to do, what to eat, what not to eat, what to make of all those crazy, seemingly random symptoms you may already be experiencing)? You'll get lots of help from *What to Expect When You're Expecting*, as well as from *Eating Well When You're Expecting*—plus, you'll be able to keep track of it all in *The What to Expect Pregnancy Journal and Organizer* and the What To Expect app—and get all the support and empathy you need from fellow moms-to-be on WhatToExpect.com. Hey, look at that—you've graduated to expecting!

followup, and is no cause for concern. Emotionally, it can be a very different story. The loss of the promise of a pregnancy, no matter how early it happens, can also be upsetting for both you and your partner—especially if you've been trying to conceive for some time. Talking to other women who've gone through the same thing may help you work through your feelings—and also help you realize that you're far from alone.

Here's the good news: There's no medical reason to wait if you'd like to TTC again on your next cycle, and experiencing one chemical pregnancy usually doesn't increase the chances of having another one. Keep in mind, too, that having conceived once makes it more likely that you'll conceive again soon (though you may want to wait a little longer to test next time)—with the much happier result of a healthy pregnancy.

Pregnancy Symptoms Without the Positive Test

"I have all kinds of early pregnancy symptoms, and my period hasn't started. But I must have taken 6 tests in the last week, and all have been negative. What should I do?"

Having spent your whole life living in it, you know your body well—possibly even better than a pee-on-a-stick test does. If you're experiencing multiple symptoms of early pregnancy, but can't get those HPTs to back up your hunch, wait a week, give your body a chance to accumulate some more hCG, then test again. Your pregnancy may be too early to call with an HPT (after all, pinpointing conception isn't a precise science). In the meantime, take optimum pregnancy care of yourself. (You know the drill, and you're probably already practicing it: Take your

There's Always Next Month

So another round of testing has arrived, along with the waiting, and hoping, and wishing, and seemingly endless anticipation. Will you be? Won't you be? You head for the toilet, heart in your stomach, emotions on your sleeve, HPT in your hand. You pee, you wait some more, you steel yourself, and you peek at the results (eyes half closed at first because you're almost afraid to look).

Negative, again, even after you retest, and retest—and wait and retest? There's no denying it—it's disappointing, whether it's the 1st month you've tried, or the 10th, or more. Frustrating, too, especially if you've been meticulous in your fertility charting and precise in your sex scheduling, and fully expected your efforts to pay off in the form of a positive HPT.

It's definitely hard to put a positive spin on a negative pregnancy test when you were so hoping this would be your lucky month—the one when all the efforts you and your partner have been putting into your conception mission would finally provide the ultimate payoff. But here's one way to try. Instead of looking back at this month's negative result, think ahead to next month's possibly positive one. Remind yourself that successful baby making, like most of life's best rewards, often takes time. But it's time that's well worth it—even if it sometimes feels like all those efforts are getting you nowhere. If you can, and if it seems to help you stay positive, try to find just one way you can improve on this month's efforts, whether it's cutting back on caffeine or stepping up your fruits and veggies, or hey, learning to love oysters. Taking another positive step can always make you feel a little better about that negative test—and can help you summon up the motivation you'll need for next month's efforts.

Most of all, in your quest for a baby, don't forget about the partner you're on the quest with. Though he may not be showing it—probably for fear of stressing you out—he's probably also feeling a little drained over all the emotional ups and downs of TTC, too. So as you look forward to next month's baby making, remember to look next to you, too.

prenatal vitamins, eat well, and don't drink or smoke.) Or, if waiting's not your game, call your practitioner and ask for a blood test, which can diagnose a pregnancy more accurately sooner.

If your hunch isn't confirmed by follow-up testing (especially if a blood test also comes back negative), it becomes much more likely that you aren't pregnant after all. Because just about every early pregnancy symptom—including a missed period—can have other triggers, it's possible to feel pregnant and not be pregnant. To screen out other physical causes for your symptoms, check in with your practitioner, especially if your period is unusually late for you. Testing again is probably also a good idea, just in case your cycle was out of whack this month and you may have conceived much later than the calendar suggests.

If your pregnancy tests are consistently negative, and your practitioner can't find a physical explanation for your symptoms, it's possible that they could have emotional roots. The mind-body connection is strong, but it can be especially strong when your mind is so eager for your body to become pregnant—and that is completely understandable, especially if you've been waiting for that happy result for a while. As many TTC moms have found, even the power of suggestion—reading about pregnancy symptoms, hearing about them from friends—can summon up everything from nausea to food cravings to fatigue when you very much want to be pregnant. Being so keenly tuned in to your body, which many TTC moms are, can also make you hypersensitive to every little possible change—which can make you see symptoms where they might not actually be. And what wishful thinking can't summon up, PMS symptoms very easily can (including bloating, breast pain, crampiness, moodiness, headache, and fatigue). What's more, being stressed out about being in pregnancy limbo (am I? am I not?) can actually keep your period from arriving, which can keep the limbo going longer—and

even exacerbate those pseudo-pregnancy symptoms.

This isn't to say that you're imagining your pregnancy symptoms—or that they're all in your head (emotionally triggered symptoms can be surprisingly convincing)—only that your mind and body may be collaborating to play tricks on you. It isn't fair, but it's very common. Most hopeful moms find themselves second-guessing symptoms, even when those pregnancy tests won't back them up—and some find themselves doing that with each and every cycle. Bring the topic up with others who are TTC, and you'll likely get an earful of empathy.

So if it turns out that the miracle didn't happen this month, realize that accepting this reality doesn't mean you're giving up on those baby hopes—just that you're giving up on this month's and moving on to the next, which will be here before you know it!

PART 3

Bumps on the Road to Baby

CHAPTER 9

Challenges to Fertility

Did you always sort of assume that getting pregnant was going to be as easy as chucking the birth control and getting busy? Often it is, but sometimes it isn't. Making a baby can take more time than you'd expect—even when everything's in working order on both sides of the bed, but especially when something (or someone) needs a reproductive tune-up, or more. For 1 in 8 couples, it's not just a matter of time, it's a matter of fertility challenges. Fortunately, most bumps encountered on the road to baby can be overcome—even if they slow the journey down or make a detour or two necessary. The right diagnosis and the right treatment can get you right back on the baby-making path and pave the way for conception.

Fertility Challenges

Often, overcoming infertility is as easy as finding out what's blocking your path to pregnancy and clearing it up. Maybe it's a condition you knew you had—but didn't realize would affect your fertility. Maybe it's a condition that you didn't have a clue about until a fertility workup uncovered it. Either way, treatment is often possible and usually successful. Here are some of the more common fertility challenges and what can be done to overcome them.

Fibroids

What is it? Uterine fibroids are almost always benign (in other words, noncancerous) tumors that grow inside or around the wall of the uterus. Fibroids can grow individually or in clusters, and each can be as small as a grain of sand or as large as a melon.

As many as 80 percent of women in the United States have fibroids, and nearly a quarter of those women have symptoms ranging from painful, extremely heavy, longer-than-normal periods and pressure in the pelvic area to constipation, urinary incontinence, and backache. Many women don't have any symptoms at all.

Though it is not completely clear what causes them, fibroids are more common among overweight women (it's believed that high levels of fat-derived estrogen contribute to the growth of fibroids). African American women are 3 times more likely than Caucasian women to develop fibroids. There's also a genetic component: If your mother had fibroids, you may be at higher risk for getting them.

How is fertility affected? Most fibroids do not affect fertility and can safely be left alone. Some, however, can interfere with conception by causing blockages in the reproductive tract and by changing the shape of the uterus, making it harder for an egg to be fertilized or for a fertilized egg to implant. Fibroids can also cause inflammation of the blood vessels of the uterus, which in turn can make implantation more difficult. Location, size, and number of fibroids influence the impact on fertility.

What are the treatment options? A number of treatment options for fibroids are available, but only one is appropriate for women who'd like to conceive. That treatment is a surgical procedure called a myomectomy, during which large or numerous fibroids are removed from the uterus. Myomectomy can be performed as an outpatient surgery with a hysteroscope introduced through the cervix or via a laparoscope (through small incisions in the abdomen). It can also be done with traditional abdominal surgery, which requires a hospital stay.

The Good News

If you're having trouble conceiving due to fibroids, research shows that treating and/or removing them can increase fertility.

Pelvic Inflammatory Disease (PID)

What is it? Any time an infection causes inflammation in the pelvic organs, the condition is known in medical-speak as pelvic inflammatory disease (PID). PID most commonly affects the fallopian tubes, but the uterus and ovaries can also be affected. It is most often triggered by untreated STDs such as chlamydia or gonorrhea—in fact, up to 40 percent of women with untreated chlamydia or gonorrhea develop PID. Far less often, PID can be caused by a ruptured appendix.

The symptoms of PID may include pelvic pain (which can come on suddenly or build up over time), smelly vaginal discharge, excessive bleeding during your period, fever, chills, painful urination, backache, nausea, and/or vomiting. Unfortunately, PID often goes undiagnosed because symptoms are typically mild or are chalked up to cycle pain or tummy troubles.

The Good News

Early and aggressive treatment of infections and STDs can decrease the chances that PID will prevent you from becoming pregnant.

STDs and Male Infertility

Men with STDs are more likely than women to exhibit symptoms soon after they are infected, which means many seek treatment right away—and that's a good thing. Even so, up to 50 percent of men with chlamydia may not have symptoms. Occasionally, untreated STDs can damage a man's fertility by causing inflammation and scarring in the testicles, epididymis, prostate gland, or urethra. But by far the greatest risk when a man has an STD: passing it on to his female partner.

Getting tested and treated for STDs early, as well as practicing safe sex, can help men protect their fertility—and their partner's.

How is fertility affected? Twenty percent of women with PID experience fertility difficulties. That's because if PID is left untreated, the inflammation can cause scar tissue to form in the fallopian tubes, making it difficult both for an egg to travel through them after ovulation and for the sperm to reach the egg. If fertilization does occur, the scar tissue in the fallopian tube can stop the fertilized egg from reaching the uterus, increasing the risk for an ectopic pregnancy (when a fertilized egg remains in the fallopian tube and grows there instead of implanting in the uterus). If the uterine lining is affected by PID, it could be difficult for a fertilized egg to implant normally.

What are the treatment options? If you notice any of the symptoms of PID, visit your doctor for a diagnosis. If PID is diagnosed, antibiotics can get rid of the infection and may protect your fertility.

Getting treated right away for STDs and following safe sex practices with partners who have STDs will decrease your risk not only for an STD, but also for PID. Unfortunately, antibiotics can't reverse damage that is already done, so if PID is not treated, and even in some cases when it is, it's still possible to suffer infertility. There are 2 treatment options for infertility caused by fallopian tube damage: surgery to try to repair the damaged tubes, or IVF. Of those choices, IVF is far more likely to lead to a pregnancy, and less likely to lead to an ectopic pregnancy.

Endometriosis

What is it? Endometriosis, a condition that affects approximately 15 percent of women of reproductive age, occurs when tissue from the uterine lining (the endometrium) grows on other parts of the pelvic area (such as the fallopian tubes, ovaries, bladder, appendix, or even intestines). This endometrial tissue acts the same way outside the uterus as it does inside. So, when estrogen and progesterone levels rise and fall as part of a normal menstrual cycle, the tissue (no matter where it is) will build up and then, if there's no pregnancy, shed (aka bleed). This can result in inflammation and scarring. Extreme pelvic pain, severe cramps during your period, painful intercourse, lower back pain, and nausea and vomiting are common symptoms of endometriosis.

Endometriosis is thought to be caused by a combination of factors, including a malfunction of the immune system, a backup of endometrial tissue during menstruation (instead of all the tissue flowing out in the form of a period, some tissue backs up the wrong way and into the abdominal cavity), and genetic factors (if your mom or another close female relative has had

The Good News

Endometriosis treatment can be tailored to your needs, and usually an effective one can be found. And there's even more good news ahead once you successfully conceive. The pain associated with endometriosis is often diminished during pregnancy, plus pregnancy provides a reprieve from new growth.

endometriosis, your chances of developing the condition are increased).

How is fertility affected? Many women with endometriosis have fewer eggs, either because the condition or surgery performed to correct it has left good ovarian tissue damaged. Fortunately, most cases of endometriosis are not severe enough to cause infertility.

What are the treatment options? Though there is no cure for endometriosis, there are several options for treating associated infertility:

- Surgery (usually laparoscopic) to remove the endometrial lesions. This procedure offers modest benefits.

- Fertility medications, used in conjunction with IUI (this also offers modest benefits).

- IVF, which offers the best chances of overcoming infertility triggered by endometriosis.

What about treating the pelvic pain that comes with endometriosis? Surgery can help, as can a variety of hormonal medical treatments, which can reduce the level of estrogen, shrinking some of the lesions. The catch-22 when you're TTC: All hormonal treatments stop ovulation, and you can't get pregnant

if you're not ovulating. The theory that hormone treatment to shrink endometriosis can provide a window for conception once the hormones have been stopped has been disproven.

Scar Tissue/ Surgical Adhesions

What is it? Scar tissue (aka adhesions) can grow in any part of your body after it has been wounded—and that goes for any part of your reproductive tract, too. These bands of fibrous material can develop in and around your fallopian tubes, ovaries, and uterus as a result of inflammation from PID, endometriosis, or previous gynecological surgery. Scar tissue from PID most commonly affects the fallopian tubes. With endometriosis, fallopian tubes are usually spared, but other pelvic anatomy, like the ovaries, can develop scar tissue. Often scar tissue doesn't cause any noticeable symptoms, though some women experience pelvic pain, pain with intercourse, and/or severe menstrual pain.

Scar tissue inside the uterus, usually the result of a dilation and curettage (D&C), is called Asherman's syndrome. With Asherman's, periods may be light or absent.

How is fertility affected? Scar tissue that closes the ends of the fallopian tubes closest to the ovaries prevents

The Good News

Pregnancy rates after surgery to remove mild fallopian tube scar tissue and mild Asherman's are very high. While getting pregnant after surgery for moderate or severe scar tissue may prove more challenging, IVF pregnancy rates are excellent.

Cervical Stenosis

Sometimes, a woman may develop small amounts of scar tissue on her cervix after undergoing a cervical surgical procedure—such as a LEEP procedure or a cone biopsy (both used to treat abnormal cells found on the cervix after a Pap test). In some cases, the scar tissue can grow thick enough to cause cervical stenosis, or a narrowing of the cervical canal. Since sperm needs only a tiny opening to swim through, cervical stenosis doesn't usually prevent conception. In rare cases, however, scar tissue completely blocks sperm from entering the uterus through the cervix. And in those cases, fertility will be affected. Luckily, intrauterine insemination (IUI; see page 183) with cervical dilation (opening up the cervix) can get the sperm where they need to go—and help you score that fertilized egg.

eggs from being plucked from the ovary. Scarring where the fallopian tubes enter the uterus prevents sperm from entering the tubes to fertilize the egg. With Asherman's syndrome, scar tissue replaces the inner lining of the uterus (endometrium), preventing embryos from implanting or triggering miscarriage if implantation does occur (a successful pregnancy requires a healthy endometrium). Rarely, scar tissue can also form on the cervix, and if it blocks the cervix completely it can impede fertility.

What are the treatment options? If you have lots of adhesions, if you have pain, or if you have trouble conceiving, surgery to remove the scar tissue may be recommended. Scar tissue involving the fallopian tubes or ovaries can be treated laparoscopically (through a tiny abdominal incision). With Asherman's syndrome, a hysteroscope (an instrument inserted through the cervix) visualizes the uterus, and if any scar tissue is found, additional instruments are inserted through the hysteroscope to remove the adhesions.

Ovarian Cyst

What is it? An ovarian cyst is a soft, fluid-filled sac that grows in the ovary. For most women who get ovarian cysts, these blister-like growths come and go with a normal menstrual cycle and are completely harmless. But for others, ovarian cysts can linger, grow large, and even cause symptoms, including pain localized on one side of your abdomen when you ovulate. They can also cause irregular periods.

How is fertility affected? If there are too many cysts, eggs could fail to develop or be released—in other words, cysts can prevent ovulation. Endometriotic cysts deep within the ovary, called endometriomas (or chocolate cysts), can destroy ovarian tissue, decreasing ovarian reserve.

What are the treatment options? Often, cysts resolve on their own, but if a cyst persists or gets larger, or if your symptoms get worse, you may need laparoscopic surgery to remove it.

The Good News

The vast majority of ovarian cysts have absolutely no effect on fertility. For those that do impact the ability to conceive, treatment almost always makes pregnancy possible.

Polycystic Ovary Syndrome (PCOS)

What is it? Eight to 10 percent of women have polycystic ovary syndrome (PCOS), and the condition is the most common cause of infertility. PCOS occurs when the body starts producing too much of the hormone LH and the ovaries start producing too much testosterone (they usually produce only a small amount) or the body becomes overly sensitive to normal amounts of testosterone. Women with PCOS are usually (but not always) overweight, are often prediabetic (or already have type 2 diabetes), typically have irregular periods or no periods (because they don't ovulate regularly or don't ovulate at all), and may experience excessive hair growth on the face and other parts of the body as well as acne (both a result of that excess testosterone). Occasionally, women with PCOS also suffer from prolonged vaginal bleeding. On ultrasound, many tiny cysts can be seen in the ovaries of women who have PCOS (thus the name polycystic ovary syndrome).

While it's not known for certain what causes PCOS, experts speculate there is a genetic component (if your mother or a close female relative has had it, your risk is higher), and that it might also have something to do with the body's inability to use insulin properly (insulin controls not only blood sugar, but also ovarian function).

How is fertility affected? It's simple: If you don't ovulate, you can't get pregnant. As a result, women with PCOS struggle with infertility.

What are the treatment options? Weight loss, regular exercise, and a well-balanced diet that's rich in complex carbs (such as whole grains and vegetables), and low in refined carbs

The Good News

There is almost always a way to treat a woman with PCOS so that she can ovulate normally and become pregnant. If not, she can move on to IVF.

(like white rice and white bread) and sugar can all help restore ovulation and regular periods in women with PCOS. If lifestyle modifications don't do the trick, adding fertility meds such as letrozole (Femara) or clomiphene citrate (Clomid) usually achieves ovulation and results in pregnancy rates of 25 to 30 percent. Another medication used in the treatment of PCOS is metformin, a diabetes drug that lowers insulin levels and improves insulin resistance, helping women with PCOS lose weight and reestablish ovulation. If Femara or Clomid, with or without metformin, doesn't work to accomplish pregnancy, careful use of more powerful injectable fertility drugs can be very effective.

Most women with PCOS conceive with the help of a combination of lifestyle changes and medication. For those who don't, IVF can help make pregnancy a reality. A surgical option, called laparoscopic ovarian drilling, cauterizes (burns) both ovaries at multiple sites. Some experts say that burning off some ovarian tissue helps improve ovulation, but results of ovarian drilling haven't been consistent so far.

Irregular Menstrual Periods/Anovulation

What is it? Irregular periods (cycles lasting longer than 35 to 40 days), no periods, or abnormal bleeding are usually signs that you're not ovulating.

Secondary Infertility

Conceiving baby number 1 was a piece of cake, but getting a second bun in the oven has been a surprising struggle? You have a lot of company. Actually, more couples experience secondary infertility (infertility that shows up after you've already had at least one baby) than primary infertility (infertility the first time around). In fact, secondary infertility accounts for 50 percent of infertility cases. Yet those stats don't seem to be reflected in attitudes about secondary infertility. Much more attention is focused on first-timers who are having a hard time getting pregnant than those who are getting nowhere on round 2. Friends and family may not feel your pain and frustration—or even understand it— if you already have a pride and joy to enjoy. Your doctor may downplay secondary infertility, urging you to "just keep on trying"—reassuring you that getting pregnant once means it'll happen again. And if you're like a lot of couples having trouble conceiving baby number 2, you may be less likely to seek help—after all, who has time for fertility screenings and treatments when you've got a little one to run after? For that matter, who has time to devote to complicated baby-planning activities— to charting, to testing, to carefully choreographed sex . . . or any sex—when you're busy scheduling an older child's activities?

Once in a while, problems getting pregnant for a second or subsequent time are related to a problem that occurred in an earlier pregnancy or delivery—like a birth trauma that damaged the uterus. But usually, secondary infertility is caused by the very same range of factors that cause primary infertility (the 2 most common: being overweight and being older).

So first, do your own assessment of your preconception prep and your TTC campaign so far (unless you've already been on top of that game). Have you been keeping track of your fertility and having sex at the appropriate times? Have you noticed any changes in your cycles that might be keeping you from conceiving? Has your lifestyle taken any major hits since your first pregnancy, and if so, is there room for improvement? For instance, has becoming a mom pushed your caffeine consumption off the charts (understandable, but too much caffeine can interfere with fertility)? Has your diet devolved significantly (less whole grain, more whole bag of chips)? Have you slipped up on smoking (smoking ages eggs, decreasing fertility)? Have there been any changes in your health—or medications you've been taking—since your first baby was born? How about your weight—have you put on some extra pounds since your first baby boarded? Or, maybe, lost a few too many since your first baby was born because you no longer have time to eat? You're obviously older than you were when you conceived the first time, but has enough time passed that your age might now be a factor when trying to conceive? Your partner should ask himself the same questions about his health, lifestyle, weight, diet, and age, too, because his fertility can also be impacted by any or all of the above. Read over Chapters 1, 2, and 3 to see if a few modifications in how you're living could help you live the pregnant life again sooner.

Then, check in with your doctor for a more professional assessment. A year of trying to conceive (or much less if you're over 35) definitely qualifies you for a fertility workup, so there's no reason to hold off if time has been ticking away. In many cases, treatment for anything that's discovered can be quick and easy, so you can finally get that second passenger on board. In some cases, treatment may take longer, but either way, moving those fertility bumps off your path to pregnancy can help put a bump back on your belly.

Of course, if you're having trouble conceiving baby number 2 (or 3, or 4), you may not only be dealing with all those typical TTC ups and downs—but also with emotional issues that are unique to those experiencing secondary infertility. First, the surprise ("I got pregnant right away last time—why not this time?") and the denial ("How can I have a fertility problem, when I've been fertile before?"). Then the guilt ("Why can't I just be happy with the child we already have?"). And the jealousy ("Everyone else can have 2 kids—why can't I?"). You may feel, strangely, more alone than other hopeful parents who are facing first-time fertility challenges—you're not a member of the primary infertility group since you have a child already, but you're not fully at home with fertile friends (or baby-toting parents at school drop-off), since you're having trouble conceiving again. This may make it harder to find the support every struggling-to-conceive couple needs. And then there's the stress of having friends, family, coworkers, even the grandmotherly woman at the dry cleaner always asking that dreaded question: "When are you having another?"

Just because you already have a child doesn't mean you aren't entitled to feel discouraged when you're having trouble conceiving another. Or that you're not entitled to all the empathy and support you need as you face this challenge. So seek it out. If friends and family just don't understand what you're going through—or if you're not comfortable broaching the subject with them—talk to those who do get it (and since secondary infertility is so common, you'll be surprised at how many do). You can find others dealing with secondary infertility on online message boards (check out WhatToExpect.com) and in support groups.

Remember, too, that you're not facing secondary infertility completely alone—you have each other. Staying connected as a twosome always takes more effort when you're also a three-some, but it's especially important, particularly as you try to become a four-some (or more). Chances are you're both feeling the same frustrations, and the same disappointment, and the same guilt, and you'll both feel better if you share those feelings with each other. But also try to make time for the kind of romance that will keep your baby-making campaign—and your relationship—going strong. If date night has lapsed—or you never got around to setting one—start dating your mate again, regularly.

One other person may be feeling the effects of your fertility struggles, even if he or she doesn't know about them: your child. Little ones, even very little ones, have supersensitive mood radar—so though your child almost certainly isn't in the loop about your conception efforts, he or she may be riding that emotional roller coaster right alongside you. To make sure those ups and downs don't leave your child feeling off balance, try to keep family life as normal as possible—even as you push forward with your efforts to add to that precious family.

Clomid to the Rescue?

Clomiphene citrate, aka Clomid, has long been the first line of treatment when a woman has trouble conceiving and the suspected culprit is an ovulation issue. And it's still considered the go-to medication for unexplained infertility. But there's another option that your doctor may prescribe: letrozole (Femara). FDA-approved for the treatment of breast cancer in postmenopausal women, Femara is often used "off-label" to induce ovulation, and has been shown to be safe and effective (with low rates of side effects and high rates of pregnancy), especially for women with PCOS. Clomid is usually taken for 5 days, beginning on the 2nd, 3rd, 4th, or 5th day of a cycle, while Femara is taken on days 5 through 9. Most women can expect to start ovulating about 7 to 9 days after the last dose of either medication. Whichever drug is prescribed, you'll likely be kept on it for only 3 to 6 months after it has started working and you've begun to ovulate. If you're still not pregnant after several months of ovulating on Clomid or Femara, next steps might be adding IUI, changing to a stronger injectable fertility drug, or moving on to IVF.

One thing to keep in mind about Clomid and Femara: Since they are medications that induce ovulation, there's a chance they'll work so well, you'll ovulate more than 1 egg. If you conceive during a cycle where more than 1 egg is released, there's a 5 to 10 percent chance you'll be seeing double in the future—as in a twin (or more) pregnancy. Other, more common (and less potentially happy) side effects of Clomid may include breast tenderness, mood swings, hot flashes, vision changes, night sweats, bloating, and weight gain.

Called anovulation, this condition can be caused by many factors, including stress, an eating disorder, being extremely underweight or overweight, too much exercise, illness, and/or a hormonal imbalance (such as a thyroid condition or PCOS).

How is fertility affected? Irregular or abnormal ovulation and menstruation is responsible for up to 30 percent of all cases of infertility. If you don't ovulate, you can't get pregnant.

What are the treatment options? First, your doctor may want to confirm that you're not ovulating. One way to confirm ovulation is with a blood test to measure progesterone levels, taken a week after your expected time of ovulation. If your progesterone levels are above a certain amount, it usually indicates you've ovulated. If they're low, anovulation is suspected. Another way for your doctor to determine whether you've ovulated is by performing a series of ultrasounds during a cycle, looking for growing ovarian follicles, for the dominant follicle, and then for a collapsed follicle in the same location, indicating that ovulation has occurred.

If anovulation is suspected, it's helpful to take a good look at your weight and your lifestyle. If you're overweight or underweight, getting your weight close to where it should be may reregulate your cycles (see Chapter 2), but don't do any extreme dieting, which can also throw your cycles off. A regular exercise program can boost your general health—and possibly, your fertility—but too much exercise (especially if your regimen has left you low on body fat) can prevent you from ovulating, so try easing up if you've been hitting the gym too hard. Eating disorders (anorexia, bulimia, or even just periodic binging) can also throw off your cycles, so if you think—or anyone around you thinks—you might need help overcoming such a problem, don't hesitate to seek it. Extreme stress can also derail your cycles, so try to relax, too (see page 29 for some tips on how). If none of these tactics seems to work, and screenings for a thyroid condition or PCOS have come up negative, your doctor may prescribe fertility drugs like Femara, Clomid, or an injectable to induce ovulation and normal periods.

Diminished Ovarian Reserve

What is it? Diminished ovarian reserve (DOR) is when the number or quality of eggs in the ovaries has begun to dwindle, decreasing fertility, sometimes significantly. It's universal, something that happens to every woman at some point in her reproductive life, usually due to normal aging but sometimes linked to other factors, such as genetics (say, early menopause that runs in the family), ovarian surgery, cancer treatment, or cigarette smoking. These factors can cause a dip in ovarian reserve that comes sooner than expected.

How is fertility affected? That depends. When egg number and quality are both low, the possibility of conceiving is low as well, even with the help of assisted reproductive techniques, such as IVF. Same is true when egg supply is adequate, but the eggs are of poor quality. But when egg quality is high—even when there are a lower number of them in reserve—fertility may be only mildly

The Good News

Though diminished ovarian reserve means a woman's egg supply is smaller than ideal, many women with DOR may still have enough eggs left to conceive, either naturally or with the help of fertility medications and assisted reproductive techniques.

affected or not affected at all. This is a more likely scenario when a woman under 35 has DOR.

What are the treatment options? Depending on how many eggs are still viable, fertility treatments like ovarian stimulation with IUI or IVF may have a high chance of success. If these aren't an option, IVF with egg donation will be necessary to achieve pregnancy. Read more about diminished ovarian reserve and how to test for it on pages 110 and 175.

Premature Ovarian Insufficiency

What is it? Premature ovarian insufficiency (POI) or premature ovarian failure (POF) occurs when a woman's ovarian follicles are completely or nearly depleted before age 40 or when her ovaries stop working properly long before they should have. POI can be caused by genetic factors such as family history (your mom or grandmother had POI), metabolic disorders, Turner syndrome, or fragile X syndrome. It can also be caused by type 1 diabetes, autoimmune diseases, or cancer treatments.

How is fertility affected? If egg follicles are nearly depleted, as they might be in POI, it becomes extremely difficult

Is It You . . . Or Is It Me?

Quick: Who's more likely to be responsible when a couple has trouble conceiving—the female partner, or the male? For centuries it was believed that the woman was inevitably the weak reproductive link when a couple came up without an heir. Even today, this long-held assumption gets plenty of popular support.

It turns out, though, that men and women can both contribute to infertility—and at about the same rates. Statistics show that 35 to 40 percent of the time, the problem lies with the man,

in another 35 to 40 percent of cases it's with the woman, and the rest of the time both partners have contributing factors or the cause is unknown.

Because either partner (or both) can contribute to a conception standstill, doctors often recommend couples start initial fertility testing at the same time: usually, blood work and physicals for both of you, plus a semen analysis for him. If all of those tests are aced, the next step would be further testing for you. See page 174 for more on the fertility workup.

to conceive. There is a small chance of spontaneous remission of POI—in other words, of spontaneously ovulating and becoming pregnant even after a diagnosis of POI. If the egg reserves are completely depleted, however, as is sometimes the case with POF, conception becomes impossible.

What are the treatment options? Hormonal treatment can help with the symptoms that arise from POI, which are similar to those of menopause, but such treatment hasn't been shown to restore ovulation and fertility. Unless the condition goes into remission (as it does 5 to 10 percent of the time), IVF

The Good News

Though POI causes a woman's egg supply to be depleted much faster than it would normally, some women with POI may still have enough eggs left to conceive. In fact, 5 to 10 percent of women with POI will conceive on their own.

using eggs from a donor or frozen eggs from an egg bank is needed to become pregnant.

Thyroid Disorder

What is it? Thyroid disorder can show up as hyperthyroidism, when too much thyroid hormone is produced, or more commonly, hypothyroidism, when too little thyroid hormone is produced. Signs of an underactive thyroid (hypothyroid) can include a goiter (a ball-like swelling in the neck), unexplained weight gain (or trouble losing weight), thinning hair, dry skin, lack of energy, depression, constipation, irregular or otherwise abnormal periods, and possibly problems getting pregnant. Those who have an overactive thyroid (hyperthyroid) can have such symptoms as fatigue, hair loss, shortness of breath, constant hunger, unexplained weight loss, sweating, weakness, and irregular periods.

Thyroid conditions often run in families. The association between female family members is particularly strong: There's up to an 80 percent

Luteal Phase Deficiency

Some suggest that abnormal luteal function (when the luteal phase of the menstrual cycle is too short and therefore progesterone levels remain too low) may contribute to fertility challenges. However, most experts believe that luteal phase deficiency (LPD) doesn't exist on its own as a fertility challenge, but that it's actually a by-product of another underlying hormonal imbalance, such as a thyroid condition or hyperprolactinemia (see page 168). Research has shown that once a thyroid condition or too-high prolactin levels are treated, normal luteal function is usually restored as well, boosting the odds for conception and a healthy pregnancy.

chance that if your mother is affected, you will be at some point in your life, too. So if anyone in your family has been diagnosed with a thyroid condition, you probably should be tested if you're planning a pregnancy. Even if there's no family history, some experts recommend routine thyroid testing during the preconception period anyway—particularly if you're having trouble getting pregnant. Testing for abnormal

The Good News

A thyroid condition is one of the easiest chronic health problems to control and to treat—and one of the easiest fertility challenges to overcome. Taking your medications daily (your dosing may have to be adjusted once you become pregnant), keeping an eye on your thyroid levels to be sure they're stable (by having regular blood tests), and getting regular medical monitoring are the keys to your fertility success. Though your regular physician or gynecologist may be able to treat your thyroid condition successfully, it may be best to have an endocrinologist oversee your care.

thyroid antibodies may also be recommended. Even women who test normal for thyroid levels sometimes have abnormal thyroid antibody levels, a sign of a related autoimmune dysfunction.

How is fertility affected? Many women with a thyroid condition, especially when it's a mild case, have no problem getting pregnant. But for some women, unbalanced thyroid hormones can throw off that delicate balance of reproductive hormones, disrupting ovulation and leading to irregular periods and fertility struggles. That's because there is a close link between the endocrine system (the team that thyroid function plays on) and the reproductive system.

What are the treatment options? Treatment for a hypothyroid condition is usually as easy as popping a daily pill to normalize thyroid function and having regular blood tests to keep an eye on your levels. Treatment for a hyperthyroid condition (also known as Graves' diseases) sometimes includes anti-thyroid medication, but this therapy isn't used for women who are pregnant or planning to be. Radiation can be used to shrink or destroy the thyroid gland, but that option (again) isn't open to pregnant women (though you can probably TTC 6 months after this therapy).

Male Infertility

When a couple has difficulty conceiving, approximately 35 to 40 percent of the time the issue can be traced to the man—easily identified in a semen analysis or sperm count. Any deficiency in sperm count (the number of sperm), sperm motility (ability to move), forward progression (quality of movement), and/or sperm morphology (size and shape) can indicate fertility challenges.

What are some of the possible causes of a sperm disorder?

- Anatomical problems, such as scrotal varicocele (in which varicose veins around a testicle and abnormal blood flow to the area hinder sperm production—about 15 percent of men have varicoceles, and most can be repaired with surgery), retrograde ejaculation (in which the ejaculate flows backward into the bladder instead of out through the penis, common in men with long-standing diabetes), an undescended testicle (in which the testicle failed to complete its descent into the scrotum by infancy and therefore doesn't function normally), and blockages of any of the tubes that carry sperm (the result of a birth defect, injury, infection, or prior surgery, such as hernia repair or prostate surgery). Sometimes medications and/or surgery can correct these problems so that fertility is restored. Assisted-reproduction techniques (such as IVF) can also help get around these problems.

- Hormonal imbalance. It's not as common in men as it is in women, but occasionally a hormonal imbalance can trigger infertility. These imbalances can originate in the testicles or in the hypothalamus, pituitary, thyroid, or adrenal glands, but the bottom line is the same: The imbalance impacts production of testosterone and sperm. Once diagnosed, these imbalances can usually be treated effectively. For example, in the case of hypothalamic hypogonadism, when the testicles do not receive an adequate signal from the brain and the pituitary, hCG injections can get those signals up and running, restoring fertility.

- Testosterone replacement therapy. An increasingly common cause of abnormal semen analysis, and one that many men who take it and doctors who prescribe it aren't aware of: testosterone therapy can seriously impair sperm production. Ditto steroid use.

- Other medications. Certain prescription and even herbal medications can impact fertility in men. See page 14 for more.

- Uncontrolled chronic disease. For instance, uncontrolled diabetes can cause erectile dysfunction, and thus infertility. Another possible (and easily treated) cause of male infertility: untreated celiac disease. Getting chronic conditions under control can increase your chances of conception.

- Infection. Inflammation of the epididymis or testicles or some STDs can sometimes impact sperm production or block the tubes that carry sperm. If damage can't be reversed, sperm can be retrieved and used for IUI or IVF. Some childhood infections may also impact fertility, such as mumps (if contracted after puberty).

- Genetic abnormalities, including Klinefelter syndrome and Y-chromosome microdeletion, may be linked to male infertility. Men who carry the CF gene may have been born without a vas defererens (a tube that delivers sperm from the testicle out the urethra), making ejaculation (and thus natural conception) impossible. In these cases, sperm may be extracted directly from the testicles and used to conceive via IVF.

- Immune problems. In rare cases (more often after a vasectomy reversal), a man may produce antibodies that treat sperm as foreign invaders. These antibodies attack the sperm, adversely affecting sperm motility and sometimes its ability to fertilize an egg. Corticosteroids can be used to decrease the production of antisperm antibodies. If that fails, fertility treatments (such as IVF or ICSI; see pages 202 to 213) can help bypass the antibody problem.

- Obesity. Men who are obese or even overweight may have infertility problems. That's because excess fat converts the male hormone testosterone into the female hormone estrogen, possibly suppressing sperm production and lowering overall sperm quality. Weight loss can reverse this type of infertility.

- Underweight. Very low weight in men can be linked to lower sperm count and decreased sperm function. Once an underweight man gains weight, this fertility issue can disappear.

- Age. While men can be fertile well into their 80s, sperm quality and motility gradually start to decline at age 40. Sometimes this downward trend begins to affect fertility, sometimes it doesn't.

- Cancer treatments. Chemotherapy and radiation targeting certain areas of the body may contribute to fertility issues in men (see the box on page 168).

Lifestyle and environmental factors may be linked to male fertility problems—in these cases, eliminating the factor can eliminate the problem:

- Prolonged overheating of testicles (in hot tubs, hot baths, from laptops, or with electric blankets, for instance) can damage sperm.

- Extreme cycling (spinning, mountain biking, and so on) that puts too much pressure on the testicles, sports trauma to the penis and/or testicles, or extremely intense exercise routines may lower sperm production.

- Exposure to toxic substances (such as pesticides or other environmental or occupational hazards) or to excessive levels of radiation may affect sperm production and quality.

- Use of drugs (including pot and prescription painkillers), excessive use of alcohol, and smoking can also impact male fertility and sperm production.

- Some lubricants can affect sperm quality and motility—and some types can even kill sperm (see page 118 for more).

- Extreme emotional stress can also depress testosterone levels and thus sperm production.

- Though the jury is still out, there is some preliminary data that excessive cell phone and wireless device radiation may possibly alter sperm cells (see page 34).

A sperm analysis is an important step in a male fertility workup. But if you have concerns about the quality or health of your sperm, or if you suspect any kind of sperm disorder or testicular dysfunction, be sure to schedule an appointment with a doctor to check it out right from the start.

Cancer and Fertility

Each year, 140,000 men and women under the age of 45 in the United States are diagnosed with cancer. Cancer diagnoses are always heartbreaking, but they can be especially devastating to men and women who plan to have children one day. Happily, thanks to advanced treatment options, cancer survival rates for young people are at an all-time high. Though these treatments are lifesaving, some of them can also lead to infertility. Educating yourself about the fertility risks and options for becoming a parent after cancer is important so you can make the choices that are best for you.

So what are your options for saving your fertility before cancer treatments?

- Egg freezing. In this procedure, your eggs are retrieved after hormonal stimulation and then frozen until needed (see page 43).

- Embryo freezing. Once your eggs are retrieved, they are fertilized with sperm (from your partner or a donor) and the resulting embryos are frozen until needed.

- Ovarian tissue freezing. If you don't want to (or can't) have hormonal stimulation to retrieve eggs, ovarian tissue freezing is a surgical procedure in which ovarian tissue is removed, frozen, and then reimplanted after treatment with the hope that it will resume normal functioning. This procedure is promising, but still experimental.

- Ovarian shielding, or moving the ovaries outside the radiation field, is a method that minimizes the dangers of radiation to your ovaries and eggs and may be an option depending on the type of cancer you have and the treatments that are necessary.

Sometimes, fertility returns after treatment, making natural conception possible. If it turns out that your fertility has been permanently affected and you're unable to conceive naturally, you can use assisted reproductive techniques with the frozen eggs or embryos. Donor eggs can also be considered as an option. You'll need to discuss your situation with your doctor and oncologist to see whether pregnancy will be safe. Most of the time, it will be.

For men, cancer and its treatment can damage fertility, too. Sperm banking before treatment can preserve the ability to father a baby. Testicular tissue freezing is an experimental option that may be available for you, too.

Surgery to remove the thyroid gland is possible but not usually recommended. When treatment involves removing or destroying the thyroid gland, thyroid replacement hormone will easily deliver this essential hormone for life.

Once any thyroid imbalance is corrected, a thyroid condition shouldn't interfere with your fertility. Since thyroid needs change during pregnancy, it will be important to have your levels monitored closely once you've conceived.

Elevated Prolactin

What is it? Prolactin, a hormone produced by the pituitary gland, is responsible for producing breast milk after the birth of a baby. But some women have abnormally elevated levels of prolactin when they're not breastfeeding—a condition called hyperprolactinemia—and this imbalance of hormones can lead to irregular ovulation, missed periods, or no periods at all. Other signs of the condition can be a milky discharge from the nipples (again, without having recently had a baby). Blood tests can reveal if you have excess prolactin.

What causes elevated prolactin? Small benign tumors in the pituitary (seen on an MRI) can cause an increase in prolactin production, as can hypothyroidism, PCOS, a kidney condition, excessive stress, excessive exercise, lack of sleep, and some foods and medications. But sometimes no cause is found.

How is fertility affected? Too much prolactin interferes with communication among the hypothalamus, pituitary gland, and ovaries, leading to irregular periods and anovulation, which in turn affects fertility. High prolactin levels inhibit secretion of the hormone FSH, which stimulates the ovarian follicles to mature. Without FSH, there's no ovulation.

What are the treatment options? Once a follow-up blood test confirms high levels of prolactin, your doctor will try to figure out what's causing the hyperprolactinemia and tailor the treatment to the cause. You might simply need to stop taking a particular medication or be treated for hypothyroidism. Or your doctor may recommend medication to help bring prolactin levels back to normal, after which your chances of becoming pregnant are excellent.

The Fertility Workup

You've done your preconception homework, become a pro at pinpointing ovulation, and have your sex timing and positioning down to a (fun) science. But as hard as you try—and try, try again—to conceive, you've yet to score that positive pregnancy test. And now you're wondering what's keeping sperm and egg from meeting and creating the baby you're so looking forward to greeting. Is it you? Is it him? Is it both of you? Or is it just a matter of time? What's causing your fertility frustrations? And when should you stop trying and place a call to the doctor—or get a referral to a fertility specialist, so you can get some help getting pregnant? Read on to find out when you should start that fertility workup—and what you can expect when you do. (Read on, too, if you've been advised to get a fertility workup right from the start because of your age or another factor.)

Do You Need Help?

If your plans to start a family have been stuck in the planning stage longer than you anticipated, you might be thinking about seeing a fertility specialist to move things along. But would that be too much help too soon? Should you give your TTC efforts another month or 2—or even 6? Or should you call to schedule a fertility workup—just in case? Does your age, an irregularity in your cycles, a hormonal imbalance, or another factor bump up the chances you'll need a reproductive jump start—or more?

When to Get Help

"We've been trying to get pregnant for 6 months already. Is it time to find a fertility specialist?"

Considering how fundamental a human function it is (there couldn't be humans without it), conception isn't typically as easy to achieve as you'd think. Sure, it can happen overnight—or even after one early morning quickie—but it usually takes much longer. In fact, under the best of circumstances, a healthy, young couple with no known fertility issues has only a 20 to 25 percent chance of conceiving in a given menstrual cycle, which means they have a 75 to 80 percent chance of coming up empty at the end of any given cycle. So no need to jump to any conclusions about your fertility—or to jump in your car and head for the nearest fertility clinic—if sperm and egg don't meet up right away.

That said, if you've reached the 6-month mark of active trying (following all the recommended TTC guidelines) without accomplishing your mission, you might want to start thinking about next steps—though, depending on your age and other factors, it might be too early to actually start taking those steps right now. Here's the usual fertility rule of thumb when it comes to when to seek help:

- If you and your partner have no known reproductive problems and you're under 35, consider trying for a year without help.

- If you're older than 35 and don't have any known fertility issues, help is usually suggested after 3 to 6 months of trying without success, though you can seek it earlier if you're concerned about running out the reproductive clock before you finish your family.

- If you are 38 or older, many doctors recommend beginning those workups after just 3 months.

- If you're over 40 or have a history of medical problems or a family history of infertility or any other factors that might impede fertility, it makes sense to arm yourself with the right help right from the start, to give your more challenging campaign the best chance for success.

- If you have a history of pelvic inflammatory disease, miscarriage, irregular cycles or very painful periods, if you are significantly overweight or underweight, or if you know that your partner has a low sperm count or an anatomical issue like an undescended testicle or a scrotal varicocele, consider getting help if you've been trying for a few months without success.

But before you start Googling fertility specialists in your area, pick up the phone and make an appointment to see your regular ob-gyn. Find out if he or she can handle your fertility needs (at least any initial workup) or whether you'll likely need a specialist on board, too. Even if your particular fertility scenario calls for a specialist—either to consult or take over your diagnosis and treatment—your regular practitioner should still be in the loop and on the team.

Keep in mind that because many doctors—particularly specialists—book months in advance, it makes sense to call ahead of time to schedule a fertility workup, before you're even sure you'll need it. The worst-case (or rather the best-case) scenario: You make the appointment, and then have to cancel and schedule a prenatal visit instead—because you're pregnant!

Does Insurance Have You Covered?

Before you call to schedule an appointment with a fertility specialist, put in a call to your health insurance company. While more and more of the major insurance companies offer some kind of fertility coverage, policies vary . . . a lot. Your policy may determine what kind of health care provider you see, and what kinds of fertility tests and treatments are covered (if any) and in what sequence.

Are you getting the sense that your insurance company is giving you the runaround (or is turning you down for coverage you're pretty sure you are entitled to)? Make sure you do some more digging. What you're entitled to may depend on where you live: Some states have laws that require insurance providers to cover some type of basic infertility treatment, while other states require that plans cover IVF. But even those states that require some type of coverage may not mandate comprehensive coverage—which means you'll have to find a way to cover the rest out of pocket, and it may take deep pockets. In states where coverage isn't mandated, many health insurance policies will cover testing and evaluation to determine the cause of infertility, but far fewer will cover any treatments.

If you find you'll need to pay out of pocket, you'll have to do some financial planning to see how far you'll be able to take your treatments. Fertility

Which Specialist Is Best?

"I don't know the first place to start with finding a fertility specialist—all I know is we're having trouble conceiving and we have no clue why."

If sperm and egg aren't connecting on their own, which type of doctor would be the best matchmaker? Your ob-gyn is a good place to start, because he or she can begin a basic fertility workup and either treat your fertility issues or send you for a more complete workup and more advanced treatment with a reproductive endocrinologist (RE)—the technical title for someone who's a fertility specialist.

Fortunately, many fertility difficulties can be resolved by an ob-gyn without an extensive fertility evaluation or treatment by a fertility specialist. And even if you're sent to a specialist, it doesn't mean you're starting down the path of high-tech and expensive fertility treatments. In fact, couples can often be treated with simple medications and/or minor surgery and possibly IUI, although many end up having to turn to the more involved IVF.

Whichever type of doctor you're seeing (or even if you're seeing more than one), come prepared with a list of questions. Knowledge is power, and the more you know about tests and treatment options you might be facing, the less daunting they'll be to face. Here are some suggestions for questions you may want to ask your ob-gyn or RE:

- What tests and workups would you recommend to figure out why I haven't conceived yet?

- Should my partner get a workup, too? What tests will be involved? Should he be tested first or at the same time?

treatments can be expensive, especially if you go down the IVF route. For many couples, it's a good investment in their future, considering the odds of getting the return they're hoping for are very high (it's estimated that 70 percent of infertile couples who undergo fertility treatments succeed in having a baby, though the numbers are lower for women over 38). Just make sure you take into account, as you take a look at your budget, that it can take 2 or even 3 IVF cycles before a successful pregnancy is achieved. If at first you don't succeed, you'll need to consider how many times you'll be able to try again (at IVF centers with average success rates, nearly half of women under age 35, about 40 percent of women between ages 35 and 37, and a quarter of women between ages 38 and 40 do hit the baby jackpot with a healthy pregnancy and baby after just a single egg retrieval).

Another financial consideration: Will you be able to afford time off from work for fertility treatments, which can end up being very time consuming? Will your employer be amenable to giving you the time you'll need off, and will you feel comfortable sharing the reason why you need it? In some situations, you may be able to take time off under the federal Family and Medical Leave Act (FMLA) while you undergo treatments (though the leave will likely be unpaid). In some cases, you may be protected under the Pregnancy Discrimination Act (though protection varies from state to state).

For more on how to finance fertility treatments, see page 230.

- How much will all the testing cost?

- How long will it take to diagnose a problem if there is one?

- Based on the results of those tests, what are the treatment options?

- How much do the treatments cost?

- How long do we try one treatment option before we move on to another?

- What is your success rate with fertility treatments? (See the box on page 214 for more on how to make sense of a fertility clinic's success rates.)

Finding a Fertility Specialist

How do you go about finding a fertility specialist if you end up needing one? Your best lead will probably come from your ob-gyn, who will likely refer you to one he or she recommends and works with often. You can also ask friends who have had fertility challenges. Or go to the Society for Assisted Reproductive Technology website (sart.org) or contact RESOLVE (resolve.org) to find doctors on their physician referral list. You'll definitely want a specialist you feel comfortable with—one who comes with a stellar success rate and unbeatable credentials, but also an exam-side manner that puts you at ease—so consider a consult before you sign up for care.

At-Home Fertility Screening

Eager to assess the state of your fertility, but not ready to head off to the doctor's office for all that poking and prodding? Is your partner eager to make a baby but less than eager to produce an in-office sperm sample (even with the door locked from the inside)? There are some his-and-her screening test options that both of you can try at home, at least to get you started.

For him, it means measuring the concentration of motile sperm in his semen using a testing device that gives a result in lines (like a pregnancy test). One line indicates a low concentration of motile sperm, 2 lines indicate a normal concentration of motile sperm. There are also smartphone apps that can determine approximate sperm count and motility using a microscope attachment to the phone's camera and break down results to low, average, or above average. And how's this for at-home entertainment: Some apps allow you to watch sperm swimming on the smartphone screen.

For you, the at-home screening tests ovarian reserve by measuring the level of FSH on the third day of a period using a urine test similar to a pregnancy test. An abnormally high level of FSH suggests a low supply of eggs (low ovarian reserve; see page 110). One caveat: FSH levels can vary from month to month, so the level you get when testing it at home one month may not be representative of the overall level. Also,

your age should be factored in to the results. If you're over age 35, you probably won't want to rely on an at-home ovarian reserve test, since the results aren't as reliable (you might be falsely reassured by a false-normal result and put off getting professional fertility help that you need). In a doctor's office, you'll also be tested for other factors that will provide a more complete and accurate picture of your ovarian reserve.

Though these at-home screenings aren't a substitute for a thorough exam and evaluation by your ob-gyn or fertility specialist (the results are not definitive), they could give you a heads-up on what you might—or might not—find if you do eventually go for the full fertility workup. But remember, these tests are far from comprehensive in what they can look for—you'll be able to test only for the very basics, not for such fertility-related issues as blocked tubes, cysts, varicoceles, and so on. Plus, if the at-home screens do hint at a potential problem, you'll still have to get medical followup and in-office testing done. Same if the screens come up clean but conception continues to elude you.

Finally, though an at-home screening is definitely cheaper than a full-on fertility screening, it's still pricey (and usually isn't covered by insurance)—so you may want to consider if you'll be getting what you pay for before placing your order.

The Fertility Workup

"What's involved in a fertility workup? And do we both get one at the same time?"

Conception is definitely a team effort—but when it comes to fertility testing, one team member is likely to put in a lot more effort: you. Trying to find out why the seemingly simple process of reproduction isn't working can be a little complicated for women, so some doctors suggest that workups start with the male partner—especially because the workup for men is so much

Screening for Ovarian Reserve

How many high-quality eggs are in your reproductive basket? A screening for ovarian reserve can determine that, and it is often one of the first steps in a fertility workup. Ovarian reserve decreases with age, but most fertility specialists screen all patients. That's because diminished ovarian reserve isn't only age-related. It can also be linked to shorter menstrual cycles, a history of ovarian surgery, a history of chemotherapy, and a maternal family history of early menopause. Ovarian reserve screening can include:

- Blood tests measuring anti-mullerien hormone (AMH), follicle-stimulating hormone (FSH), and estradiol (E2). Read more about these hormones and tests for them in the box on page 110.

- Ultrasound to measure antral follicle count (or AFC; see page 176).

- The Clomid challenge test. This test, officially called the clomiphene citrate challenge test (or CCCT) measures day 3 FSH and estradiol in addition to day 10 FSH after your ovaries have been stimulated with a low dose of Clomid (100 mg daily on cycle days 5 through 9). CCCT is rarely used anymore unless it's required by an insurance provider. It has largely been replaced by AFC and AMH.

Has your screening shown low ovarian reserve? Discuss the results with your doctor, but try not to sweat the numbers too much. Keep in mind that a diminished ovarian reserve doesn't necessarily mean you won't be able to conceive either naturally or with assisted reproductive techniques. Ovarian reserve screening is one way to get a picture of your fertility and can help you and your doctor develop the best treatment approach for you. There are other screenings and tests that will contribute to that picture and that might be more helpful in determining why you're having trouble getting pregnant.

Since a woman's egg-creating days are over by the time she's born, eggs can't be replaced once they're lost. Though the hormone supplement DHEA has been touted as a possible way to boost ovarian reserve, studies haven't backed that up.

easier (as is the treatment of any diagnosed fertility issue). Other doctors suggest working up a couple simultaneously. Talk to your practitioner about the best way to proceed, and ask whether you should be worked up one at a time or in tandem. See the box on page 176 for all the details about what's included in the male fertility workup.

The female fertility workup can include multiple exams and tests. Here's what your workup may include:

A physical exam, if you haven't had one recently. Hop onto the exam table, because it's time for a physical, a comprehensive pelvic exam, a Pap test to rule out abnormal cervical cells, cultures or other tests to rule out infection, and a full medical and gynecological history. If you've had all these done recently, they won't need to be repeated (though if you're seeing a specialist instead of your regular ob-gyn, you'll probably be asked for a full medical and gynecological history again).

Blood tests. Roll up that sleeve and get ready for a variety of blood tests, including ones for:

The Male Fertility Workup

Though your partner is the one hoping to get pregnant, it takes 2 healthy people to make the dream of a baby a reality. If you and your partner are having trouble conceiving, you'll need to be tested, too, to make sure everything is working the way it should on your end. The male fertility exam can include all or any of the following:

Physical exam. A general physical as well as an evaluation of your health and medical history—including but not limited to sexual history, illnesses and infections, surgeries, medications, lifestyle habits such as smoking and alcohol and marijuana use, plus questions about exposure to radiation, steroids, chemotherapy, and toxic chemicals.

Genital exam. A thorough examination of the testes, scrotum, and penis, and perhaps a culture from the opening of the penis to rule out infection

(don't worry—it's quick, easy, and usually painless). Since one fairly common cause of male fertility difficulties is varicoceles (enlarged veins in the scrotum; see page 166), the doctor will carefully examine your testicles, too.

A semen analysis. While it's inherently unfair that the female workup involves needles and ultrasounds and the male workup involves masturbation, a semen analysis is a crucial first step in figuring out where the fertility problem might be originating. A sperm analysis checks the quantity and quality of sperm in your ejaculate (there should be more than 15 million sperm per milliliter of semen, more than 40 percent of them should be moving, and at least 4 percent should have a normal shape, aka morphology). If the numbers come back low, the test is repeated (sperm count varies from ejaculate to ejaculate).

You'll need to avoid ejaculation

- Progesterone. Detecting progesterone in your blood around day 21 of your cycle involves a simple test to confirm that you're ovulating.

- FSH and estradiol. Testing on day 3 of your cycle for the hormones FSH and estradiol can help determine your ovarian reserve (how many eggs you have available in your ovaries).

- Anti-mullerian hormone (AMH). Testing for AMH, which measures ovarian reserve, can be done at any time during your cycle. It's especially useful because it can identify a low ovarian reserve before FSH can.

- Other hormones. Thyroid and prolactin may also be checked, since abnormal levels of these hormones can affect fertility. If PCOS is suspected, testing for male hormones such as testosterone and DHEA-S may be ordered.

Ultrasound. Pelvic ultrasound (usually performed transvaginally) can help determine the number of egg follicles (called antral follicles) in the ovaries and how they are growing. An antral follicle count (AFC) is most accurate when performed within a few days of the start of your period. An ultrasound can also visualize the uterus and cervix, looking for anatomical abnormalities (such as fibroids or ovarian cysts). The 3-D

(from sex or from masturbation) for 2 to 5 days before the semen analysis so that sperm count will be at its highest. If multiple samples will be necessary, it's best to obtain them using the same spacing (in other words, if your first sample was produced 3 days after your last ejaculation, the next should also be produced after a 3-day wait). To produce the semen sample, you'll be asked to ejaculate into a clean sample cup—either in a private room in the doctor's office or, if you live close enough to the office, at home just before bringing it to the office for testing. If it's possible to produce the sample at home, be sure to get it to the office within an hour, carrying it in a bag or coat pocket, depending on the weather (it shouldn't get too hot or cold—room temperature is best). If the thought of masturbating into a cup isn't appealing to you, ask the doctor if you can use a special condom during intercourse to collect the sample instead. That sample, too, would have to be rushed to the lab (so much for the post-sex cuddling). If the sample must be produced in-office instead of at home, keep in mind that the staff at the facility will be completely professional and discreet. They'll also give you all the time and privacy you need—as well as an impressive choice of adult videos to get your mind off your sterile surroundings (and the fact that you're romancing a cup).

A blood test (especially if sperm concentration is low) to measure testosterone and prolactin levels.

A genetic blood test if genetic or chromosomal abnormalities are suspected.

A biopsy. If the semen analysis shows no sperm at all, the doctor might recommend a testicular biopsy (done using anesthesia) to see whether there is sperm in the testes. The presence of sperm production in the testes and an absence of sperm in the semen could indicate a blockage in the reproductive tract.

version of ultrasound can be even more helpful in some cases, such as when an abnormality of the uterus is suspected.

Hysterosalpingogram (HSG). This test is used to assess the uterus and fallopian tubes to make sure there is no scarring or any blockages that might be preventing conception. A small catheter is inserted into the cervix to allow liquid dye that can be seen on x-ray to fill the uterus and fallopian tubes. Once the liquid is injected, an x-ray is taken, showing the outline of the uterus and fallopian tubes. This test, performed 6 to 10 days after your period, is done with you awake, lying on an exam table. You might feel crampy when the liquid is injected, but that should go away after 10 minutes or so.

Hysteroscopy. In this simple procedure, a narrow endoscope is placed through the cervix into the uterus to visualize growths, such as polyps or fibroids, that might prevent conception or lead to a miscarriage.

Sonohysterogram. In this essentially painless test, the uterus is infused with saline (through the cervix) so it can be clearly visualized on ultrasound and checked for any anatomical abnormalities.

Pelvic MRI. Though expensive, this test can screen for fibroids, endometriosis, and congenital anomalies (defects you were born with)—possibly pinpointing the cause of your fertility challenges.

Genetic tests. Your doctor might recommend genetic testing if there's a suspicion that genetic or chromosomal abnormalities are contributing to infertility. A small blood sample is sent to a lab for evaluation.

Does it sound like you and your doctor have your work cut out for you during this workup? You definitely do. It will take about 6 to 8 weeks for all the tests to be completed and the results compiled and evaluated. Once that's all finished up, your doctor will discuss with you the best plan of action to help you conceive.

Subfertile vs. Infertile

"My doctor used a term I've never heard of before. She said I may be 'subfertile.' What does that mean?"

Often the terms "subfertile" and "infertile" are used interchangeably, but there are subtle differences between the definitions, and it sounds like your doctor is being extra precise about the state of your fertility.

What's the difference, precisely? An infertile couple (for example, the woman has lost both fallopian tubes or the man has no sperm) is completely unable to become pregnant without the help of reproductive technology. A subfertile couple is capable of getting pregnant (there's at least 1 open fallopian tube, eggs in the ovaries, and sperm available) but for some reason they aren't getting pregnant, at least not easily or quickly.

Sometimes, it might take a subfertile couple a few extra months (or even longer) than other couples to conceive. Or it might take more work for a

subfertile couple to conceive (with extra attention given to ovulation tracking or a little nudge to nature in the form of Clomid or another fertility med). Or it might mean that a subfertile couple is facing a hormonal challenge (like PCOS, for instance, or prolactin levels that are too high), but that once the condition is treated, they may be able conceive naturally. Or that conception the first time was easy but the second time isn't (known as secondary infertility, though it could more accurately be called secondary subfertility).

Some experts prefer to use the term "subfertile" instead of "infertile" because it doesn't seem to come with the same emotional baggage and the unfair stigma. It gives a couple hope—hope that all couples with fertility challenges should have—that though the road might be a little longer and perhaps a little bumpier, a baby will likely be in their future.

Bottom line: When your doctor says you're subfertile, he or she is likely convinced that you and your partner can conceive and probably will conceive —just that you might need some extra patience and, maybe, some extra help in the meantime.

Unexplained Infertility

"My partner and I haven't been able to conceive, so we both had fertility workups, and the doctor says he can't find anything wrong with either of us. Now what?"

So you've both been worked over, maybe more than once. You've done plenty of waiting—and more waiting— for the results. But it's all worth it, you figure, because finally, you'll have the diagnosis that will solve the mystery of why you haven't conceived yet, and with it, the treatment that will bring you one

Taking the Emotional Leap

You've put your all, and then some, into making a baby—devoting months to exhaustive fertility charting, exhausting sex-on-demand, and emotionally draining ups (it's time to test again!) and downs (it's negative again!). You and your partner have done absolutely everything you physically can to conceive on your own—but emotionally, you're not sure whether you're ready to look for help.

Beginning the fertility treatment process is an emotional leap. Making a baby is supposed to be a natural process, and a beautiful one—one that brings 2 people in love together in the most intimate of physical acts, so they can create a child who will forever be a symbol of that love. Taking that process out of the bedroom and into sterile exam rooms and treatment centers, making it a clinical experience instead of a personal one, can seem to steal some of its wonder and innocence. It's also, once and for all, an admission that you have a fertility problem, and no amount of trying and waiting is likely to change that. And that can be tough for you both to accept.

Not only are you not alone in your situation (about 12 percent of couples experience infertility) but you're not alone in feeling this way. Just about every couple experiences a wide range of conflicting emotions—from sadness to anticipation to guilt to ambivalence to jealousy of those who conceive with ease—as they contemplate ending one

path to conception and beginning another. But the truth is, the sooner you overcome this emotional hurdle, the sooner you can begin the treatment that can make your baby dreams come true.

Which isn't to say that getting the help you need will bring you the results you're hoping for right away (depending on the cause of your infertility, treatment may be quicker than you'd imagined or take even longer than you feared). There may be plenty of ups and downs ahead of you—just as there were when you were trying to conceive naturally. And considering the even higher stakes (especially if you're paying a premium for the treatments), any downs may be harder to handle. But the first step, deciding to take the leap and make that first round of appointments, is the most important one. You're on your way—and you're on your way together.

The more support you gather for your journey, the better. Look to each other, of course (open communication will help you both get through the experience and also help strengthen your bond), but turn, too, to those who know exactly what you're going through. Join a support group locally (click on Support at resolve.org) or online (try the message boards at WhatToExpect.com) to gain insights, reassurance, validation of your feelings, a chance to vent, and the pep talks and perspective you'll sometimes need.

step closer to filling your belly—and, ultimately, your arms—with the baby you've been hoping for.

Sometimes, it is as simple as that—diagnosing is straightforward and treatment is an easy fix. A correctable

condition is discovered, and all that's needed is minor surgery to remove some scarring or a cyst, some thyroid replacement therapy to jump-start your cycles, or a simple procedure to fix his undescended testicle. But that discovery isn't always easy, especially once the usual suspects of infertility are ruled out. Sometimes, a seemingly unrelated condition (for instance, celiac disease, which may lead to infertility in both females and males if it goes undiagnosed or untreated) is ultimately detected as the cause. But often, not even that exhaustive—and exhausting—full battery of tests and screenings (and needle pokes and embarrassing sperm collections) uncovers the exact cause of a fertility problem. Many couples, like you, end up with the finding "unexplained infertility." But isn't that where you started in the first place, before all the testing began?

You have lots of company. About 30 percent of couples seeking help because they've been unable to conceive are told they have unexplained infertility. There are plenty of eggs, lots of healthy, swift-swimming sperm, a fully functional uterus and fallopian tubes open for business, and hormone levels that are right on target. But for some unexplained reason, those healthy eggs and sperm aren't connecting to create the baby they've been trying for.

Fortunately, in most cases you don't need a definitive diagnosis to treat a fertility issue. No matter what the cause—and even if there is no known cause—there's usually at least one treatment option open. It could be as simple as making some lifestyle changes (you losing weight, him losing weight, both of you getting more exercise), or perhaps it may require a little nudge from medicine (for instance, with Clomid to stimulate ovulation). Or maybe you'll need to go a step further (to IUI) or even beyond that (to IVF). Read more about the available treatments for fertility (explained or unexplained) in the next chapter.

And try to keep this in mind, too: When you're eventually holding your baby in your arms, it probably won't really matter that modern medicine couldn't explain your infertility. All that will matter is that modern medicine helped put that baby in your arms.

CHAPTER 11

Fertility Treatments

I f you're like most couples, you probably didn't start out thinking that getting pregnant would be more than a 2-person job (and almost certainly didn't consider it might involve a team of other people wearing sterile exam coats and latex gloves). Or that there would be anything high-tech about the process (not counting the ovulation predictor kit or the fertility app). Maybe you knew that conception might not happen overnight, but you were pretty confident it would happen—and that just the two of you could make it happen, in the privacy of your own bedroom.

For about 12 percent of couples, however, getting pregnant does require some outside help, sometimes a little (from a regular ob-gyn writing a prescription for fertility medication), sometimes a lot (from a team of specialists performing procedure after procedure). And often it also comes with plenty of waiting (for appointments to be made, cycles to come and go, results to come in) and a high cost to pay—both financial and emotional. But (fertility fingers crossed) it will all be for the ultimate payoff: that beautiful bundle of baby you've been hoping for.

This chapter covers the most common fertility treatments. Read up

so you'll start the process with some idea of what you can expect—even if you're not sure yet what procedures you have ahead of you. Talk openly with your doctor or team of doctors about your concerns and questions, about risks, benefits, and odds of success. And talk, too, with your partner about the steps you're both about to take. Just remember as you do: Even if you're moving on to a whole new strategy (taking the baby making out of the bedroom and into the lab), even if you're signing on another baby-making team member or two (or more), your game plan is the same. Go out there and make a baby.

Artificial Insemination

Overcoming fertility challenges doesn't always mean complicated surgeries or high-tech procedures. In some cases, a couple needs just a little extra help to make the miracle of conception happen. Artificial insemination (AI) may be one of the oldest assisted reproduction techniques, but it's still a successful one. Because most couples who turn to AI don't do so because of female fertility problems, pregnancy rates are high—about 40 percent for younger women after up to 6 tries. AI is also one of the simplest techniques.

How simple? As simple as placing your partner's (or a donor's) sperm inside your reproductive tract when you're ovulating and letting conception take place naturally.

AI is usually performed when sperm count is on the low side, when sperm have poor motility, or when there is just no known infertility cause but it's clear that nature could use a nudge. It can help, too, when the cervical environment or cervical mucus is hostile to sperm, making it hard for them to swim. Same-sex couples can also turn to AI for

Sperm Washing

Maybe you've already heard that sperm being used for IUI have to be washed first—and chances are you're wondering: Why would sperm need washing, and how does it get washed? In IUI, your partner's sperm (or donor sperm) is inserted directly into your uterus. That's good for those little swimmers, since it cuts down on travel time to Destination Egg. But there's a major potential downside for them, too. Sperm that bypass the vagina and cervix don't come into contact with cervical mucus. You already know how important cervical mucus is for figuring out where you are in your cycle. But it also plays another role—getting sperm ready for fertilizing action. When sperm comes right from the source (aka "raw" sperm), it hasn't undergone this vital preparation. Enter, sperm washing—a process that does the job cervical mucus can't do when sperm is being injected directly into the uterus, as it is during IUI.

Why can't raw, unwashed semen be used in IUI? First, that seminal fluid contains prostaglandins—chemicals that cause muscle contractions. If those prostaglandins were to find their way into the uterus, they could cause severe cramps, which not only could prove uncomfortable, but also might keep a fertilized egg from implanting. Second, straight-from-the-source semen contains bacteria, white blood cells, and assorted substances that could be toxic to your waiting egg or cause infection. Finally, when semen enters your reproductive tract the traditional way, through the vaginal canal, the cervical mucus helps sperm release enzymes in a process called capacitation. These enzymes enable the sperm to eventually burrow into an egg. Without the capacitation process, the sperm would be unable to perform its most fundamental of functions: fertilization.

help starting their family (either themselves or with a surrogate), as can single women who want to become moms on their own.

AI can be used without fertility medication, assuming all is well in the ovulation department, or in conjunction with meds if ovulation issues have been identified as well (see page 187). The success rate of AI is twice as high when combined with Clomid or other ovulation inducers compared with AI alone, but not all women need both to achieve pregnancy. Fertility drugs are usually not needed when using donor sperm for AI.

Intrauterine Insemination (IUI)

Intrauterine insemination aims to give sperm a better chance of reaching their target by bypassing the initial hurdles they would encounter in the vagina and cervix—sort of a running (or swimming) head start. The majority of couples using IUI have unexplained infertility or mild male factor fertility problems.

How does IUI work? Around the time you're ovulating (either on your own—called natural-cycle IUI—or with the help of Clomid or another ovulation induction medication) and using a

---

Sperm washing (no matter how it's done) takes on all of the responsibilities nature generally reserves for cervical mucus, optimizing the sperm in an effort to maximize the odds of fertilization. The process of washing separates sperm from the semen and separates nonmotile sperm from motile sperm. It purifies the sperm, removing potentially toxic substances and fluid. And it improves sperm capacitation, a necessary part of a successful conception.

But how is sperm washing done? In one of these ways:

- Simple sperm wash. Thawed frozen or fresh ejaculate is placed in a test tube and diluted in a solution of antibiotics and proteins. The test tube is then placed in a centrifuge—a machine that spins around at rapid speeds (think of it as the spin cycle for sperm). As the semen mixture is spun, sperm cells fall to the bottom of the test tube. These sperm are then removed from the test tube and used in IUI.

- Density gradient sperm wash. Considered the "premium" of sperm washes, this technique is also the most popular. Thawed frozen or fresh ejaculate is placed in a test tube filled with multiple layers of liquids of different densities. The test tube is then placed in a centrifuge where it is spun, separating the healthy, swimming sperm (which fall to the bottom layer of liquid) from dead sperm, white blood cells, and seminal debris (which end up in the top 2 layers). Once the top layers are removed, only the healthy, active sperm remain, ready to be put to use in IUI.

- Swim-up technique. This technique uses a layering technique that separates the healthiest and strongest sperm. A special liquid called a culture medium is placed on top of thawed frozen or fresh semen in a test tube. The super-high-quality sperm are attracted to this culture medium and swim up into it. These healthy, potent sperm are collected and used for IUI.

concentrated sperm sample that has been "washed" (basically, preparing sperm for fertilization; see the box on page 182), your doctor will insert a thin, flexible catheter through your cervix (which will already be slightly open since the procedure is done when you're ovulating) and inject the healthy sperm directly into the uterus, close to the fallopian tubes, where fertilization takes place. Hitching this ride through the vagina and the cervix cuts down on the swimming sperm have to do, making it more likely that they'll reach their target on time. The same process occurs whether your partner's sperm or donor sperm is being used. The whole procedure—with

you lying on the exam table and with your feet in stirrups as they would be for a pelvic exam—takes only a couple of minutes, and there isn't much discomfort (about as much as you'd have during a Pap test). Once the insemination is complete, you'll be asked to lie on your back for a brief period. Most women can return to regular activity right after the procedure (no need to worry if you experience light spotting for a day or two after your IUI). The goal: to get those sperm close to the fallopian tube so they can be at the right place at the right time to fertilize your egg.

If you're using fresh sperm (see page 226 for more on fresh vs. frozen

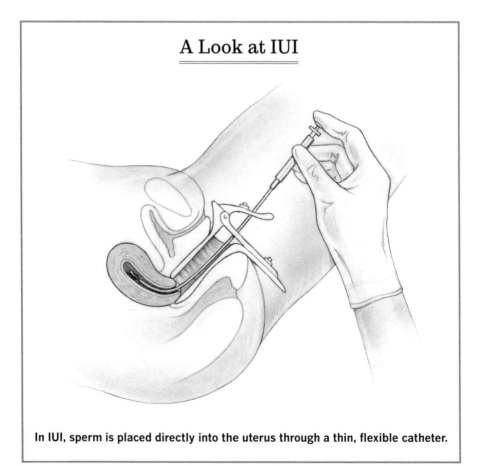

A Look at IUI

In IUI, sperm is placed directly into the uterus through a thin, flexible catheter.

sperm), your partner or donor will need to abstain from ejaculation for at least 48 hours before the procedure (ask the doctor for guidelines) and then provide his sperm sample (either in the clinic's collection room or at home) the same day as your IUI, making sure that the sperm is handed over about 1 to 1½ hours before the IUI. The sample should not be produced more than 2 hours before your scheduled IUI procedure. The insemination takes places as soon as the sperm washing is complete.

Though the IUI success rate depends on a host of variables (your age, your fertility profile, sperm quality, whether fertility medication is used, and so on), you can expect a success rate of anywhere from 5 to 20 percent per IUI. If you still haven't achieved conception success after 3 to 4 rounds of IUI, you'll likely be advised to move to the next step: IVF.

IUI isn't recommended for women who have significant fallopian tube blockages or conditions, a history of pelvic infections, or significant endometriosis. IUI is also not usually attempted in women over 40. Finally, if your partner has a very low sperm count, or significant problems with sperm motility or morphology (the percentage of sperm that appear to be of normal shape and size), IUI is not likely to be successful.

Fallopian Sperm Transfer Insemination (FAST)

If placing sperm close to the fallopian tubes gives them a better shot at reaching and fertilizing their egg target, would depositing them directly into the fallopian tubes give them the best shot of all? That's the theory behind

---

Is It Wet in Here, or Is It Me?

Some women report feeling "wetter" after IUI. If that happens to you, don't worry. While some sperm may drip out, your cervix does a pretty good job of keeping most of the sperm in. Besides, the healthy sperm are already swimming upstream to your fallopian tubes, en route to their target. So why so wet? Sometimes the catheter used to deposit the sperm in your uterus loosens cervical mucus, allowing it to leak out more easily. Remember, too, that IUI is performed when you're ovulating, which means there's already mucus aplenty. Take a look at that wetness, and you'll likely see that it's of the fertile variety—egg-white-like in texture—indicating that you're ovulating exactly when you want to be!

---

the FAST technique, in which washed sperm is inserted directly into the fallopian tube so it can meet up with the egg just after ovulation. However, studies show that FAST offers no advantage over standard IUI when it comes to conception success (in other words, it's not so FAST after all).

At-Home Artificial Insemination

While there are definitely more effective fertility treatments, there are none as low tech as at-home AI. Some TTC couples opt to give AI a shot at home before moving on to the bigger fertility guns available in a clinic setting—either because they'd like to skip the fertility doctor (and fertility doctor bills) if possible, or they'd like to keep fertilization a more intimate experience ("just the two of us"), or have other privacy concerns. Single women or lesbian couples may also consider at-home AI first, before turning the insemination process over to a professional. But keep in mind that for heterosexual couples DIY AI offers no fertility edge over DIY sex.

As with IUI, sperm for at-home AI can be provided by a woman's partner or by a donor (fresh sperm or thawed frozen can be used). Also as with IUI, timing is everything: You'll need to inject the sperm as close to ovulation time as you can possibly calculate. And at-home AI, like IUI performed in a clinic, won't be effective if you have ovulation problems. It will also be met with less success if your partner has a low sperm count or poor-quality sperm. Unlike IUI, at-home AI places sperm close to the cervix, not in the uterus, which is why sperm doesn't have to be washed first.

Thinking of going DIY with your AI? There are a few ways you can try this fertility technique at home:

- One commonly used DIY AI technique is often referred to as the "turkey baster method." Using a needleless syringe or medicine syringe, you'll inject freshly ejaculated semen that has been collected in a clean plastic cup or collection condom or frozen donor sperm that has been thawed according to the sperm bank's directions. Place the end of the syringe in the pool of semen and draw the plunger back, sucking up as much of the semen as you can. Turn the syringe so that the opening is facing upward, tap out any air bubbles, and depress the plunger just enough to get rid of the air (you don't want to inject air into your vagina). Then lie down, preferably with your hips raised, and

gently guide the syringe into the vagina until it is close to, but not touching, the cervix. Then slowly inject the sperm.

- Another option is using a birth control cervical cap or diaphragm (both are available by prescription only) or a period collection cup (which is available over the counter). Fill the cup, cap, or diaphragm with the fresh or thawed frozen semen, then insert it over your cervix, leaving it in place for 2 to 3 hours.

- You can also use an at-home AI kit that comes with a condom-like sheath attached to a cervical cap where the sperm collects. Then, using the included insemination tool, the cervical cap is placed against the cervix so the sperm get as close as possible to the uterus.

Before you give DIY AI a try, think about both the risks and the rewards. The rewards are obvious if you succeed inseminating at home: conception, at a relatively low cost. The risks are less obvious, but there are some. Some medical experts warn that at-home insemination (because it's not performed by medical professionals or in a medical setting) can cause tissue damage, uterine perforation, and even infection if insertion is too deep or done improperly. And then there's the legal risk if you're using donor sperm, since the legal protections afforded by medically supervised donor sperm used for IUI in a fertility clinic—things like the automatic termination of the donor's parental rights—don't always cover women who artificially inseminate at home (the laws vary from state to state, so do check your state's statutes). In other words, insemination that is done without the supervision of a licensed medical professional can end up with the sperm donor legally claiming parenthood.

There are risks, too, if you're using a friend as the sperm donor for your DIY AI, especially if you haven't had that donor medically tested and/or had the sperm tested and screened to make sure it's safe and healthy. Plus there are the legal risks. Sure, you may all be friends now and all on the same page about the arrangement, but what happens without legal protection for your child or the donor friend? Who claims paternity? Who is responsible for child support? What if you can't agree to agree down the road on issues like these?

If you think at-home insemination is for you, have a conversation with your doctor to make sure you'll be doing it properly to minimize health risks. And if you're using donor sperm, be sure to talk to a lawyer to make sure all the legal i's are dotted and t's are crossed.

Inducing Ovulation with Medication

If your fertility workup shows you're not ovulating regularly, you've got plenty of company. About a third of all women struggling to get pregnant have ovulation issues, sometimes explained, often not. But for many, there's an easy fix in a little pill. Clomiphene citrate (brand name Clomid) and other oral fertility drugs (such as Femara) stimulate your ovaries to release eggs and correct irregular ovulation. Oral fertility meds can also be given to women who are already ovulating on their own, but for some reason are not conceiving. The medications can help stimulate extra follicles to develop in the ovaries, boosting the chances of conception.

Clomid

Clomid works by making your body think estrogen levels are low (who said you can't fool Mother Nature?). When your body believes estrogen levels are low, it compensates by producing more FSH and LH, stimulating the development of the follicle and egg and causing ovulation to occur. After that, it's a sort of domino effect—but the good kind (the kind that's meant to knock you up, not knock you down). The development of the eggs kicks up your estrogen, which in turn helps produce better-quality cervical mucus (for most, but not all women—some women find their CM becomes dry and sticky while on Clomid), making it easier for those sperm to hitch a ride toward the egg or eggs now being released. And there's more to this chain of happy events: More eggs mean more progesterone (produced by the corpus luteum that's left behind after an egg is released). More progesterone also helps build a strong uterine lining for that fertilized egg to latch on to, plus helps maintain a new pregnancy. Clomid may be used alone or with IUI.

Here's what to expect if your doctor decides to try to induce or boost ovulation with Clomid. You'll begin by taking 50 mg of Clomid per day for 5 days, beginning on day 2, 3, 4, or 5 of your cycle. If you don't begin to ovulate right away during your first cycle— usually between day 14 and day 19 as determined by an OPK—the dose will be increased by 50 mg per day each month up to 150 mg (some doctors will go as high as 200 mg, or even 250 mg).

Clomid for Men?

You probably wouldn't be surprised to hear that your partner may need to take some fertility drugs to help improve the chances of conception success. But did you know that you might possibly be on the receiving end of fertility drugs, too? The truth is, just as women need the right balance of hormones to ovulate regularly, men need the right balance of hormones to produce enough healthy sperm to fertilize an egg. And if fertility testing shows that you have a low sperm count because your hormones are out of whack, it's possible you'll be the one popping those fertility pills.

Clomid, used mainly to induce ovulation in women, can be used in some cases to boost a hopeful dad's sperm production. Some men with low sperm counts have low levels of the primary male hormone, testosterone. Clomid—25 mg taken daily or every other day—increases the production of FSH and LH (yes, even in men). The increase in FSH leads to an increase in sperm production, and more LH leads to an increase in testosterone production. Men with a low sperm count may also benefit from Femara (it boosts testosterone levels; see the facing page), Anastrozole (a drug similar to Femara), hCG or hMG injections (see page 191).

Still, treating men with fertility drugs isn't common, at least not yet. That's because even though there is evidence that certain fertility drugs may work for men, the findings are limited. If you're wondering if your infertility issues might be helped with fertility drugs, ask your fertility specialist.

Once the drug is working and you've begun to ovulate, you'll likely be kept on Clomid for 3 to 6 months. Your doctor will probably give you blood tests (on top of the OPKs) to make sure ovulation is occurring and may monitor you with regular ultrasounds to make sure you're stimulating enough eggs but not too many eggs (called hyperstimulation; see the box on page 192). If you haven't conceived by the 6th month on Clomid (whether you're taking it alone or in conjunction with IUI), you'll move on to other medications (see the facing page) or hormone shots (see page 190) and/or assisted-fertility techniques. Approximately 80 percent of women will ovulate, and 30 percent will become pregnant within 3 months of being started on Clomid.

Something to keep in mind: Since Clomid increases LH, which is the hormone detected by OPK testing, it is important not to start OPK testing too early in the cycle, or you may get a false positive result. It's best to wait until cycle day 10 or 11 before starting OPK testing.

Happily, there are few side effects with Clomid, and if you do experience them (bloating, nausea, headache, hot flashes, breast pain, mood swings, and in rare cases, ovarian cysts), don't worry—they're only temporary. Some women also experience vaginal dryness.

Taking Clomid does increase the chance that more than 1 follicle and egg will be stimulated. In fact, you'll have a 7 percent chance of conceiving twins using Clomid compared with a 1 percent chance of conceiving twins naturally. The chances of higher order multiples (triplets or more) are low with Clomid. Because extra babies equal extra risks to your pregnancy, your health, and the health of your babies (as well as the very low chance of ovarian hyperstimulation), your doctor will keep you on the lowest dose of Clomid possible.

Femara (Aromatase Inhibitor)

If you haven't met with ovulation success on Clomid, you may have better luck with another class of fertility drugs called aromatase inhibitors—especially if you have PCOS. Though the FDA has not approved these meds for infertility (they're used in breast cancer treatment), many fertility doctors prescribe Femara (the brand name for letrozole, an aromatase inhibitor) to help induce ovulation, with positive results. One advantage to Femara over Clomid is that it stimulates fewer follicles and results in lower estrogen levels, theoretically reducing the chance of conceiving multiples. It also has a shorter half-life (meaning it stays in your system for a shorter time) than Clomid.

Metformin and Fertility

Is metformin the answer to your PCOS-triggered fertility problems? It is true that women with PCOS who take Clomid plus metformin do ovulate more regularly than those skipping the metformin. But studies show that the diabetes drug doesn't improve the rate of successful pregnancy, whether it's taken alone or along with Clomid. For that reason, though metformin may be used as part of your PCOS treatment plan, it isn't considered a first-line fertility drug.

Clomid or Femara: Which Is Right for You?

Femara is probably the best choice if you have PCOS and do not ovulate regularly.

Clomid remains the preferred choice for unexplained infertility, particularly if you'll be doing IUI.

And if your fertility problems have been caused by PCOS, here's the really good news: Femara is more likely to induce ovulation in women with PCOS than Clomid—and to result in a successful pregnancy and a healthy birth, too.

Like Clomid, Femara suppresses estrogen, which in turn increases FSH production—stimulating the ovarian follicles to mature and triggering ovulation. If your fertility specialist recommends Femara, you will likely be given 2.5 mg per day on days 5 through 9 of your cycle. In some cases, a higher dose—5 mg or 7.5 mg per day—is given. Women treated with Femara have significantly fewer hot flashes than those treated with Clomid, but often report mild dizziness and fatigue.

Not all doctors feel comfortable using Femara to induce ovulation—both because it is considered "off-label" (not FDA-cleared for fertility use) and because of some concern that it might be linked to an increase in birth defects (the link hasn't been proven). If you're concerned about using Femara or wondering why Femara hasn't been offered as an option for you (especially if you have PCOS), be sure to have a conversation about it with your fertility specialist, one that includes a discussion of potential risks and benefits.

Inducing Ovulation with Hormone Shots

If oral fertility drugs like Clomid or Femara (on their own or with IUI) don't do the trick, your doctor may opt to kick it up a notch with hormone shots, which pack a more powerful fertility punch. These injectable hormones (you'll inject them at home) contain a high concentration of FSH and LH, so they work directly on the ovaries to help mature the follicles and eggs and stimulate ovulation—basically triggering the same reproductive chain reaction as oral fertility drugs do, but with much more bang. Hormones shots may be used if you're not ovulating regularly and haven't responded to Clomid or Femara, but would still like to TTC with timed sex or via IUI. Injectable hormones will also be prescribed if you'll be undergoing IVF.

Are you using hormone shots to boost ovulation, and plan to TTC through timed sex or IUI? Then low and slow will be the way to go. With low and slow, the dose of hormone shots starts out very low and is increased gradually every 4 to 7 days until the ovaries start to respond (as measured by blood estrogen levels and ultrasound changes). The goal with a low and slow approach: to produce only 1 to 2 mature eggs at a time—and ultimately, hopefully, only 1 baby. After all, multiple mature eggs encountering sperm in your fallopian tubes or uterus can result in multiple embryos and a high-order multiple pregnancy, which comes with multiplied risks. Carrying a single baby is much safer than carrying twins, triplets, quads, or more.

Taking hormone shots because you're planning IVF? You'll need more eggs, not fewer (an average egg retrieval in an IVF cycle aims for 10 to 15 eggs). So while your fertility specialist will still proceed carefully when using hormone injections to stimulate your ovaries (to avoid overstimulating them; see the box on page 192), the doses of hormones will be higher when you're having IVF.

Some common side effects of hormone injections include breast tenderness, mood swings, headache, abdominal pain, and nausea. In rare cases, ovarian hyperstimulation may occur. In most cases, women taking hormone shots notice more cervical mucus. This happy side effect might actually aid in your conception quest if you'll be trying a side of natural baby-making sex even as you pursue IVF.

Are you the squeamish type? Your partner can learn how to do the injecting, so you won't have to. Both of you are needle-phobic? You likely won't be after a few practice runs (see page 194 for more).

Types of Hormone Shots

Here's the rundown on some of the hormone shots (also known as gonadotropins) you might need, but keep in mind that depending on your situation and your doctor's preferences, you may be prescribed only 1 or 2 of these medications, or several. Keep in mind, too, that it may take several cycles and adjustments in your medication cocktail (adding on, changing it up) before you hit your optimal fertility prescription. Since every woman's fertility needs are different, every woman's fertility treatment plan will be different. To save yourself some stress and confusion, try not to compare your hormone injections with those of other hopeful moms you know (or meet in the doctor's waiting room, or hang out with on your TTC message board) who are undergoing similar treatments.

Follicle-stimulating hormone (FSH). These injections (brand names include Bravelle, Follistim, and Gonal-F) act like your own natural FSH to stimulate the growth of follicles and maturation of your eggs. You'll need to inject FSH once or twice daily, usually starting on days 2 to 4 of your cycle.

Human menopausal gonadotropin (hMG). While "menopausal" doesn't sound promising when you're trying to get pregnant, these hormones can deliver. The injections (brand names include Menopur and Repronex) contain both FSH and LH—2 important hormones necessary for stimulating the development of the follicles and the maturation of the eggs. You'll take the injection daily or twice a day, usually starting on days 2 to 4 of your cycle for about 12 days.

Human chorionic gonadotropin (hCG). This sounds more like it (after all, hCG is the pregnancy hormone). The brand names of this type of hormone injection include Ovidrel, Novarel, and Pregnyl, and they are used in conjunction with FSH and hMG injections, or even in

Monitoring While You're Stimulating

Since your eggs require both LH and FSH, most stimulation protocols include a combination of FSH and hMG, given for anywhere from 10 to 13 days. To keep an eye on your response to the medicines while you're on them, you'll need 5 to 7 blood tests to measure hormones and repeat ultrasounds to measure the growth of ovarian follicles. Your doctor might tweak the schedule and type of hormone shots, depending on the results of these tests. A lot of monitoring, but hopefully well worth it!

conjunction with Clomid. Known as the "trigger shot," hCG will help to trigger ovulation, mimicking the natural LH surge. When 1 or more follicles reach the point of no return (ready to release a mature egg), you'll inject the hormone hCG to push the final maturation steps and trigger ovulation. Ovulation will usually occur 36 to 40 hours after hCG is injected. Another bonus from the hCG: It improves the quality of the uterine lining, effectively plumping and fluffing it for the arrival of an embryo.

One thing to keep in mind if you're getting hCG injections is that early home pregnancy tests won't be accurate. HPTs look specifically for hCG in the urine, since it's a hormone that shows up in the body naturally only once an embryo implants. If you're receiving hCG through injections, any pregnancy test you take while hCG is still in your system (at least 10 days after it's injected) will be considered a false positive.

Taking the Plunge

Needle-phobic by nature? Afraid to take the plunge . . . into your soft, delicate skin? Some needle novices find it helps to start with some fruit for practice. Using an empty syringe (no need to shoot up a plum with hormones), stab away until you're feeling like a pro—at least when it comes to produce.

Ovarian Hyperstimulation Syndrome

All those hormones you inject yourself with are designed to stimulate your ovaries just enough to allow the right number of follicles and eggs to grow and mature—definitely a good thing if you've been having trouble in the ovulation department. But in a small number of women using these medications (less than 5 percent), that stimulation becomes too much of a good thing, resulting in ovarian hyperstimulation syndrome (OHSS). OHSS occurs when ovaries hyperstimulated by FSH or hMG are exposed to hCG. Early OHSS, which happens within days after an hCG injection and lasts only a few days, is usually mild. Late OHSS develops after a successful implantation (when the body starts to produce hCG naturally), usually a week or more after egg retrieval in an IVF cycle, and sometimes as late as 3 weeks after a positive pregnancy test. Late OHSS often lasts much longer, and may be more severe and more dangerous than early OHSS.

If you develop mild OHSS, you'll notice ovarian and abdominal swelling, mild pain, mild nausea, vomiting, and/or diarrhea. With moderate OHSS you'll experience the same symptoms, and an ultrasound will show a collection of fluid inside your abdomen.

If you notice any symptoms of OHSS, call your doctor or the fertility clinic the same day. If the symptoms are severe, call right away, since there is a risk of serious complications, including kidney problems and blood clots in the lungs. Symptoms of severe OHSS include:

- Rapid weight gain (2 or more pounds a day)
- A collection of fluid in the abdomen
- Severe bloating
- Severe abdominal pain
- Ovarian tenderness
- Diarrhea
- Severe nausea and vomiting
- Decreased urination
- Shortness of breath

Gonadotropin-releasing hormone (GnRH) agonist. Sometimes FSH or hMG injections can stimulate the release of eggs before they are mature. Enter a GnRH agonist (fortunately you don't have to spell or pronounce any of these medications, you just have to inject them—plus brands include the easier-to-ask-for-by-name Zoladex and Lupron). GnRH agonist works on the pituitary gland to help prevent immature eggs from being released too soon. It does so by first increasing and then suppressing FSH and LH, preventing the LH surge (which triggers ovulation) and allowing additional time for more high-quality eggs to develop. It also helps produce a greater number of high-quality eggs. You'll probably start injecting GnRH agonist between a couple of days and a couple of weeks before FSH and hMG shots are started if you're doing an IVF cycle.

Gonadotropin-releasing hormone (GnRH) antagonist. Like GnRH agonists, this hormone injection (its brand names include Ganirelix and Cerotide) is used in IVF cycles to prevent a too-soon LH surge—ensuring that eggs are

- Low blood pressure

- Blood test abnormalities (elevated potassium, low sodium, elevated white blood count, elevated hematocrit)

Mild OHSS usually resolves on its own within a week or two. To help speed recovery, get plenty of rest but continue with light activity, keep your feet elevated when you can, and drink plenty of electrolyte-rich fluids. You can also take a mild pain reliever (acetaminophen) if necessary. If you become pregnant, the pregnancy is likely to proceed normally. However, keep in mind that if you develop OHSS in the middle of an IVF cycle, your fertility specialist may opt to cut the cycle short to avoid pregnancy (the eggs or embryos will be frozen for transfer at a later date) so that your OHSS can resolve more quickly.

If your OHSS is moderate, treatment might include painkillers, antinausea meds, adequate electrolyte-rich fluid intake, support stockings to prevent blood clots, and monitoring with ultrasounds, blood tests, measurements of urine output, daily weigh-ins, and physical exams.

If your OHSS is severe, you may need to be admitted to the hospital for more aggressive treatment, including IV fluids, draining excess abdominal fluid (via a needle into the abdominal cavity), and medication to relieve your symptoms and prevent the risk of blood clots.

What puts a woman at higher risk of OHSS? There are a number of factors that may contribute, including having PCOS, being under age 35, being underweight, having high levels of estrogen during fertility treatments, and having had OHSS before. Fortunately, if you fall into a high-risk category, your doctor can reduce the chances of OHSS by making several adjustments to your stimulation treatment. These include using the lowest possible dose of hormones needed to stimulate the ovaries, using a GnRH antagonist rather than an agonist to prevent premature ovulation, using Lupron (leuprolide) rather than hCG to trigger ovulation, and freezing your embryos rather than doing an immediate embryo transfer (see page 218).

released when they are mature and not before. GnRH antagonists work much faster than GnRH agonists, so they don't have to be started before FSH and hMG shots. Instead, they're likely to be started at least 5 to 7 days after starting FSH and hMG. Who's a good candidate for GnRH antagonists? On one end of the spectrum, they're used in some women who respond poorly to FSH and hMG. On the other end, they're prescribed for women at risk of responding too well to those hormones—and ending up with ovarian hyperstimulation syndrome (OHSS; see

the box above). OHSS is less common when using a GnRH antagonist.

Progesterone. The hormone progesterone (known as the pro-pregnancy hormone) keeps you pregnant once you've conceived—preventing miscarriage and helping ensure your pregnancy (and that newly conceived baby) thrives. In natural cycles, the ovary produces progesterone until you are about 2 months pregnant, at which point the placenta takes over the responsibility. Not so in IVF cycles, where GnRH agonist and antagonists prevent the ovary from

Do Fertility Drugs Come with a Cancer Risk?

Can fertility drugs and shots increase your risk of cancer? Happily, the answer to that question is no. Studies have shown that there is no increased risk of ovarian or breast cancer in women taking fertility drugs. Ditto for an added risk of other cancers, such as melanoma, or cervical or colon cancer. So no need to worry that extra help getting pregnant will result in an extra risk to your health. Put that stress to rest while you're following your doctor's orders on fertility meds.

making progesterone. Consequently, your IVF pregnancy needs supplementary progesterone to pick up the baby-sustaining slack until the placenta is ready to assume the job. Progesterone can be taken as an intramuscular injection (see page 197) or via the vagina as a gel or suppository.

Injecting Yourself with Hormone Shots

So, chances are you've been on the receiving end of your fair share of needles over the years—but unless you're a medical professional or diabetic, it's not likely you've ever given an injection, particularly not to yourself. Yet if hormone injections are going to be a part of your fertility treatment plan, inject you must (that is, unless you can talk your partner into wielding the needle—if so, have him read over this how-to, too).

Don't try your first stab at real injections at home, though. You'll feel more comfortable if you (or your partner) tackle that first shot attempt at your doctor's office, under close supervision and with supportive guidance. You'll be given specific instructions on when, where (in the muscle or under the skin), and how to give the injections. It's best to follow doctor's orders, of course, but just in case you've forgotten the basics by the time you get home (or you blank on everything that the doctor or nurse showed you yesterday), here's a step-by-step guide. Keep in mind that the first few times may be stressful (especially for the squeamish), but before you know it, you'll be injecting with ease.

1. Pick a spot in your home. Ideally, you'll want to find a quiet area where there will be minimal distractions (and away from any clamoring kids or curious pets). Also important is that the area is clean, for obvious reasons. The bathroom or kitchen are good choices because of the countertop space, and because they're easy to sanitize (compared with the living room sofa).

2. Set up. Wash your hands and set up a clean zone on a countertop to spread out your injection supplies (medication, syringes, alcohol swabs, needles, and disposal container). If you're going to want to numb your skin first, you'll need some ice handy, too. Make sure the needles do not touch anything other than the medication containers or the injection site—otherwise they'll become contaminated and unusable (in other words, keep the cap on the needle until you're ready to use it—just like the professionals do).

3. Choose the right syringe and needle (as directed by your doctor). If you're injecting the drug into your muscle (intramuscular), you've probably been told to use a 1-mL or 2-mL syringe. If you're injecting the drug under your skin (subcutaneous), you'll probably use a 1-mL syringe. Needles for subcutaneous injections are shorter (usually only ½ inch long) than ones for intramuscular injections (1 to 2 inches long). If you need to mix the solution, you'll have to attach the large "mixing needle" firmly to the syringe first (illustration A).

4. Prepare the medication. Depending on the type of medication, you may need to dissolve powder into a solvent (liquid) before you inject. (Note: If your syringe comes prefilled, or if your medication comes in a prefilled "pen," skip ahead to step 6.) First remove the cap (illustration B), wipe the top with an alcohol swab, and pierce the rubber-stoppered cap of the solvent container

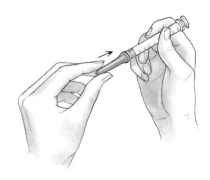

A. Attaching needle to syringe

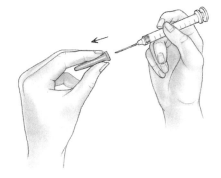

B. Removing needle cap

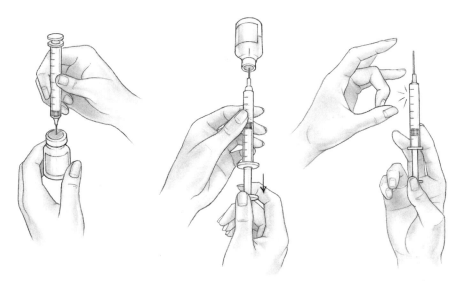

C. Piercing rubber stopper

D. Drawing up medication

E. Tapping out air bubbles

with the larger mixing needle (illustration C, page 195). Draw up the solvent to the prescribed amount (you'll see the measurements on the side of the syringe; illustration D, page 195). You might have been instructed to turn the syringe so the needle is facing upward and then to tap out the air bubbles (illustration E, page 195). Then squirt the solvent into the container containing the powdered medication by piercing the rubber-stoppered cap with the same needle. Repeat until the proper dose of solvent is in the powdered solution. The powder, by the way, should dissolve on contact with the fluid, and the solution should look clear. If it doesn't, you can gently roll the vial between your hands to mix. (If the medication comes in glass vials—or ampules—you'll have to break off the tops and then prepare the medication as described.)

5. Replace the large needle that you used to prepare the medication with the finer needle necessary for the injection, and load the prescribed amount of medication into the syringe by drawing up on the plunger.

6. It's shot time. You can do this!

For subcutaneous injections (most injections designed for use with assisted reproductive techniques are this kind):

- Identify your location. The best place to inject the medication is a few inches below and to the side of your belly button (see illustration F). You can also inject it on the top of your thigh or in the back of your upper arm.

- If you like, numb the area with ice.

- Sterilize the area with the alcohol swab and let it air dry.

- Remove the needle cap (illustration B), hold the syringe straight up, tap the sides of the syringe so no air bubbles remain (illustration E), and push the plunger slowly until you see a drop of the medication come out.

- Pinch the area you'll be injecting with your fingers.

- Holding the syringe as shown in the illustrations below, quickly insert the needle at a 45-degree angle until it's

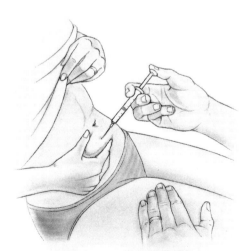

**F. Injecting below and
to the side of the belly button**

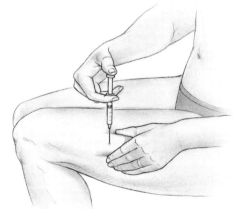

**G. Injecting on the outside
of the thigh**

completely submerged, then release the fingers doing the pinching.

- Slowly depress the plunger, and when all the medication is injected, quickly (but gently) pull the needle straight out.

- Apply pressure to the injection site with a gauze pad to stem any bleeding.

- Dispose of the syringe in a biohazard container or another container that you can seal. Never reuse needles or syringes.

Intramuscular injections (usually hCG and progesterone) are a little harder to DIY, so you may want to enlist your partner or a friend to help, if possible:

- First, identify your location. The best place to inject is in the upper outer quadrant of your buttocks (just below the hip bone but above the butt crack; illustration H) or on the middle of the outside of the thigh (illustration G; alternate sides for each injection so your muscles won't get sore).

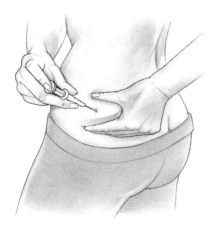

H. Injecting in the upper outer quadrant of the buttocks

- Lie down, sit, or stand with your weight off the side you'll be injecting.

- If you'd like, numb the targeted area with an ice cube.

- Give the area to be injected a swab of alcohol and then let it air-dry.

- Remove the needle cap (illustration B), hold the syringe straight up, tap the sides of the syringe so no air bubbles remain (illustration E), and push the plunger slowly until you see a drop of the medication come out.

- Take a big pinch of the area to be injected—taking both the skin and muscle—with your fingers. Some doctors recommend pulling the skin taut instead of pinching—ask which would work best or you.

- Holding the syringe as shown in the illustrations, quickly insert the needle at a 90-degree angle completely into the pinched skin and muscles, making sure none of the needle is exposed.

- Draw back on the plunger slightly. (In the unlikely case blood appears in the syringe, remove the needle, replace it with a new needle, and repeat the process.) Then *slowly* push the plunger all the way to inject the medication.

- When you're done, quickly (but gently) pull the needle straight out.

- Gently massage the injection site for 30 seconds afterward to spread the medication. Ice can help minimize the pain.

- Dispose of the syringe in a biohazard container or another container that you can seal. Never reuse needles or syringes.

7. Give yourself a pat on the back (after you've disposed of the syringe, that is).

Pregnancy Tests and Fertility Meds

Wondering if the fertility medications you're taking can mess up the results on that HPT you're itching to put to the test? Some of them can. If you've received an injection of hCG (or any fertility medication that contains hCG; ask your doctor for the details of your hormone cocktail if you're not sure), testing too early can give you a false positive. That's because pregnancy tests screen for the presence of hCG, which is normally produced once an embryo implants. You'll need to wait 7 to 14 days after your last injection of hCG to be sure all the hormones from the shots are out of your system. If you're taking other fertility medications (either oral like Clomid or via injection), you don't have to worry about them interfering with an HPT.

Surgery

Surgery was once considered the go-to treatment for an infertile couple. Today, doctors are more likely to turn first to ovulation induction (see page 187) and, as needed, assisted reproductive technology (ART; see page 202). But if tests show that you have an anatomical problem (in your ovaries, fallopian tubes, uterus, cervix, or vagina) that's keeping you from getting pregnant or staying pregnant, surgery might be the quick fix (or the initial step) you need to overcome your fertility challenges. Happily, most surgery is simple, done as an outpatient procedure (you'll be able to go home a few hours after the surgery), and with little downtime for recovery. In many cases, once the problem is fixed, Mission Conception can be accomplished—naturally or through ART—soon after surgery.

Uterine Surgery

A healthy uterus provides the perfect environment for a baby to grow in. But there are a number of conditions of the uterus that may contribute to—or be the cause of—infertility. Congenital malformations (defects present at birth) such as a uterine septum, where excess tissue forms a wall in the uterus, partially dividing it and possibly affecting its shape or size, can prevent it from providing a safe and secure home for a developing baby. Fibroid tumors in the uterus can also contribute to problems staying pregnant after conception, as can uterine adhesions (scar tissue that can result from pelvic inflammatory disease or from previous gynecological procedures, such as a D&C). Polyps are another common condition that can prevent an embryo from implanting. Surgery to correct these conditions may help bring you closer to the baby of your dreams.

Often, uterine surgery is performed with a hysteroscope, a narrow fiber-optic telescope inserted through the cervix and into the uterus that visualizes the uterine cavity. If any abnormalities are found (such as polyps, fibroids, scar tissue, or a septum), additional instruments can be inserted through the hysteroscope to remove or repair the problems.

Another procedure, known as laparoscopy, can also be used to view the uterus, and as needed, to remove scar tissue or fibroids. With laparoscopy, your doctor inserts a narrow fiber-optic telescope (or laparoscope) through an incision in your belly button to take a look at your uterus. If surgery is necessary, surgical tools will be guided through small incisions near your bikini line.

If you need surgery to correct a uterine condition, ask the doctor about the benefits and risks of the surgery. Ask, too, when you can start trying to conceive again. Some procedures require a 3-month waiting period before TTC efforts resume, primarily to give the uterus time to heal properly. Something else to be aware of: Depending on the type of uterine surgery and/or condition, you might need a cesarean delivery once it's time for your baby to arrive.

Fallopian Tube Surgery

The fallopian tubes play an all-important role in conception. It's through one of the tubes that an egg passes on that journey from ovary to uterus and where conception takes place. If you have scar tissue in one or both of your fallopian tubes (from an infection, for example), if you've had tubal ligation (to "tie" your tubes), or if there's fluid buildup in the tubes (the result of blockage, often caused by infection), the chances that sperm and egg will meet up and/or that a fertilized egg will reach the uterus are low to none. Damaged fimbriae (the finger-like ends of the tubes that catch the egg after the ovary releases it) could also contribute to infertility.

Tubal factors account for about a third of all infertility cases. In many cases of tubal factor infertility, the best course of action is to proceed straight to IVF. Still, because not all couples can afford costly IVF and because some tubal blockages and conditions can be easily fixed with surgery, your doctor may recommend a surgical procedure to help make the dream of pregnancy a reality.

Some examples of fallopian tube surgeries are:

- Salpingolysis. This is when scar tissue surrounding the fallopian tubes is removed laparoscopically.

- Salpingoneostomy. If a tube is blocked, and the fimbriae are damaged or absent, a new opening is made in the far end of the tube, near the ovary, in order for the egg to enter the fallopian tube after ovulation.

- Salpingectomy. In this procedure, performed laparoscopically or abdominally, the doctor removes the blocked or scarred portion of the tube close to the ovary.

- Fimbrioplasty. This laparoscopic procedure may be used to correct damage to the fimbria.

- Tubal reimplantation. When the damaged part of the fallopian tube is significant and closer to the uterus, this surgery—which removes the damaged portion of the fallopian tube and then reconnects the healthy part of the fallopian tube to the uterus—can help restore the fallopian tube to working condition. It's usually done abdominally.

- Tubal reanastomosis. If you had your tubes tied but now would like to TTC, this surgery can be performed to reconnect the 2 ends of the fallopian tubes (see the box, page 200, for more on reversing tubal ligation). Reanastomosis can also be used to

Tubal Reversal Surgery

Did you have your tubes tied—and now you wish you hadn't, so you could pick up filling your nest where you last left off? Luckily, those tied tubes won't likely stand between you and your renewed baby dreams. One option is to bypass the tubes altogether and go directly to IVF. Because fertilization takes place outside of your body with IVF, and the resulting embryo (or embryos) is placed directly into Destination Uterus, the fallopian tubes (the tubes that are "tied") aren't needed.

If you'd like to try conceiving the old-fashioned way, you may be able to have surgery to reverse your tubal ligation (depending on whether your fallopian tubes were cut, tied, cauterized, or nonsurgically blocked). Tubal reversal surgery is most commonly performed through an incision in the abdomen (though some doctors perform it laparoscopically or robotically).

The surgery is not a walk in the park, unfortunately (you'll need to stay in the hospital for a few days), and recovery can take a few weeks. Still, it could definitely prove worthwhile: For women under 35 with no other fertility problems, there is a 75 percent success rate within a year post-surgery (though the procedure slightly elevates the risk of ectopic pregnancy). Tubal ligations with clips or rings, performed at the time of cesarean delivery or the day after you delivered your last baby, all have good chances of being reversed. Tubes that were extensively cauterized (burnt), or completely removed, can't be fixed.

Before you opt for surgery, your spouse's sperm should be tested to make sure it's top-notch. After all, you wouldn't want to undergo tubal reversal only to find out later that his sperm count is low and IVF is your only conception option.

remove scar tissue or cysts from inside the tubes. This surgery is usually done abdominally.

- Tubal recanalization. Though not technically surgical, this procedure can be useful to clear blockages in the fallopian tubes close to where they enter the uterus. During this procedure, the doctor inserts a small catheter into the fallopian tubes through the cervix and uterus to find the blockage in the tubes. Once the blockage is found, a thin wire is threaded through the catheter and moved back and forth to dislodge the blockage—kind of like unclogging a drain. The procedure clears the tubes temporarily—usually for up to 6 months, giving you a short window

to try to get pregnant. The good news is that you'll likely be able to TTC as soon as the mild spotting from the procedure has stopped (you don't even have to wait a whole cycle). The not-so-good news is that the tubes typically become blocked again after a few months.

If your doctor has suggested tubal surgery, ask about the risks and success rates for the particular procedure being recommended, and also consider getting a second opinion. In many cases (especially when the blockage is significant and the surgery will be extensive and likely unsuccessful), women with tubal issues may be better off going straight to IVF. In fact, more and more fertility specialists are recommending

Surgery for Male Infertility

For men struggling with infertility because of a sperm flow problem, there are a number of surgical procedures that may offer some help:

- If you are among the 15 percent of men who have a varicocele (essentially, varicose vein of the scrotum; see page 166), your doctor may recommend a varicocelectomy to treat the problem, hopefully restoring fertility. The surgery is relatively simple, involving 1 or 2 small incisions in the lower abdomen that allow the doctor access to repair the abnormal veins. Once the repair is made, sperm production should return to normal. Whether the surgery helps resolve infertility problems is still being debated. Some experts say there is little improvement in pregnancy rates after the surgery, while others maintain it's an easy and proven treatment for male infertility.

- If you've had a vasectomy but now want to have it reversed so you and your partner can TTC, surgery can help. Your doctor will perform a vasovasostomy (or, depending on how many blockages you may have, a less common procedure called an epididymostomy). In a vasovasostomy procedure, the doctor restores sperm flow simply by reconnecting the ends of your previously cut vas deferens. In an epididymostomy, the doctor connects the vas deferens directly to the epididymis to allow the sperm to flow through. Nearly all men who have a vasovasostomy (and around 70 percent of those who have an epididymostomy) produce sperm after the surgery. Sperm can be banked at the time of vasectomy reversal surgery, in case the surgery is not successful.

- If tests have found that you have blockages in the vas deferens or the epididymis (often caused by STDs, infections, or trauma) or in the ejaculatory duct (usually the result of cysts in the prostate or scarring), surgery (either a type similar to a vasovasostomy or sperm duct microsurgery) can help the sperm bypass the blockages and get to where they need to go for fertilization. Another treatment option for these rare blockages: Sperm can be removed directly from the epididymis (in a procedure called microsurgical epididymal sperm aspiration, or MESA) or directly from the testicle (called testicular sperm extraction, or TESE) and then used in IUI or IVF.

skipping fallopian tube repair surgery and turning first to IVF. That's because the vast majority of women—80 to 85 percent—do not benefit from tubal surgery. An additional reason why: The risk of an ectopic pregnancy (a pregnancy that implants in the fallopian tubes instead of the uterus) is higher in women with tubal issues. IVF bypasses the fallopian tubes, lowering the risk.

Ovarian Surgery

Without healthy, functioning ovaries, it's hard to get pregnant. For instance, cysts on the ovaries can keep eggs from maturing and being released, making conceiving naturally close to impossible. Scar tissue from previous gynecological procedures or deposits from endometriosis could even encase an entire ovary, completely preventing the fallopian tube from grabbing the egg as it is released from the ovary. Surgery to correct certain ovarian problems can make conception possible for some women— though it definitely doesn't offer a fertility guarantee. Ovarian surgical procedures are minimally invasive, performed using laparoscopy, with a same-day discharge and recovery within a week.

One surgical option that has shown some promise for women with PCOS is called ovarian drilling. In this procedure, several holes are burned into the ovaries. Though some women experience improved ovulation after ovarian drilling, fertility drugs or IVF may still ultimately be needed to achieve conception success. Another surgery—ovarian tissue transplantation—is an experimental procedure. Pregnancies have resulted after this type of surgery, but the numbers worldwide are still small.

Assisted Reproductive Technologies (ART)

For as long as there have been men and women, sperm and egg have been meeting up the old-fashioned way: through sex. And more often than not, they still do. But sometimes, physiological factors intervene to make that amazing meeting impossible, or at least, highly improbable. Or partners of the same sex want to have a baby together— but can't make that miracle happen the traditional way. When alternatives like IUI or surgery are off the table or have been tried unsuccessfully, conception is turned over to higher-tech science and becomes an ART. Assisted reproductive technologies (ART) is the umbrella term for fertility treatments that bypass most fertility obstacles altogether by bringing sperm and egg together in the lab to create an embryo, and then transferring that embryo directly into a woman's womb. The most common ART procedure is in vitro fertilization (IVF). There are nearly 200,000 IVF cycles done per year in the United States, resulting in more than 60,000 IVF babies born each year. And that means approximately 1.6 percent of all infants born in the United States every year are conceived using ART. Now, that's a whole lot of ART!

In Vitro Fertilization (IVF)

IVF is considered the most effective of the ART techniques, and there are plenty of reasons why your fertility specialist may recommend it if fertility drugs and/or IUI haven't worked or aren't likely to help you. Among those reasons are severe blockages in the fallopian tubes, ovulation disorders, diminished ovarian reserve, poor egg quality, endometriosis, or insurmountable sperm deficiencies. IVF is also the go-to option for many same-sex couples (using a surrogate when both partners are male or when one lesbian partner wants to be the egg donor and the other partner carries the pregnancy, aka reciprocal surrogacy; see page 220 for more), couples using donor eggs, or for any couple who might need to use preimplantation genetic diagnosis or screening (PGD/PGS) to screen embryos when there are concerns about possible genetic problems (see page 212).

The upside of a successful IVF cycle is clear—having the baby of your dreams. The downsides include the high cost (which may not be covered or covered fully by insurance), the higher chances of multiples (if more than 1 embryo is implanted), the need for procedures and medications that carry a small risk, and a possible slight increase in pregnancy-related complications or problems with the baby. Be sure to have detailed discussions with your doctor about what you should expect from IVF, what your chances for a successful pregnancy could be, and what the risks to you and/or your baby might be.

Here's the basic outline of how an IVF cycle works:

Ovarian suppression. Your IVF cycle begins, ironically, with birth control pills (and sometimes also Lupron), taken to suppress your natural hormonal and menstrual cycle in order to control the timing of the IVF cycle. Research also suggests that using birth control pills prior to ovarian stimulation may help the ovaries respond better to the hormone injections about to come. Not all clinics or specialists start with this step, so if yours doesn't, not to worry.

Ovary stimulation and trigger. Hormone injections (see page 190) are used to help stimulate your ovaries to produce eggs. The precise cocktail your fertility specialist uses will be unique to you, but most women can expect to start off with daily FSH and LH injections. During this ovary stimulation phase, you will be asked to come in to your clinic every few days (or more often) so the doctor can check, via ultrasound, how many follicles are growing and how well they are developing. The ultrasounds will also monitor how well your uterine lining is thickening. You will probably also be given blood tests to monitor your hormone levels. Once it's determined that your follicles are mature enough for egg retrieval, you'll inject a trigger hCG or Lupron shot

to finish egg maturation and begin the ovulation process. You won't be allowed to ovulate on your own, since your eggs will be retrieved prior to ovulation; see below.

Something to keep in mind, in case you're wondering: Stimulating the ovaries does not deplete eggs for the future, since those being stimulated for an IVF cycle would have grown or died that month anyway.

During the ovary stimulation phase, you'll be told to avoid unprotected sex (sex with a condom is okay). That's because the hormone injections you're taking will be stimulating many eggs to mature. If those eggs "ovulate" on their own and you have unprotected sex, there's a chance all or many of them might be fertilized naturally. The potential risk—becoming pregnant with 6 or even more embryos—is something you'll need to avoid.

Egg retrieval. After 9 to 14 days of stimulation with fertility drugs and approximately 36 hours after your trigger hCG shot, the stimulated eggs will be mature and ready. But instead of letting them be released on their own, your doctor will remove them from your ovarian follicles so that they can be fertilized in the lab. The doctor will retrieve the eggs transvaginally with an ultrasound-guided needle that reaches your ovaries and aspirates the fluid and egg from each follicle. Most doctors try to retrieve up to 15 eggs per cycle. The number of eggs retrieved will depend on how many are available—it may be as few as 2 to 3 or as many as 15 or more.

The egg retrieval takes 20 to 40 minutes on average, and is done under monitored anesthesia care—IV medications to sedate you and relieve pain (so you won't feel anything). Because you'll be groggy and sleepy after the procedure, you won't be able to drive, so

A Look at Standard IVF

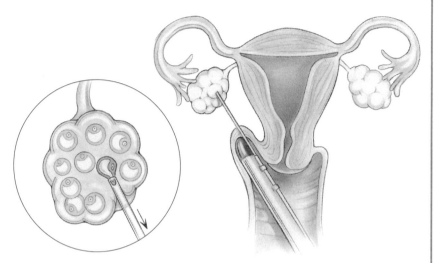

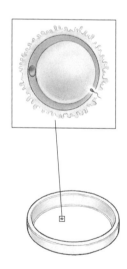

Under transvaginal ultrasound guidance, eggs are aspirated from the ovary.

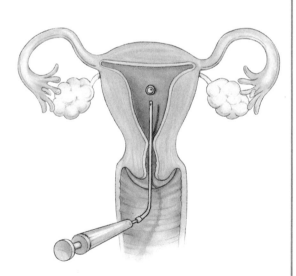

The egg (or eggs) and sperm are placed together in a petri dish for fertilization.

The fertilized egg, or embryo, is placed in the uterus through a thin flexible catheter.

make sure someone will be there to give you a ride home. Once you're home, plan on spending the rest of the day off, resting and relaxing.

Cramping and bloating for a few days after egg retrieval is normal, and your doctor will probably prescribe Tylenol or Tylenol with codeine to take as needed for post-procedure pain. You'll also be told to avoid sex and any high-impact activity until after your pregnancy test.

Sperm sample. While you're busy with the egg retrieval, your partner is busy producing a sperm sample (he will have been asked to avoid ejaculation for 2 days prior to giving the sample). If you're using donor sperm or your partner's previously frozen sperm, the clinic is getting it ready, thawing it if necessary. The sperm is then "washed"—sperm is separated from the semen and the nonmotile sperm are separated from the motile sperm in a centrifuge (see the box on page 182).

Fertilization. The eggs are now ready for fertilization, either through standard insemination or with ICSI (see page 213). With standard insemination, now performed in fewer than 50 percent of all IVF cycles, the retrieved eggs are placed in a petri dish with 50,000 to 100,000 sperm, and allowed to mingle and (hopefully) meet up. The dish contains a culture medium, a special fluid that resembles what's naturally found in the fallopian tubes and uterus. With ICSI, now used in over half of all IVF cycles, an extra step is taken to jump-start fertilization, with a single sperm injected directly into each egg first. The culture dishes are left in a special incubator and checked 12 to 24 hours later to see if fertilization took place. Estimates are that about 80 percent of mature eggs become fertilized during IVF.

Embryo evaluation. An embryologist will monitor each developing embryo over the next 3 to 6 days, looking for healthy growth and development. By day 3 after fertilization, the goal is to have a 6- to 8-cell embryo, sometimes called a cleavage stage embryo. By day 5 or 6, the embryo should become a healthy blastocyst (see the box on page 206). Approximately 30 to 50 percent of all embryos make it to the blastocyst stage.

If preimplantation genetic testing is planned, the embryos are biopsied (see the box on page 212).

Progesterone supplementation. Around 24 to 48 hours after fertilization, you'll receive a progesterone supplement that will optimize your uterine lining in anticipation of the embryo transfer and implantation. Progesterone can be given by injection, vaginal suppository, or vaginal gel. Adding hCG to the progesterone supplement is no longer recommended, because it increases the risk of ovarian hyperstimulation syndrome. The supplement is usually continued at least until a positive pregnancy test result and often through week 8 to 10 of a pregnancy.

Embryo transfer. Approximately 3 to 5 days after the eggs are successfully fertilized (though it could be shorter or longer than that, depending on your doctor's preference; see the box on page 206), or if you're using frozen embryos (see the box on page 218) whenever your uterine lining is ready for implantation, the embryo or embryos are slowly and carefully transferred into your uterus (see the box on page 216 for information on how many embryos are usually transferred). Under ultrasound guidance, your doctor will insert a thin, flexible catheter through your vagina and cervix into the uterus, and then gently depress the attached syringe

Day 3 or Day 5 Embryo?

When will your growing embryos be ready to be transferred to your eagerly waiting womb? Some fertility clinics prefer to transfer 3-day-old embryos (at the cleavage stage, with 4 to 8 cells) in an IVF cycle, while others transfer only 5-day-old embryos (called blastocysts and resembling a ball of cells). Does an embryo's age make a difference? It may. Some research suggests that blastocysts (aka 5-day-old embryos) have higher implantation rates than younger embryos, while other research doesn't back that up. Ultimately, your fertility specialist will decide on the optimum day to make the transfer, based on your unique situation.

Why might a day 5 transfer be best? By the time an embryo has been growing for 5 days, it has already divided into 2 different cell types—surface cells that eventually become the placenta, and inner cells that become the fetus. It has also already activated genes that will allow it to continue growing and dividing. Since only about one-third to one-half of embryos grow to blastocysts, reaching that stage is an important survival test—one that indicates that an embryo is more likely to

continue growing into a healthy baby once it's transferred. Transferring a 5-day-old embryo into the uterus also more closely mimics nature's timeline, since a naturally conceived embryo typically reaches the uterus on day 4 or 5 after having grown and divided on its journey down the fallopian tube after fertilization.

Why might your transfer take place with a day 3 embryo? One possible reason: Your cycle has produced few eggs and embryos. Your doctor may determine that waiting until day 5 may run the potential risk that none of the eggs or embryos will survive and grow into blastocysts in the lab. Transferring on day 3 may, in your case, give an embryo or embryos the chance to grow and ultimately implant inside your uterus.

The bottom line: While timing may not be everything, your fertility specialist will opt for a day 3 or day 5 transfer depending on clinic protocol and which option is most likely to maximize your chances for a successful pregnancy. But if you're unsure why your doctor has chosen one transfer timeline over the other, ask for an explanation. The more you know!

---

containing the embryo(s), placing it in your uterus with the hope that it will implant and continue to grow just as it would with unassisted conception. Any extra embryos that aren't transferred can be frozen for future use.

You'll need to have a full bladder for the procedure so that the doctor can visualize the lining of the uterus with ultrasound and place the embryo(s) in the best place for implantation. You will be wide awake for the transfer (no anesthesia necessary), and you'll likely

be able to watch it all on the ultrasound monitor—that is, if you'd like to.

Some fertility clinics coat the embryo in "embryo glue" before transfer to help it adhere to the uterine wall during implantation. The "glue" is a specially developed solution that contains hyaluronic acid, a substance that naturally occurs in your uterus, fallopian tubes, and ovaries and makes the secretions from these organs stickier. Research on whether embryo glue helps boost the odds of a successful embryo

Mock Transfer

Embryo transfer seems simple enough (for an experienced doctor, at least): Thread a thin, flexible catheter through your vagina and cervix into the uterus, and then insert the embryo(s) into your uterus. But embryo transfer is a delicate procedure, even in the most experienced hands. It's not just about dropping the embryo(s) into the uterus—it's about placing it precisely in the optimal spot for implantation. If the placement misses its mark, the entire IVF cycle could be lost. Which is why many fertility clinics perform a mock transfer before the real deal transfer.

A mock transfer is basically a practice run that allows your doctor a chance to scout out the best route to the best spot in your uterus for your embryo to implant—all without that precious embryo cargo on board. The doctor will use the mock transfer to measure your uterus, too, and determine what type and size of catheter would be best to use during the actual embryo transfer process. This practice procedure also lets your doctor know if there might be any potential difficulties or anatomical obstacles to overcome when it's time for the real embryo transfer.

A mock embryo transfer is performed like the real deal (though without any of those embryos, of course). You'll be in a pelvic exam position, and a catheter will be inserted into your vagina, through the cervix, and into the uterus. You might feel some slight pain and experience mild cramping after the mock transfer.

Some doctors choose to do a mock transfer well in advance of the actual embryo transfer (at least a month in advance—for instance, when you're already undergoing an HSG or hysteroscopy). Other fertility specialists set up a mock transfer right before you start your hormone shots for your IVF cycle. Still others perform a mock transfer at the same time as the egg retrieval.

But does a mock transfer actually improve the chances that your real embryo transfer will be successful? The research is still unclear. The jury is also still out on the optimum time to perform a mock transfer.

Not every fertility clinic requires a mock transfer. So check with your specialist ahead of time and ask whether one will be part of your IVF plan, and why (or why not if one isn't planned).

transfer and pregnancy has been conflicting so far. Still, some clinics encourage its use, particularly when a woman has had repeated implantation failure.

Recovery. You'll likely rest for a short time (about half an hour) in the recovery room and then head home. You might notice some discharge (bloody or clear) after the transfer, usually the result of the cervix being swabbed and manipulated slightly during the procedure.

That kind of spotting, bleeding, or discharge is totally normal and not a sign that the embryo(s) is being lost. Mild cramping and bloating are also not unusual, and some women experience slight sharp pain in the few days post-transfer, possibly from the ovaries as they return to normal size after stimulation. Definitely contact your doctor if you have moderate or severe pain (something that is rare and usually isn't related to the embryo transfer itself).

IVF and Your Baby's Health

For couples otherwise unable to conceive, IVF can deliver the happiest news of all—that the baby of their dreams is finally a reality. And there's more good news: Not only can IVF deliver babies, but it delivers an excellent long-term safety track record for mom (see the box on page 194). And the good news continues: Studies have shown that children conceived via IVF are not at greater risk for developing learning disabilities, autism, or speech and language disorders compared with children conceived naturally.

That said, IVF does present risks to a baby's health. The greatest risks, however, come from the possibility that there will be 2 or more babies—something that can be completely avoided by transferring only 1 embryo. Multiples come with multiple risks—twins are far more likely to be born prematurely, which in turn increases a variety of other significant risks, short and long term.

The risks for single IVF babies are much lower. Still, babies (even singletons) conceived via IVF are nearly 2 times more likely to have a low or very low birthweight, even if they're born full term. There is also a very slightly higher chance of preterm birth (again, even for single babies), asthma, epilepsy, and birth defects for IVF babies, as well as a slightly increased risk of childhood cancer. ICSI seems to increase the risk of birth defects slightly.

An IVF pregnancy also comes with a slightly increased risk of complications for mom, including miscarriage, gestational diabetes, hypertension, preeclampsia, placental abruption (separation), and a 6 times higher risk of placenta previa (a complication where the placenta is near or actually covers the cervix, making a vaginal birth impossible). Cesarean delivery is also more likely in an IVF pregnancy than a naturally conceived one. But since common contributing factors in infertility (such as being older or being overweight) are also common contributing factors in pregnancy complications, it's hard to sort out whether an increased risk of complications is due to IVF or to the underlying conditions that led to infertility. Either way, the increased risk is small to begin with—and any mom-to-be can lower the risk of pregnancy complications even further by getting good prenatal care, eating well, exercising regularly (as recommended), and cleaning up any baby-unfriendly lifestyle habits, like smoking.

So, bottom baby line: The news about IVF is good, and only looking up. Experts are learning more and more about how to lower the already low risks. The best way: transferring a single embryo instead of 2 or more. Stimulating fewer eggs during an IVF cycle seems to lower the risk for mom and baby, too, and that's something that fertility doctors are already doing—which means your chances for a successful IVF cycle that results in a healthy pregnancy and a healthy baby are getting better each day.

Resting at home beyond the first day after the transfer isn't medically necessary, though if it's feasible and you're feeling spent, you may want to consider taking a day or two off from work. Heading off to the gym or hitting the jogging trail right away, however, is a different story. Even though studies haven't shown that strenuous physical activity after an IVF transfer decreases

IVF Cancellation

You prepped, you've prepared, you've been poked, you've been prodded, and you're more than ready—make that eager—to get your IVF cycle well under way or completed. But then you get the dreaded call—the fertility clinic telling you your blood test results or ultrasound scan aren't looking good to go, or the embryos you've pinned so much hope on aren't viable, and this IVF cycle needs to be canceled.

Most IVF cycles proceed according to plan, but about 10 to 20 percent of the time—more often in women over 35—IVF is canceled for a number of possible reasons. Sometimes the follicles don't grow, despite all those injections. Sometimes they grow too much, so the trigger shot and the rest of the cycle are canceled to prevent ovarian hyperstimulation syndrome (see the box on page 192). Or ovulation happens on its own before the eggs can be retrieved. Or maybe there were no eggs able to be retrieved from those growing follicles. Or perhaps the eggs that were retrieved never became fertilized, or the fertilized eggs never grew into viability.

It's understandably disheartening when a cycle is canceled—you've spent money, time, and emotional energy. But the good news is, one canceled cycle doesn't predict that the next one is likely to fail as well. You and your doctor will discuss the reason for this cycle's cancellation and determine what changes might need to be made to the IVF protocol for your next cycle—one that will hopefully result in a successful pregnancy.

---

the chances of a successful pregnancy, most clinics and doctors take a play-it-safe approach and recommend taking it easy for the first 5 days. That's to minimize the chances of uterine contractions that might prevent the embryo from implanting. For the same reason, you'll likely be advised against having sex—sometimes until after the first pregnancy test. Another reason to take it easy post-transfer: This will protect your still enlarged ovaries.

The pregnancy test. Around 9 to 12 days after embryo transfer (sometimes a little sooner or a little later), you'll have a blood test that will confirm whether or not the procedure was successful. As eager as you'll be to get an early heads-up, don't be tempted to use an HPT before you get your blood test results—testing too soon can give you a false positive (if you had a shot of hCG) or a false negative (because it's too soon for the pregnancy to generate its own hCG). If the first pregnancy blood test is positive, another check of blood hCG levels is done to make sure the pregnancy is continuing to develop. If the initial pregnancy blood tests look good, your clinic will probably schedule you for a pregnancy ultrasound about 2 weeks later. The timing of all these tests may differ slightly, depending on your clinic's protocol.

If the testing shows you're not pregnant, you will likely be told to stop taking progesterone. Then you, your partner, and your doctor will discuss possible next steps (to try another IVF cycle, for instance, or to take a break for a few months). Remember, as heartbreaking as a failed cycle is, having one cycle fail doesn't mean you won't be successful if you try again.

What Are Your Odds for IVF Success?

Even with the tremendous technological advances in fertility treatments over the last few decades, there are still some individual factors that increase the chances that your IVF cycles will result in a healthy pregnancy and a healthy baby. Those factors include:

Younger age. IVF is often very successful in women under 35, but success rates decrease with age. The chance that a woman younger than 35 will become pregnant and deliver a baby after an IVF with egg retrieval is almost 50 percent. For a woman age 35 to 37, the chance of a live birth is 38 percent, at age 38 to 40 it's 24 percent, at age 41 to 42 it's 12 percent, and over age 42 it's less than 4 percent. The reason the odds decrease as a woman gets older is directly related to the fact that older ovaries don't typically respond as well to hormonal-stimulating drugs, and that means there are fewer eggs available for IVF. What's more, older eggs are typically of lower quality, resulting in lower-quality embryos that may have a harder time implanting in the uterus. Another reason for lower live birth success rates the older you get: Older moms-to-be have a higher risk of miscarrying, so even when IVF results in a pregnancy, that pregnancy has a somewhat lower chance of sticking. Remember, though, that these statistics are just that—statistics. Though the odds of having a healthy pregnancy and a healthy baby through IVF are significantly lower at 42 than at 32, there's still a chance it could happen.

Good ovarian reserve. You've heard about the importance of ovarian reserve to conception success in general, so it's no surprise that the better your ovarian reserve, the higher the chances for IVF success. Women who have 2 or more significantly higher levels of day 3 FSH and estradiol (meaning a poorer ovarian

Natural Cycle IVF

IVF may seem like the least "natural" way to conceive a baby, but there may be a way to make the process more natural for you. So-called natural cycle IVF skips the hormone injection phase (other than the hCG shot that triggers ovulation and progesterone to help sustain the pregnancy), allowing your body to do what it does naturally as it gets ready to ovulate during your regular menstrual cycle. How does it work? Your fertility specialist will use blood tests and ultrasound scans to monitor the growth of the cycle's dominant egg follicle and the maturation of the egg destined for ovulation (the one preselected by nature). Right before you would naturally ovulate that single egg, you'll head to the clinic to undergo single egg retrieval. Since the retrieval is quick, you may not need any anesthesia—a definite plus, since you won't be groggy afterward. That single egg will then be fertilized and transferred as it would be during a regular IVF cycle. A caveat: Not every follicle contains a retrievable egg, so if you're relying on 1 dominant follicle, there's an 80 percent chance that you'll end up with an egg—and a 20 percent chance that you won't.

Are you a candidate for natural IVF? While the procedure is used more often in older women who are still ovulating, women with low ovarian reserve (aka high FSH levels), and those who are so-called poor responders to fertility

reserve) can still become pregnant using their own eggs for IVF—it's just that the chances of success are lower. Another option for women with very low ovarian reserve: using donor eggs for their IVF cycle (see page 219).

Healthy fallopian tubes. Even though IVF bypasses the fallopian tubes altogether, studies show that women who have fluid-filled blockages in the fallopian tubes (called hydrosalpinx) have lower success rates with IVF. The good news is that having a salpingectomy procedure (see page 199) before IVF can significantly improve pregnancy chances.

Healthy lifestyle. Women who are smokers have significantly lower IVF success rates. So if you smoke, don't wait until your baby is on board to quit—especially if you're planning to try IVF.

Healthy weight. Women who are very obese are less likely to become pregnant after an IVF cycle than normal-weight women. The same is true for underweight women, who also have a lower chance of becoming pregnant after an IVF cycle compared with normal-weight women.

The right clinic. Your fertility clinic's general IVF success rates can also have an impact on your individual success rate. See the box on page 214 for more.

Wondering about other factors that you've heard increase or decrease IVF success? Here's the lowdown: Having endometriosis does not lower your chances of achieving pregnancy through IVF. Neither does having had 1 or more miscarriages or a previous unsuccessful IVF cycle. And though you may have heard that taking aspirin during an IVF cycle increases the chances of a successful pregnancy, the latest studies don't back that up. What about CAM techniques for boosting IVF success rates? See the box on page 217 to get the facts.

drugs (either the drugs don't stimulate enough eggs or stimulate too many eggs, causing ovarian hyperstimulation; see the box on page 192), some clinics will consider it for any woman who has relatively regular cycles but has unexplained infertility (though the success rates are lower than standard IVF; see below).

The upside to natural cycle IVF: You don't have to use hormone injections to stimulate your ovaries, thereby eliminating that uncomfortable and stressful step, and avoiding the side effects of ovarian stimulation and the potential risk of developing ovarian hyperstimulation. A natural cycle IVF is less expensive because there are no costly hormone shots to pay for and because retrieval is faster and potentially less complicated. And since there's only 1 egg retrieved and fertilized per cycle, you won't end up with multiple embryos to screen (which means lowered testing costs) or extra ones to store (also lowered costs). It also means there won't be any "leftover" embryos that you'll have to figure out what to do with, as you might in a stimulated IVF cycle.

Ending up with 1 embryo per cycle, however, is also a potentially considerable downside (and one reason why not all fertility clinics offer natural cycle IVF). If the single retrieved egg in a cycle doesn't end up being fertilized or doesn't continue to develop, there's no backup—you'll have to start from square one next cycle. With traditional

Preimplantation Genetic Testing

The technology involved in IVF is nothing short of miraculous—allowing embryos to be created outside a woman's body. But if that's not incredible enough, today's technology also allows for those embryos formed in vitro to be screened for chromosomal and genetic abnormalities, giving fertility specialists the opportunity to select the healthiest embryos—those with the greatest potential to grow into fully healthy babies—for implantation. This technology is called preimplantation genetic diagnosis (PGD) when it's used to test embryos for a specific genetic disorder (such as cystic fibrosis), and preimplantation genetic screening (PGS) when it's used to count the number of chromosomes in an embryo (to rule out chromosomal abnormalities). Either way, it's essentially an embryo biopsy. The embryology team removes 5 to 7 cells from the part of the blastocyst that will eventually become your baby's placenta. In most cases, the embryos are frozen for future transfer (pending test results) as soon as the biopsy is done. The collected cells are then transferred to a genetics lab for evaluation.

Once the report is in and an embryo is found to be free from identifiable chromosomal and genetic abnormalities, it can be transferred to your uterus with the hope that it implants and develops into a healthy pregnancy and healthy baby. If there are multiple healthy embryos, the extras can remain frozen (or be frozen if they haven't already been) for future use.

Of course, complicated procedures often come with complicated decisions. Before choosing PGD/PGS, you and your spouse will want to have a conversation with your doctor so that you're clear about the pros and cons of the procedure, as well as the potential risks involved. You'll also need to be comfortable with its implications (there might be embryos that show chromosomal anomalies, and you'll need to think about what will be done with those). It's also important to consider the added cost (the procedure's not cheap, and IVF is already expensive) and to keep in mind that not all abnormalities can be detected by PGD/PGS. It's also not yet clear whether PGD/PGS improves pregnancy success rates or reduces miscarriage rates. Still, for many couples—especially those who have been suffering from recurrent pregnancy losses—PGD/PGS may tip the healthy-pregnancy scales in their favor.

IVF, there are multiple eggs retrieved and fertilized, which means there are multiple options to screen and select from (to pick, essentially, the best of the cycle for transfer). That's why live birth rates from traditional IVF are much higher than from natural cycle IVF. So while each natural IVF cycle might be less costly, each cycle is also far less likely to be successful. You also won't have leftover embryos to freeze for the next cycle and beyond—a perk you'll probably have with traditional IVF. Another downside of natural cycle IVF is a higher cancellation rate. That's because ovulation that's natural is less predictable than ovulation that's stimulated by fertility drugs.

Thinking about going natural for your IVF? Speak to your fertility specialist to see if the procedure is offered at your clinic, and whether it's recommended in your case. If so, you'll have to weigh those pros and cons, and, in discussion with your specialist, figure out whether natural cycle IVF is right for you. If your doctor feels that natural cycle IVF isn't recommended in your case but you're still concerned about all those fertility shots in a standard IVF cycle, ask about minimal IVF, in which lower levels of hormones are used (sometimes just oral meds like Clomid plus an hCG trigger shot) to stimulate the ovaries to produce more eggs than in a natural cycle.

Realistically, the only advantages of natural IVF or IVF with minimal stimulation are that they're less invasive and come at a lower cost. As embryo-freezing technology has improved—allowing you to retrieve and fertilize many eggs at a time—there's not much upside to one-at-a-time retrieval for those opting for IVF.

Intracytoplasmic Sperm Injection (ICSI)

ICSI, pronounced ICK-see, takes IVF one step further. Pioneered and often used as a solution for male infertility—such as when there is a very low sperm count, low sperm motility, or poor-quality sperm—ICSI is now performed in more than half of IVF procedures and is growing in popularity. That's because many experts believe it offers a better shot at conception success compared with standard IVF, even when fertility challenges aren't linked to the male partner. With ICSI, instead of merely mixing your eggs and your partner's sperm in a petri dish and hoping they get together, seal the deal, and make an embryo, the doctor actually injects a single sperm directly into an

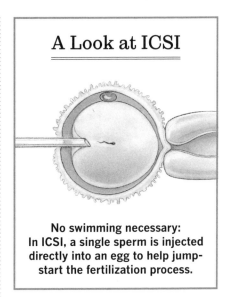

A Look at ICSI

No swimming necessary: In ICSI, a single sperm is injected directly into an egg to help jump-start the fertilization process.

egg to assist with fertilization—basically eliminating all of the challenges that the little guy would otherwise have had to face.

Here's how it works: Egg retrieval is the same as it is for a regular IVF cycle (see page 203). Once the eggs are retrieved, they are "washed" to loosen their protective outer coating. Collected, washed sperm are then slowed down with a chemical solution so it's easier for the technician to "catch" one. Then that microscopic sperm's tail is immobilized so the sperm head can safely puncture the egg's membrane and be injected deep inside the egg. Once the sperm is injected into the egg, fertilization hopefully occurs. The same process is repeated with the rest of the retrieved eggs, each receiving a single sperm. As with standard IVF, the fertilization occurs, the embryo (or embryos) is transferred into the uterus, and less than 2 weeks later, you discover whether Mission Conception has been accomplished. Extra embryos can be frozen for future transfer.

Ranking Your Clinic

How can you tell if the ART clinic you're considering is likely to deliver (and not just promise) the healthy baby you're hoping for? Most reputable IVF clinics are members of the Society for Assisted Reproduction Technology (SART) and submit their pregnancy and live birth rates to both SART and the CDC for tracking. The best thing about this extensive database: You can view it online (at sart.org) to size up the success rates of your prospective ART clinic before signing up for your treatments. To glean the most helpful information, focus on the number of live births per retrieval as opposed to pregnancies (which doesn't factor in the miscarriage rate). Equally important is the clinic's multiples rate. Multiples come with the potential for multiplied risks. Some centers achieve their high success rate by transferring more embryos, despite the possible risks—and that's a red flag. If you're over 35, look at the clinic's stats for your age bracket, since some lump live birth rates for young women together with rates for older women in order to boost their ranking—and that could be misleading.

If your clinic doesn't show up on the database, it could mean its success rate is so low that they're not reporting their numbers at all (and that's not a good sign). It could also mean the clinic you're visiting is too new to show up on the database (there's about a year or two delay with the reporting to allow for the pregnancies to conclude and to compile all the data). Still, you might want to think twice about going to a clinic without a proven track record. If the clinic you're contemplating is quoting a high success rate yet the numbers don't show up on the SART database, prospective parents beware. The clinics with the best numbers have the best reputations—and they're proud to have their data on the SART website.

Assisted Hatching

Though assisted hatching sounds like something you'd find going on in a chicken coop, it's actually a highly specialized ART technique designed to make the implantation process less challenging for a fledgling lab-grown embryo. For an embryo to implant inside the uterus, it must "hatch" out of its protective shell (called the zona pellucide). When you conceive naturally, the trip the embryo takes down the fallopian tube enables the shell to thin, making it easier for the embryo to implant successfully in the endometrium. Embryos grown in a lab, however, don't have the benefit of that trip down Fallopian Lane, so some—though certainly not all—embryos created in vitro have a thicker than normal shell and may need an extra push to break out of it. In some women, this extra-thick shell may be the reason previous IVF attempts have failed. Enter assisted hatching—a procedure in which a laser is used to make a microscopic hole in the zona pellucide right before the embryo is transferred to the uterus. This tiny opening enables the cells of the embryo to escape the shell and attach more easily to the uterine wall. The benefit of assisted hatching is probably modest, at best. So far, research hasn't shown improved live birth rates when the technology is used.

The Emotional Pain of the Waiting Game

If you've been trying to conceive for a while (and if you've turned to ART, it may have been a pretty long while), you've already done more than your share of waiting. Waiting for ovulation. Waiting to do an HPT—and then waiting to retest. Waiting for medications to work. Waiting for test results. Waiting for appointments with specialists and treatment centers. But probably the toughest wait is the one you have ahead of you after a round of IVF. Though you might feel hopefully pregnant the moment your embryo or embryos are transferred into your uterus, you'll have to wait 9 to 12 days after the transfer for confirmation of a pregnancy (testing with an HPT before the blood test at your doctor's office won't be accurate because of all the hormones you've been taking).

Just because you've become a pro at playing the waiting game doesn't mean waiting won't be hard to handle. The days can pass agonizingly slowly, and the mounting anticipation can make it difficult to focus on anything else (work, romance, relationships, eating, sleeping). As always, relaxation techniques may help you stress less while you're waiting. Eating well, as hard as it might be when you're so nervous, may also help reduce stress (and at the same time, reducing stress will help you eat well—which is so important for a healthy pregnancy). Keeping a journal—writing down all of those conflicting feelings (excitement that you might be pregnant, dread that you might not be)—can help pass the time and also help contain the emotional overload. Venting in a blog will accomplish the same goal, and opening up a dialogue with others confronting fertility challenges can be enormously helpful all around. And speaking of dialogues, if you haven't already found an online support group, check out the fertility treatments message board at WhatToExpect.com. No one knows what the waiting's like better than others playing the same waiting game.

Endometrial Scratch

If you're itching for a baby, endometrial scratching may help you get there. Typically reserved for women who have had 2 or more IVF cycles that were unsuccessful even though the embryos implanted were of high quality, endometrial scratching has been shown to improve IVF implantation rates by at least 20 percent—with some research showing up to 70 percent increased likelihood of pregnancy. The procedure involves gently "scratching" the uterine lining using a thin catheter threaded through the cervix and into the uterus. The scratching is performed around day 21 of the cycle—just before an IVF cycle begins. The procedure is quick (just a few minutes) and usually painless—you'll have it done in the doctor's office without anesthesia, and there's no down time. You may experience some cramping and mild bleeding after the procedure.

How can endometrial scratching help? Experts aren't sure exactly, but they suspect that irritating the lining of the uterus releases certain growth factors, hormones, and chemicals to help "repair" the lining, and that in turn helps improve embryo implantation. Another theory is that sometimes the genes that are responsible for implantation aren't

One Embryo or Two . . . Or More?

The more embryos transferred in an IVF cycle, the better to up the odds of a successful pregnancy—right? Well, not always. Too many embryos can turn into too many babies—and that could lead to a riskier pregnancy for mom and brood. Which is why most doctors recommend a single embryo transfer (SET) instead of transferring more than 1 embryo. It's also the reason why the American Society for Reproductive Medicine issues these guidelines to help doctors and couples decide how many embryos to transfer:

- No matter what her age, a woman who has undergone PGD/PGS should have only 1 embryo transferred.

- A woman under age 37 who hasn't had PGD/PGS but has all signs pointing to IVF cycle success (she has produced more than 1 high-quality embryo, for instance, or has had a previous live birth after IVF) should have only 1 embryo transferred.

- Women ages 35 to 37 without clear evidence of IVF cycle success should receive no more than 2 to 3 embryos.

- Women ages 38 to 40 should have no more than 3 cleavage stage embryos or 2 blastocyst stage embryos transferred.

- Women over age 40 should have no more than 4 cleavage stage embryos or 3 blastocyst stage embryos transferred.

Of course, these guidelines—based on the latest research—are a good place to start when making the decision of how many embryos to transfer. But not all specialists agree with them or follow them for every woman, every time. Some will agree to transfer 2 embryos in a younger woman, even though the guidelines recommend implanting no more than 1. Some will transfer no more than 2 embryos in an older woman, even though the guidelines allow for more.

Hoping for a more-is-more approach to your IVF transfer? That's understandable. After all, getting to this point in the process takes a lot of hard work, and often, a lot of cash—and you're hoping upon hoping that it will pay off in baby dividends. But the truth is, transferring more embryos may not only increase risk, but it's possible that it won't increase benefits, either. In fact, preliminary research suggests that for women ages 35 to 37, the rate of implantation with the transfer of a single embryo is higher than with transfer of 2 or more embryos. So don't be surprised if your doctor recommends a single embryo transfer.

---

automatically switched on in some women. Endometrial scratching may switch on these important genes, increasing the chances of implantation.

Gamete Intrafallopian Transfer (GIFT)

There's no greater gift than a baby— and gamete intrafallopian transfer (GIFT) is a procedure that can help

deliver that gift to some hopeful couples. GIFT is a more expensive and more invasive ART treatment than IVF, which is why it's used much less frequently (less than 1 percent of the time), but it allows fertilization to occur naturally inside your fallopian tube instead of in a petri dish. Eggs are stimulated and retrieved, and sperm is collected as with IVF, but instead of having them meet up in the lab for their fertilization date, the newly retrieved egg (or

Can CAM Lend a Hand?

There's definitely no shortage of high-tech techniques—from surgery to medications to IVF and more—that can help couples overcome fertility challenges big and small. But can complementary and alternative medicine (CAM) techniques lend a reproductive hand to those eager to conceive as well?

The answer is . . . it's unclear. For instance, while some studies suggest that women receiving acupuncture treatment while undergoing IVF have higher rates of pregnancy than women who don't have acupuncture, most studies show no difference in IVF success. Some research shows that women who are hypnotized before IVF embryo transfer are more likely to become pregnant than those who aren't—but other research doesn't show the same effect. There's also research showing that elecroacupuncture (the application of a pulsating electrical current to acupuncture needles, further stimulating the acupoints) may help induce ovulation in women with PCOS. But, guess what? Other studies don't show similar benefits.

Adding to the confusion of whether CAM provides a complementary boost to ART or not: Even in cases where studies show a CAM benefit, it's hard to tell if the benefit is the result of physiological factors or of a mind-body connection (I think, therefore I will be, pregnant). But does that matter? And do CAM techniques really need to be backed up by science before you use them to back up your high-tech assisted reproductive efforts? Probably not. Since there's no harm done with acupuncture or hypnosis, and since it's hard to argue with the potential of even slightly greater success, there's no reason not to try these types of CAM techniques if you'd like to and they're accessible to you.

Just keep in mind: There may be CAM treatments that not only don't help but might even hurt your ART treatment. Not all CAM therapies are created equal, and not all CAM therapists are, either. So before you go down the CAM path, talk to your doctor about how such therapies might be integrated into your conception campaign, which are safe bets (and which aren't), and if there are specific therapists he or she recommends. Also check in with your insurance company before you book your CAM therapies—some are covered by some plans, and others are not.

---

eggs) and sperm are laparoscopically placed together into your fallopian tube through a small incision in your abdomen. The hope is that fertilization of the egg or eggs will take place (usually within hours) and the resulting embryo(s) will then travel down to your uterus for implantation.

Because fertilization (hopefully) happens inside your body instead of inside a lab, the success rate with GIFT is relatively high. Experts speculate that the journey through the fallopian tube nourishes the new embryo and thins the shell, giving it a better chance of being healthy and able to implant in the uterus. Another reason for the increased success rate could be that the embryo arrives in the uterus at the "right" time for implantation (as opposed to IVF, in which the embryo arrives in the uterus when your doctor places it there—and that might not be exactly the time frame nature had in mind). Recovery from a GIFT procedure is similar to recovery from IVF, with perhaps a few more

Fresh or Frozen Embryos?

There's nothing like fresh—or is there? For decades, using freshly stimulated and retrieved eggs, freshly mixed with sperm to create fresh embryos (all within a few days) was considered the most effective and safest way to go, especially when the technology for freezing and preserving embryos was in its infancy. But that technology has come a long way, baby—resulting in substantial advances in more efficient cryofreezing and thawing, thanks to the use of vitrification or ultra-rapid flash freezing. And with this new technology, teamed with new data looking at the outcomes of both fresh and frozen embryo transfers, the choice to use fresh over frozen isn't as obvious as it may once have been. In fact, some research now finds that implanting thawed frozen embryos is just as safe as using fresh ones and may even be more effective, yielding healthier babies and more viable pregnancies. Because of the changing research, there's a definite trend in the United States toward more frozen embryo transfers and fewer fresh transfers. Almost all treatments involving preimplantation genetic testing also involve embryo freezing.

So what are the benefits to frozen embryo transfer (FET)? While IVF babies (whether they started out as fresh or frozen embryos) are, in general, healthy (see the box on page 208), studies have found that women who use frozen embryos are less likely to have a preterm birth and a baby with a low birthweight. Babies from frozen embryos are also less likely to need breathing help after birth compared with babies born from fresh embryos, and are less likely to have birth defects. And exciting research shows that frozen embryos are more likely to result in a pregnancy—and, most importantly, a live birth—than fresh embryos. This is especially true in women with PCOS. Frozen embryo transfers also seem to have slightly lower rates of ectopic pregnancies than fresh embryo transfers,

---

hours spent in recovery before you're sent home and told to take it easy for a few days.

As IVF technology improves, GIFT is used less and less, despite its high rate of success. Because it requires laparoscopy, it's a once-cutting-edge technology that's becoming increasingly obsolete.

Zygote Intrafallopian Transfer (ZIFT)

With zygote intrafallopian transfer (ZIFT), the method is similar to GIFT, but the eggs are fertilized in the laboratory before being placed (often within hours after fertilization) laparoscopically into your fallopian tube.

Why opt for ZIFT over GIFT? The advantage to ZIFT is that it's clear fertilization has taken place. With GIFT, the hope that fertilization occurs is there, but there's no way to know right away if egg and sperm are actually getting together to make a zygote (an early embryo). In effect, ZIFT gives a pregnancy a running start. ZIFT, like GIFT, is used very infrequently now that success rates for IVF are so much higher.

and there's a lower risk of ovarian hyperstimulation syndrome, too.

Even with all of those frozen embryo pluses, there are some statistical pros to fresh embryo transfer. There's a lower risk for developing placenta accreta (when the placenta attaches too deeply in the uterine wall) with fresh embryo transfer. A fresh embryo transfer also lowers the risk for having a large-for-gestational-age baby compared with frozen embryo transfer.

So should you have a fresh vs. frozen preference when it comes to your embryos? Definitely talk to your doctor to find out which is best in your case. Some things to consider: If you happen to need multiple IVF cycles to achieve a pregnancy, you'll realize some cost savings if you're able to use your previously frozen embryos. A frozen embryo transfer cycle also uses less medication (you'll still need some hormones to get your uterus ready to receive the embryo, but you won't need to inject yourself with ovary-stimulating medications), and there's data to suggest that an IVF cycle without all those hormone injections is more likely to result in a successful pregnancy. Another potential bonus: no stressful waiting to find out if the embryos conceived in the lab are healthy (that process was already done before the freezing, so you know the frozen embryo you'll use for transfer is of the highest quality).

If you and your doctor choose an FET, you'll go through the egg retrieval process as you would for a full IVF cycle, but you won't continue with the rest of the cycle. Your eggs will be fertilized and the healthiest embryos will be frozen. Whenever you are ready—in a month or in a year or in 5 years or more (frozen embryos can stay frozen for years and years)—you'll start a new IVF cycle that bypasses all the hormone shots and egg retrieval. Instead you'll take estrogen (via pill, skin patch, or injection) for about 5 to 7 days before the planned transfer. You'll also take progesterone starting on cycle day 5 or 6. The embryo(s) will be thawed the morning of the scheduled transfer and the transfer process will proceed in the same way as a fresh transfer.

Egg Donation

Time was, a woman who wanted to experience pregnancy and childbirth had no choice but to use her own eggs, conceiving either naturally or with the help of IVF. Which meant that women without viable eggs (because of age, ovarian failure, or a genetic disorder, for example) were out of fertility options. The same went for women who were known carriers of serious diseases that they didn't want to pass on to their offspring. But all that has changed with egg donation technology. With this ART procedure, an egg (or eggs) from a donor (either fresh or frozen and thawed) is mixed with sperm provided by the hopeful father or a sperm donor to produce an embryo. The embryo(s) is then placed in the uterus of the hopeful mom, where it will (hopefully) grow into a healthy pregnancy. (Are you considering using a gestational surrogate to carry a baby conceived with a donor egg? See page 227.)

The rate of successful pregnancies using donor eggs is high, primarily

My Two Moms (or Dads)

The path to parenthood for same-sex couples (even if they're healthy, young, and individually fully functional in the reproductive department) is never as easy as it is for a fertile heterosexual couple. But happily, it has become easier and more accessible than ever. Here are some of the options, with more likely on the near horizon.

Lesbian couples. There are 2 options for biological parenthood if you're a lesbian couple:

- Artificial insemination. This is the lowest tech option: One of you is artificially inseminated (while you're ovulating) with donor sperm, usually via IUI (see page 183) in the doctor's office or via at-home AI (see page 185). Fertility drugs may be used if the hopeful mom has ovulation issues.

- Reciprocal IVF. This increasingly popular option for lesbian couples allows you both to be involved in the creation of your baby. In this procedure, the egg or eggs are retrieved from one mom and fertilized with donor sperm in an IVF cycle. Then, in the ultimate team effort, the resulting healthy embryo (or embryos) is transferred to and hopefully carried successfully by the other mom (as it would be in a gestational surrogacy; see page 227). Extra embryos can be frozen for future cycles. Which mom plays which role in the process may be a personal preference, or may be at least partly dictated by age, fertility, general health, and other factors. Of course, traditional IVF can also be used for lesbian couples, with one mom providing both the egg and the uterus (again because of preference or because one mom isn't fertile and can't carry a pregnancy).

Gay couples. There are a couple of options if you're a gay couple hoping to start a family:

- Traditional surrogacy with artificial insemination. This is the simplest and potentially least expensive option, particularly if you're using a friend or relative who has volunteered to carry your baby (though there may be strings attached; see page 229). Sperm from one of you will be inserted into the surrogate when she's ovulating, via IUI (see page 183), where it will hopefully meet up with her egg and

because the donors are generally young and therefore have healthy eggs. Currently, about 12 percent of all IVF cycles—about 20,000 a year—are donor egg cycles. Donor eggs are especially helpful for much older women. In fact, most women in their 40s who do become pregnant via IVF do so using donor eggs (the odds of a woman in her mid- to late-40s conceiving during an IVF cycle with her own eggs are less than 1 percent).

Finding an Egg Donor

The first step if you're considering egg donation is to factor in the costs involved (those for the donor's medical care, travel costs if the donor lives out of town, fees for the donor's and agency's services, and legal fees—plus the standard IVF costs). Then it's time to find an egg donor. A close friend or relative may offer to be your egg donor, and if she's a relative such as a sister, your baby

develop into a baby she will carry to term. If you'd like your child to be as biologically close to both of you as possible, one of you can provide the sperm and the other can choose a close relative—say, a sister—to be your traditional surrogate.

- Gestational surrogacy with IVF. There are several ways to accomplish this, but all require a gestational surrogate and donor eggs (see page 219). You can use sperm from one of you to fertilize the donor egg or eggs, or you can each provide sperm, which will be used to separately fertilize different batches of the donor eggs. For example, you can use embryos fertilized by one of you to have a first baby, and then freeze the other dad's fertilized embryos for a second baby. It's possible for a pair of embryos—one fertilized by dad A and one by dad B—to be transferred to the surrogate at the same time, but that might result in a twin pregnancy, and twin pregnancies come with increased risks for the surrogate and the babies.

And with all these options for same-sex couples who'd like to become pregnant comes even more good news. Even though you'll be conceiving your child with the help of fertility treatments,

your chances for success are high—higher, in fact, than they are for heterosexual couples undergoing fertility treatments. Though some same-sex couples end up having fertility issues (at about the same rate as heterosexual couples), most are fully fertile and seeking help not because they aren't reproductively functional, but because they can't reproduce in the traditional way. If you'll be an active participant on Team Baby (you'll be providing sperm, or an egg, or a uterine home for your baby), you can boost those excellent odds of reproductive success further by following (or maintaining) all the healthy preconception lifestyle changes outlined in this book: taking prenatal vitamins, not smoking, checking your meds, eating healthy, taking precautions to avoid exposure to Zika virus, and so on.

No matter how you go about building your family, be sure you hire an attorney who is knowledgeable about reproductive law and the statutes in your state so that you can be assured your parental rights are protected. And look for a fertility clinic that specializes in helping LGBTQ couples become parents (ask other couples for recommendations and check reviews online).

will contain genes resembling yours. Or you might decide to choose an egg from an anonymous donor through your fertility doctor or through agencies that match donors with recipients. Using an egg from a donor you don't know provides more confidentiality and a clearly defined relationship with the donor (you'll define the parameters of that relationship with the agency, your doctor, and your lawyer)—something that may be a pro or con for you, depending

on your perspective and desires. Be sure to find out, however, how much donor information the agency releases now and in the future (in the event your child ever develops a condition that might require you to obtain information about the donor's genetic health).

No matter where you get your donor eggs from, the potential donors are screened for genetic disorders, psychological conditions, STDs and other infectious diseases, drug use, blood

Donor Eggs and Zika Virus

When choosing an egg donor, you may have specific traits in mind—height, intelligence, musical ability, green eyes. But probably the single most important characteristic for your baby-to-be's egg donor: good health. And that's true whether you're seeking an egg from an anonymous donor, a good friend, or a family member. That's why the FDA and other experts have issued guidelines saying that egg donors are considered ineligible if they have been infected with Zika virus, live in or have traveled to an area with a CDC Zika travel notice in the last 6 months, or have been sexually active within the last 6 months with someone who is infected or lives in or has traveled to affected areas. While Zika virus causes mild to no symptoms in most people, it can be devastating in pregnancy (see box, page 10), and that's why it's important to make sure your donor eggs haven't even potentially been exposed to Zika. These same guidelines apply to sperm donation as well (see page 227 for more on donor sperm screening). That said, there has been no known case of Zika virus transmission through the use of donor eggs, and it's highly unlikely that a donor, even if she had Zika, would have the virus in her eggs.

Far more important, however, is protecting yourself from the virus. Even if you know (or are pretty sure) that your donor egg (or sperm) has no possibility of being infected with Zika, you're the one who will be pregnant. So you'll still need to protect yourself from the virus before and during pregnancy. The same goes for a surrogate, if you'll be using one to carry your baby.

type, and general health. In fact the FDA has a stipulated set of guidelines and regulations for infectious disease screening that includes testing for HIV, hepatitis B, hepatitis C, syphilis, Chlamydia, gonorrhea, West Nile Virus, Creutzfeldt-Jakob disease, and Zika virus. If you're choosing an anonymous donor egg, you'll also be able to screen for other genetic factors that matter to you (perhaps because they are similar to your traits), such as height, hair color, special talents, personality, and so on (think of it like online dating, but instead of looking for traits in a mate, you're looking for your future baby's genetic traits).

Another choice to make when considering using donor eggs is whether to use fresh eggs from a live donor cycle or frozen eggs bought from an egg bank. Here's the lowdown on both:

Fresh eggs from a live donor cycle are eggs that are essentially retrieved to order. You (or the donor agency, if you're using one) schedule the egg retrieval when you (and your uterus) are ready to receive the embryos that the donor eggs and your partner's sperm have created. What are the benefits of fresh donor eggs? For one, there's a higher chance of a live birth from fresh vs. frozen—in the 50 to 55 percent range. Some research shows that fresh eggs edge out frozen-and-thawed eggs in quality—and higher quality eggs result in higher quality embryos. What's more, literally: You're likely to net more eggs from a live donor cycle, especially if your donor is young and healthy. Extra eggs can be fertilized, resulting in extra embryos—which can be frozen for later use, ensuring that your future babies (if you opt to have more than one) will be biological siblings. Which means you can potentially build your entire family from just one egg retrieval.

There are downsides to using fresh eggs from a live donor cycle, however. For one, they cost more—often a lot more. That's because you'll be paying the donor, the agency (if you're using one), the cost of evaluating the donor, transportation fees for the donor, and the donor's medical expenses—all on top of the price of IVF. Another challenge: You and your donor will have to synchronize your cycles, so that she's ready to offer those eggs when your uterus has been primed for the resulting embryos (in other words, hormones all around).

Frozen eggs from a bank are ready when you are. The bank has already done the heavy lifting—screening and evaluating the donor, having her ovaries stimulated, and having the eggs retrieved. There's no transportation cost beyond shipping the frozen eggs to your clinic—and your donor's location isn't a consideration. No synchronizing your cycles either—you choose when to have the eggs thawed and fertilized and the embryo(s) transferred. All for about half the price of using fresh eggs.

The downsides to using frozen eggs: They're somewhat less likely to result in a live birth—in the 38 to 40 percent range. You're also less likely to net as many eggs (since banks usually only sell 6 to 8 at a time) or embryos. So depending on how many high-quality embryos you end up with, you may or may not have spare ones to freeze for later use. And if you end up needing/wanting more eggs from the same donor, there's definitely no guarantee that they'll be available. Still, since egg-freezing technology has come so far in recent years, results with frozen eggs are improving all the time. Along with the low cost and convenience of using frozen eggs, this makes them an attractive option for many couples—and for some couples, they're the only affordable option.

Once you've chosen a donor (or even better, while you're looking for that donor), you'll need to involve a lawyer, since there are certain legal issues surrounding egg donation and you'll want a formal written contract with your donor and/or the donor egg agency. The egg donor contract is usually explicit about the donor waiving all parental rights and makes it clear that any children born from the donated eggs are legally the recipient couple's children. The contract may also spell out specifics on what to do with any extra embryos (such as freezing them for later use). Keep in mind that laws vary from state to state.

Most clinics also recommend that couples meet with a therapist experienced in the emotional side of egg donation. You'll discuss the pros and cons of meeting the donor (more and more egg donation agencies enable the donor and recipient couple to share identities and even to meet over the phone, via video call, or in person), talk about whether to be open with your child later on about his or her genetic origins, and also dive into the emotional issues that may come up when using a donor egg: Will I love my baby as much as I would if he or she had my own genes? Will I have mixed emotions—say, feel detached from the baby—during pregnancy? When thinking about those emotional questions, remember that even if your DNA isn't being passed to your child, your partner's is—and that it will be your blood and your body that will nurture your baby, linking you together forever. Talking out any concerns you have—before pregnancy and during—with a therapist, your doctor, and your partner can help smooth the emotional path going forward. Also turn to insight from other couples who've had a baby using a donor egg.

Preparing for a Donor Cycle

Once you've chosen an egg donor and the contracts are signed, it's time to get ready for a pregnancy—one that involves 3 people at this point. Both you and your donor will have to undergo hormonal treatments to coordinate your cycles and to prepare each of you for your individual job responsibility (though if the eggs or embryos will be frozen for future use, synchronizing your cycles isn't necessary). Your donor will take fertility drugs (similar to the cocktail of drugs anyone undergoing IVF would use) to stimulate her ovaries to produce multiple eggs, and you'll use estrogen and progesterone to build up your uterine lining so it'll be ready for implantation. When your donor's eggs are mature, they will be retrieved and then mixed with your partner's sperm in a culture dish, and the best embryo or embryos will be transferred to your uterus within 3 to 5 days (assuming you coordinated your cycles) just like in a regular IVF cycle. If there are high-grade embryos left over, they can be frozen. If all the embryos are to be frozen for future use, preparing your uterus and transferring the embryos can be done at any time.

Sperm Donation

Thanks to advances in sperm-enhancing fertility treatments, the need for donor sperm has decreased somewhat. Still, there are a number of reasons why donor sperm might be considered or needed—for instance, if a male partner has an extremely low sperm count, no sperm, sperm of low quality, or sperm that carry a genetic defect. Lesbian couples or single women who will be using artificial insemination or IVF to conceive a baby will also need donor sperm.

Finding a Sperm Donor

Obtaining donor sperm is easier—and less expensive—than obtaining a donor egg for one simple reason: The sperm donation process requires so much less effort than the egg donation process. There are no cycles to consider, no hormones for the donor to take, no medical care for him to undergo (at your expense)—and of course, the actual retrieval of sperm could not be simpler (especially compared with egg retrieval).

Still, you're choosing half of your future baby's DNA when you're choosing a sperm donor—so you'll definitely want to choose with care. You'll also want to be picky when picking a sperm bank if you'll be using one—and there will be legal details to consider, too. So instead of jumping in to sperm donation, plan to take some baby steps first:

- Consider counseling first. Picking the biological father for your baby-to-be is about as major a life decision as you can make. That's why many experts recommend that you and your partner

Embryo Donation and Adoption

What happens when a couple can't conceive with their own egg and sperm? Does that mean their hopes of becoming pregnant are over? Not necessarily.

Embryo adoption, while not as common as using donor eggs or sperm, is an option more readily available for couples looking to build a family when other assisted reproductive routes have failed. With embryo donation, a previously frozen embryo from another couple is donated to you and implanted into your uterus—where it hopefully grows into a healthy pregnancy, just as with any IVF cycle.

Why would a couple give their embryos to another couple? It could be because they have surplus embryos from an IVF cycle after having already achieved one or more pregnancies and completing their family, or have opted against using the embryos they've created (say, because they have run out of IVF funds or are splitting up and no longer want to have a baby together) and have given the fertility clinic the right to donate them. And for some couples, stipulating that the extra embryos be given to another hopeful couple is preferable to storing them indefinitely (at a substantial cost), donating them for scientific research, or having them destroyed.

The odds are good that a frozen embryo transfer will result in a birth—about 37 percent according to recent data. Still, it's important to consider that donated embryos often come from older couples or from couples who were experiencing fertility challenges themselves, which make them less likely to result in a healthy pregnancy and live birth than an embryo created from an egg donation from a young, healthy donor.

(if you have one) see a counselor or therapist who's experienced in the field before going ahead with sperm donation. Talk about any concerns or questions you have about parenting a child conceived with donor sperm—whether the donor will be anonymous or a friend (and talk through the pros and cons of each option if they're both open to you). Discuss openly and frankly whether you'd want the biological father to be a part of the child's life—from the start, or years later, if your child ultimately wants that connection (and the sperm donor is willing).

■ Consider the bank. If you're thinking of using a sperm bank, do your homework first. All banks must be registered with the FDA, but ask if yours is accredited with the American Association of Tissue Banks, too. Accreditation is voluntary and costly, so many reputable banks may choose not to get accredited. Still, it's good info to have. Another thing to ask when looking for a sperm bank: how much information they will release now and in the future (in the event your child ever develops a condition that might require you to obtain information about the donor's genetic health). Ask, too, how thorough their screening process is. Most reputable banks will screen donors for diseases, get a complete family and medical history, and test for genetic disorders (it'll be important to know if the donor is a carrier for any genetic disorders, especially if you're also a carrier). Donors with a history or evidence of alcohol or drug abuse, as well as ones with some mental health conditions (like bipolar disorder or schizophrenia), are usually excluded from the donor pool. Also ask how much screening you'll be able to do when choosing a donor from their bank (keep reading).

■ Consider what you're looking for. You won't be living with this person, but you are making a baby together—so you'll want to spend some time thinking about what traits and characteristics will be at the top of your donor wish list. Most banks have comprehensive profiles on their prospective donors, a snapshot (often literally) of the man behind the sperm—everything from height to hair color, IQ, education, hobbies, ethnic background, and so on—so you can do some screening of your own. Some banks have both adult and childhood photos of the donor—giving you a clear picture of what your donor looks (and looked) like. You might also consider choosing your donor's blood type if you have Rh-negative blood and want your donor's to match (to avoid the potential for Rh incompatibility) or you'd like your baby to have the same blood type as your partner. One other pertinent bit of information you'll probably want to know: how many times a particular man has become a biological father through donation—and whether the donor has agreed to share identifying information with any children conceived with the use of his donor sperm (once they are over age 18). Fine with any eye color or ethnicity—just want your baby's sperm to come from a healthy source? The bank can select screened sperm randomly for you.

■ Consider whether you'll want more of the same. If you're thinking about having more babies and you'd like them to share the same biological father, make sure there will be additional batches of sperm from the same source available when you're ready.

■ Consider the strings attached when choosing a donor you know. Using a friend as your baby's sperm donor might be ideal for you and your partner—just remember that even your closest friend will have to be screened just as carefully as an anonymous donor would be. There are legal issues to consider, too, when using a known donor. If your goal is that the donor will have no parental rights or responsibilities, have the sample provided directly to a physician. Though state law varies, inseminations performed with a physician generally protect the rights of the donor to have no financial or parental obligations toward the child conceived with his sperm. If you think you might want the donor to have some relationship with your child, be sure to involve an attorney who will draw up a contract clearly outlining the donor's parental rights and responsibilities (but understand that, depending on your state laws, the court may not recognize the agreement).

■ Consider the legal ramifications. Be sure to learn the sperm donor laws in your state, because they are different in every state.

When you choose to use donor sperm from a bank, you'll be getting frozen sperm. An obvious bonus of using frozen sperm: no need to use a local source, since it can be safely shipped. But that's not the only reason why donor sperm is provided frozen. It's because most banks quarantine the sperm sample for several months and then retest the sample to make sure there are no infectious diseases that may not have been apparent at the time of donation. In fact, the American Society for Reproductive Medicine recommends that only sperm that has been frozen and stored for at least 180 days be used for donor insemination. Sperm banks carry out infectious disease screening and testing for syphilis, gonorrhea, chlamydia, HIV, hepatitis B, hepatitis C, West Nile virus, Creutzfeldt-Jakob disease, HTLV, Cytomegalovirus, and Zika virus both at the time of quarantine and when sperm is ready to be released.

Sperm bank websites should provide clear information on their policy regarding infectious disease screening, including for Zika virus. Genetic screening for cystic fibrosis and, depending on the donor's ethnicity, other genetic screening is also carried out.

Once you've made your donor choice, his frozen sperm will be delivered to the clinic and thawed and used to inseminate you either via IUI or an ART technique like IVF. In case you were wondering, most clinics will not allow a couple to mix the donor's sperm and the husband's/partner's sperm during insemination.

Surrogacy

What if you're longing for a biological baby but can't carry a pregnancy? Or you're a gay couple who wants to have babies of your own? You and your partner can turn to a surrogate—a woman who can carry your pregnancy for you, making your baby-making dreams come true. The right surrogate provides the nurturing uterine home your baby will need to develop from fertilized egg to ready-to-cuddle newborn. Then she delivers your bundle of joy—right into your loving arms. The perfect solution to your fertility challenges? It definitely could be—and in some cases, it's the only solution if you'd like your baby to have a genetic connection to at least one of you (it's definitely the only genetic option for a pair of hopeful fathers). Just be prepared to face a number of complex legal issues and intense emotions if you choose the surrogacy route. Expect the entire surrogacy process to take at least a year to a year and a half.

Types of Surrogates

You can grow your family using one of these 2 types of surrogates (though keep in mind that not all states allow surrogacy of any type and some allow only one type of surrogacy and not the other):

Gestational surrogacy. Gestational surrogacy is when a woman (called the gestational carrier) carries a baby who is not biologically related to her. This might be an option if you have viable eggs and want a biological child, but can't carry a baby yourself (because you can't sustain a pregnancy, don't have a uterus, have a medical condition that makes pregnancy dangerous or impossible, or for another reason). The embryo is formed in vitro with your eggs (which are retrieved as they would be for IVF) or with a donor's eggs and your partner's or a donor's sperm and is transferred to the gestational carrier's uterus, where it grows until the baby is ready to be born.

Fertility Treatments: To Tell or Not to Tell

As if the challenges of infertility don't shake you up enough, the emotional roller coaster of fertility treatments can be plenty unsettling—and one you and your partner may be riding alone, without the grounding support of family and friends. After all, seeking help for infertility is a very personal decision, and you (like many couples) may be reluctant to share your struggles, even with those you're closest to. Completely understandable, but it might not be the best approach. Researchers have found that couples who seek out social support from friends and family have a much healthier response to the emotional journey of IVF and other fertility treatments compared with couples who keep all those ups and downs on the down-low. And because the reduction of stress that comes from talking openly about your infertility and the efforts you're making to overcome it can have a positive physical effect, a healthier emotional response may translate into a better response to treatment. Trying to hide your struggles from those closest to you can put extra stress on you and your partner—stress that can lower the odds of IVF success. So even if you're

not feeling very sociable with all you're going through, think about surrounding yourself with supportive family and friends. No need to tell your hairstylist or the guy in accounting (unless you really want to, or they've shared similar challenges), but consider reaching out and sharing those highs and lows with those you love and who love you.

Opening up to others about something so intensely private may be hard at first, especially if you're not usually a sharer by nature. And feeling compelled to constantly offer updates can be wearing, too. Still, unloading that overload of emotions may be just the release you need to relax—which may, in turn, bring you closer to that baby you're longing for.

Still uncomfortable talking it out with friends and family? You can also turn to online support from others seeking fertility treatment: hopeful moms and dads who can relate, who can commiserate, who share your concerns and fears, and who know what you're going through. But, because these boards can be nearly anonymous, they don't know who you are, allowing you to express yourself without identifying yourself.

Since the baby is yours, there's no need for adoption after birth. In many states, you'll be able to get a pre-birth order so that your names go directly on your baby's birth certificate, though in some states, the birth certificate is amended after your baby's birth.

Gestational surrogacy is a popular choice for gay couples—as well as for lesbian couples, who can choose a twist on gestational surrogacy known as reciprocal surrogacy (see the box on page 220). In some states same-sex

couples will both be able to put their names on the birth certificate. In other states, the nonbiological parent will have to go through a second-parent adoption.

Traditional surrogacy. In traditional surrogacy, the surrogate is artificially inseminated with sperm from the male partner of an infertile couple, hopefully resulting in a pregnancy. The pregnancy can also be achieved through IVF. The couple may then legally adopt the child after birth (laws can vary from state to state, so be sure you consult with a reproductive rights attorney). Traditional surrogacy might be an option if you don't have any viable eggs, can't carry a pregnancy, and still want a baby who's biologically related to your partner. Gay couples can also choose traditional surrogacy (see the box on page 220).

There may be logistical obstacles when choosing traditional surrogacy. Because there have been legal challenges surrounding parental rights when traditional surrogates are used, many IVF programs will work with a gestational surrogate, but not a traditional surrogate. Legal consultation is important for any third-party reproduction relationship, but particularly when contemplating a traditional surrogate.

Choosing a Surrogate

There are a number of guidelines that experts recommend should be followed when choosing a surrogate. Your potential surrogate should be between ages 21 and 45, have a healthy BMI and a healthy lifestyle (no smoking, no drugs, and a willingness to abstain from alcohol during the pregnancy), be in a stable living situation with the support of a husband or partner, and have already given birth to at least one healthy baby. This is to make sure that the birth mother is familiar with the emotional and physical stresses of pregnancy and childbirth and understands what it means to carry, give birth to, and bond with a newborn (and therefore can appreciate how potentially difficult it might be to part with a baby after delivery).

A surrogate can be a close friend or family member—or one can be found through a surrogacy agency or an online matching site (though you'll get less support from online sites compared with an agency). Be sure to check the laws in your state regarding surrogacy, since they differ from state to state and can include restrictions on certain aspects of the process. If you live in a state that doesn't allow surrogacy, you may have to find a surrogate from another state where it's legal.

If you choose an agency. Going through an agency will be costly, but the agency will help you navigate this very complex process, recommending fertility clinics and mental health professionals who are experienced in surrogacy, as well as steering you to attorneys who specialize in surrogacy and are familiar with the legal issues particular to your state. The agency will also provide profiles of screened surrogate candidates to sift through and mediate initial conversations.

Your surrogate will undergo a thorough screening process that includes a psychological evaluation (this is to ensure she won't have any emotional difficulties handing your baby over to you after delivery), a full medical exam, an assessment of her ability to carry a pregnancy, infectious disease screening, and a check to make sure she's up to date on all necessary immunizations. Also an important consideration: The same guidelines about Zika virus that apply to any woman considering TTC apply to a surrogate before and during pregnancy (see page 10). A criminal background check will also be part of the screening.

Before being paired with a surrogate, you and your partner will also undergo a screening process to make sure you meet the agency's requirements for intended parents. Such a screening may include a medical exam and a mental health check, a home assessment, a criminal records check, and so on. The agency will create a profile of you and your partner that will be shared with the

Financing Fertility

The happy news if you're a couple unable to become parents the traditional way is that there are plenty of treatments and family-building options you can tap into. But once you figure out the best option or options for you, sticker shock may follow. The unhappy reality is that fertility treatments can cost a lot of money, more than most couples can easily pay, ranging from a few thousand dollars (for IUI) to tens of thousands of dollars (for IVF) and far more (for surrogacy). If you're lucky, you might be able to dip into savings to pay the high price of assisted fertility or borrow the funds from a family member (one, preferably, who's less interested in seeing interest on the loan and more interested in seeing the cuddly dividend it brings). But few hopeful parents (or hopeful grandparents or aunts or uncles) have that kind of cash on hand.

So are you out of luck if you can't afford the hefty out-of-pocket bills? Not necessarily. Here are some possible ways to finance fertility:

Health insurance. Though only a minority of states mandate some sort of insurance coverage for infertility treatments, a growing number of insurance companies offer coverage or partial coverage. Check with your employer or insurance company to find out whether any coverage applies to you, and see the box on page 40 for more on insurance.

Health savings/flex spending account. Consider looking into your flex spending account at work, if you have one. Such accounts allow you to use pretax dollars to pay for health care (though you might have to wait until the once-a-year signup time to allocate the funds). If you have access to a health savings account, you can use the tax-deductible dollars set aside in that account to pay for medical costs not covered by insurance—whether that's the high deductible, the co-pays, or even the full cost of fertility treatments.

Fertility clinic financing. Some fertility clinics will work with couples to come up with a financing plan to help make treatments more affordable through payment plans or treatment packages. Many clinics also have a guarantee or refund program for their treatments, meaning that if the treatment is unsuccessful, you'll get your money back.

Fertility financing companies. There are many fertility financing companies that offer low-interest financing, fertility savings programs, or other financing packages to help couples facing daunting fertility treatment costs. RESOLVE,

---

surrogate you've chosen to make sure there's a match on both sides.

Once both you and your intended surrogate agree to move forward, it's time to get to know each other. After all, you will likely be spending a lot of time together during the 9 months of pregnancy, and you almost certainly will be attending the birth. You can start with an initial call or face-to-face—a chance for you both to interview each other and gauge your compatibility. Ask questions: What are the potential surrogate's motives—is it for the financial benefit, or is she motivated by sympathy for your fertility struggles? Are her partner and family members supportive of her plan to be a surrogate? What is her background, and what are her interests? Does she work outside the home, and is her job pregnancy-friendly? Before you start the actual process, also schedule at

an organization dedicated to helping couples dealing with infertility, has a list of companies that offer these programs (go to resolve.org and search for "infertility financing programs").

Grant-giving organizations. There are a number of nonprofit organizations that provide financial assistance to select couples facing infertility. These include babyquestfoundation.org, cade foundation.org, payitforwardfertility .org, and others. There are also grant organizations specific to certain states. Check resolve.org for a list.

Crowdfunding online. Many couples are turning to the internet for financial help with their quest to become parents through fertility treatments, launching online fund-raising crowdsourcing campaigns through a growing number of websites. Such campaigns motivate friends and family (and even strangers) to donate money to your baby-making efforts, spurred on by watching even their small contributions add up to help you get closer to the baby of your dreams. And as an added bonus, many of these crowdsourcing sites are designated 501(c)3—which means the contributions are considered a charitable deduction on the giver's tax return.

Personal loans. Securing a personal loan from your bank or a home equity loan from your mortgage company may not be the easiest option, but if your credit is good, it's an option to explore. Putting the tab on credit cards (depending on your limits) can also be feasible, but check your interest rates first and calculate what the treatment plus the fees and charges will run you all-in.

Military help. If you or your partner are wounded active-duty military, you can tap into Tricare to cover fertility treatments. Other active duty military can take advantage of fertility treatments available at certain military treatment facilities. These treatments aren't completely covered, but they are offered at a discount, with the out-of-pocket costs lower than they would be at a nonmilitary fertility clinic. Wounded veterans can turn to the Department of Veterans Affairs for coverage of fertility treatments.

One source you should avoid dipping into when trying to finance fertility treatments: your retirement savings, such as IRAs or 401(k) plans. Not only will you likely be slapped with hefty early-withdrawal fees, but you'll also be harming your long-term financial stability and depleting funds you'll need when it comes time to pay for retirement (a time that, as hard as it is to believe now, will come!).

least one meeting that brings together you and your partner, the surrogate and her partner, and a therapist. These counseling sessions can help all the parties explore issues such as managing the surrogate-parents relationship, figuring out the type of relationship all parties want with each other, and thinking about the impact of the surrogate arrangement on the surrogate's family, spouse, children, and friends, as well as any other emotional and logistical issues that may come up.

If you choose a friend or relative. Choosing a friend or relative to be your surrogate may end up being less costly than going through an agency, and you'll already know a lot about the woman who will be carrying your baby, plus have a rapport with her. Even so, it's still important to go through all the necessary screening steps, follow all the mental health evaluation guidelines, and meet all the health requirements that an agency would advise and that laws may mandate.

Once you've chosen your surrogate (no matter if it was through an agency or if she's a close friend or relative), you'll need to hire two lawyers (one for you and one for your surrogate, but you'll be paying for both) to make sure all the legal paperwork is in order. A surrogacy contract should outline your rights and responsibilities and those of your surrogate. Issues to work out in advance include contact during and after the pregnancy, confidentiality, views on abortion (if testing reveals a problem with the pregnancy), and how many embryos you plan to transfer if you're doing IVF or how many artificial insemination attempts you plan to do if you're doing IUI. You'll want to lay out your expectations of the surrogate in terms of healthy eating, taking vitamins, not smoking or drinking or using drugs, the safe use of OTC and prescription medication, and so on, avoiding areas with CDC Zika travel notices, as well as expectations for prenatal care, prenatal and genetic tests, and other pregnancy-related care. There is also compensation to consider and document: surrogacy fees, IUI or IVF fees, prenatal care and other medical expenses (including, possibly, health insurance), food (you'll want her to be eating well while she's expecting your baby), travel to and from appointments, maternity clothing, and so on. The final tally can easily run in the high tens of thousands of dollars, and even into six figures.

The Surrogate Process

The process of creating a healthy baby is the same no matter which type of surrogate you choose, and whether or not your surrogate is someone you knew before embarking on the surrogate journey.

If you are using a gestational surrogate, your surrogate will go through the following steps:

- The surrogate may be asked to take birth control pills to sync her cycle with your cycle or the egg donor's cycle.

- The surrogate then takes estrogen and progesterone to get her uterus ready for a pregnancy.

- Regular blood draws and ultrasounds will ensure that the surrogate's cycle is on target and ready for the embryo to be transferred.

- The embryo is transferred into the surrogate's uterus as it is in an IVF cycle (see page 205) with the hopeful result of a healthy pregnancy and a healthy baby.

If you are using a traditional surrogate, she can become pregnant through IVF (in which case the steps are the same as for the gestational surrogate) or through IUI. If IUI will be used, the surrogate's cycles will be monitored and the donor sperm from the intended father will be used for insemination when she's ovulating (see page 183).

CHAPTER 12

Beginning Again After a Loss

No matter how long you've been trying to conceive, the excitement of a positive pregnancy test is overwhelming. But when the pregnancy ends abruptly in loss, the heartbreak can be overwhelming, too. The blow can be harder still if this is not your first miscarriage, or even your second, or if your path to conception was a long and bumpy one.

A loss can leave you longing for that baby more than ever, but it can also leave you with far more questions than answers as you consider your future fertility: Why did I lose the pregnancy? Are there any treatments that can help prevent a repeat miscarriage? And when can I start trying to conceive again? Whether you've suffered a single miscarriage or several, this chapter may help provide you with the answers and reassurance that you're looking for, so you can look forward to a new beginning.

Wondering About a Repeat

It's only natural to wonder—or worry—about having a repeat miscarriage after you've already suffered one loss or more. Fortunately, in the vast majority of cases, a miscarriage is followed by a healthy pregnancy. Knowing that this happy ending is most likely around the corner for you can make turning that corner much easier.

Chance of a Repeat Miscarriage

"I had a miscarriage last year, and we've finally gotten up the nerve to TTC again. Do I have a higher chance of having another miscarriage?"

Will It Happen Again?

If you've had a miscarriage, you're likely wondering—understandably—what the chances are that you'll have another. In most cases, they are probably a lot lower than you'd think (assuming you don't have any risk factors that contributed to the loss and depending on your age), and the chances of your next pregnancy having the happiest ending possible are excellent:

- If you have had 1 miscarriage, your chances of another miscarriage are pretty much the same as they are for someone who hasn't miscarried before—which means you have an excellent chance of a healthy pregnancy the next time around.

- If you've had 2 miscarriages, there is about a 75 percent chance that you'll carry the next pregnancy to term. The chance of loss is even lower if you've had 1 or more live births.

- If you've had 3 or more miscarriages, there is a 65 percent chance that you won't miscarry again.

Keep in mind that your age also contributes to miscarriage risk (the older you are, the higher the risk of miscarriage), but the chances of a successful pregnancy next time around are in your favor. You can further reduce your chances of miscarrying a second or subsequent time by treating any underlying causes that contributed to your first miscarriage or by improving any lifestyle risk factors that may have played a role in your first miscarriage.

All moms-to-be worry about miscarriage at some point in early pregnancy, and because you've already suffered a pregnancy loss, it's only natural that your stress level is stepped up. But fortunately, it doesn't have to be. Having 1 miscarriage does not increase your risk of having another—and in fact, you have the same excellent chances as someone who's trying for the first time that your next pregnancy will bring you the baby you've been hoping for. It's even possible that you can up your odds for a healthy pregnancy by reducing any miscarriage risks that apply to you (see page 237). So relax and enjoy your TTC activities—and your future pregnancy.

Testing After Miscarriage

"I just had my second miscarriage in a row. Should I get tested to figure out why this is happening?"

While a single loss isn't usually worth investigating (because most are random, one-time events, most practitioners won't work up a woman after a first miscarriage), trying to get to the bottom of recurrent losses definitely makes sense before you try to conceive again. About 50 percent of the time an explanation can be found through testing, which usually involves simple blood tests. Some of the tests you may be offered after your repeat miscarriages include:

- A karyotyping blood test for both you and the baby's father to see if either of you carries a balanced translocation—an altered chromosome arrangement—which may be the cause of the miscarriages

Looking to the Future

Just because a pregnancy doesn't take place in your body doesn't mean its loss doesn't hurt you deep inside. And just like your partner, you may approach another TTC campaign with mixed emotions. On the one hand, you're more eager than ever to produce that healthy baby. On the other hand, you're worried that another try might lead to another loss. If you and your partner have had multiple miscarriages (especially if no cause has been uncovered, making a targeted treatment trickier), hope may be hard to come by, because your hopes were dashed in the past.

But the truth is, there is a lot of hope that your baby dreams will come true. Even when miscarriages have been unexplained and there's no pinpointed cause to easily treat, a couple who has had 2 miscarriages before has a 75 percent chance of carrying the next pregnancy to term. For a couple who has had 3, the rate of success—without any kind of medical intervention—is still 65 percent.

Realistically, even the most optimistic statistics may not help you stress less about another miscarriage. So think positive (the more positive you stay, the more positive your partner will stay), but also try venting any lingering fears. Talk to each other, but also to friends who've experienced a pregnancy loss in the past (if you don't know any, look online for blogs or message boards devoted to dads who've experienced a loss). Making positive lifestyle changes, if there's any room for improvement (for instance, cutting back on alcohol, quitting smoking, losing weight, or eating better), can also help by making you feel like you're contributing to the success of the next pregnancy. Making lifestyle changes together with your partner as a team can strengthen your resolve. And as always, mood-lifting strategies (such as getting regular exercise and learning to relax) can help you see past the past—and keep your eye on the future, a future that will hopefully include that beautiful baby very soon.

- A blood test for antiphospholipid antibodies (antibodies that attack a woman's own tissues)

- An ultrasound of the uterus to check for anatomical problems

- An analysis of the chromosomal makeup of the miscarried embryo or fetus to see if there are any genetic factors that might have contributed to this loss (and perhaps your first one as well)

- Tests for vitamin deficiencies

- Tests of hormone levels (see page 239)

For more details on what all these tests might uncover, see the information starting on page 238.

Once the cause or causes are uncovered, you can talk to your practitioner about treatment options—as well as how to best care for your next pregnancy. In some instances, patients with a history of early miscarriages can benefit from hormone therapy: progesterone (begun after ovulation and before a pregnancy is even confirmed) for women who appear to be producing too little of this important pregnancy hormone, or a medication to reduce levels of the hormone prolactin in the mother's blood (if tests show that excess

Think Positive

A miscarriage—as devastating an event as it is—is a sign that you're capable of conceiving, and that's a very good sign. Even better, it's also a strong indication that you'll most likely conceive again. And even better still, like the vast majority of women who experience a miscarriage, you will very likely go on to have a normal pregnancy and a healthy baby in the near future. All very good reasons to think positive as you move forward in your efforts to become pregnant again.

It's understandable if you're having a hard time seeing a bright side in your baby future. And you may feel afraid to try again, for fear of losing again. As always, turn to your partner for support (remember, you're in this together), as well as to friends and family who've also suffered pregnancy losses and then gone on to have healthy babies. Joining a message board for moms who are TTC after a miscarriage or other pregnancy loss can also help boost your morale immeasurably (you'll find plenty of sharing on the WhatToExpect.com Grief and Loss forum).

Anything that helps you relax—and manage your emotions—can also help you think positive. Yoga, meditation, visualization techniques, deep-breathing techniques, hypnosis, and acupuncture (among other CAM approaches) can ease anxiety; exercise and eating well can lift your mood and brighten your outlook.

prolactin is the cause). If a thyroid problem is detected, it can be treated easily.

Sometimes no definitive cause turns up. Even then, reducing risk as much as possible may lower the chances of a reoccurrence (see facing page). It can also offer an important sense of empowerment: You're not just worrying about having a healthy pregnancy, but doing everything possible to help ensure that you will. No room for improvement? Just remember that the chances that you'll achieve pregnancy success next time around are very good, even if nothing in your preconception profile changes.

Ectopic Pregnancy Repeat

"I had an ectopic pregnancy 3 months ago. Does that put me at risk for a repeat?"

Your baby future is likely very bright. The vast majority of women who experience a single ectopic (or tubal) pregnancy go on to have a completely normal pregnancy next time around. If you've had 1 ectopic, the repeat risk in your next pregnancy is somewhere between 7 and 15 percent. If you've already had a successful pregnancy after an ectopic, your chances of having another tubal pregnancy are the same as for the general pregnant population, with no increased risk at all. Having no fertility issues also lowers your risk of a repeat, since most women who have repeat ectopics (which are rare) usually have other tubal or underlying fertility issues.

As for your fertility, that will depend on how your ectopic was managed (medically or surgically). If both of your tubes were preserved, your fertility is likely to be, too. More than half of all women who've had an ectopic go on to conceive a normal pregnancy within a year.

Preventing Pregnancy Loss

If you've had a miscarriage, you're undoubtedly wondering what you can do to prevent it from happening again. For most women, a miscarriage is a one-time event and the chances are excellent that the next pregnancy will deliver a healthy baby, without any intervention at all (though it doesn't hurt to increase those odds even more by minimizing, modifying, or eliminating any risk factors that apply). If you've had 2 or more miscarriages, trying to uncover the cause and then working to prevent repeats can help put a baby in your future a lot sooner. And luckily, with today's technology and advanced treatments, there are more and more ways to figure out what caused prior miscarriages and how to prevent future ones.

Reducing Risk

"I've had one miscarriage and my doctor says it probably won't happen again. Is there anything I can do now, before I start TTC again, to reduce the risk for next time?"

Your doctor's right—it probably won't happen again. Most single miscarriages are a chance occurrence, and the likelihood that you'll have a second loss is very low—in fact, as low as it is for someone who hasn't miscarried before. Still, it's always smart to maximize your chances for a healthy pregnancy. You're probably very familiar with this pro-pregnancy protocol—and you may already be following it carefully—but it doesn't hurt to check it over to see if you've got any room for improvement in your preconception prep:

- Your weight. Being significantly overweight or underweight can slightly increase the risk of miscarriage, but getting close to your ideal weight before you conceive can eliminate that risk.

- Your caffeine intake. Heavy caffeine intake early in pregnancy slightly increases the risk of miscarriage. Stick to no more than 200 mg of caffeine (about 12 ounces of brewed coffee or 2 shots of espresso) while you're TTC and once you become pregnant.

- A smoking habit. Don't worry about smoking that's in your past—but if

Could It Be You?

While a hopeful dad's health, diet, and lifestyle can all have a significant impact on fertility (as well as on the future health of your baby), they don't appear to play a role in miscarriage. Age, on the other hand, may be a factor. Because chromosomal abnormalities are somewhat more likely in an older man's sperm, dads over 40 may contribute to a slightly increased risk of miscarriage. But since the cause of most repeat miscarriages can be linked to the mom's health, dads aren't usually tested when multiple losses are being investigated unless a chromosomal problem is suspected (and then preimplantation genetic testing can be an option; see the box on page 212). So chances are you won't be rolling up your sleeve for testing, just supporting your partner as she undergoes any necessary workup.

you're currently a smoker, quit as soon as possible to cross this risk off your profile. Try as best you can to steer clear of secondhand and third-hand smoke as well (so if your spouse smokes, it's time for him to call it quits, too).

- Any drinking you do. As you've most likely heard, alcohol and pregnancy don't mix—and there's growing evidence that too much alcohol can increase the risk for miscarriage. So if you do drink, quit once you start TTC—that way, you'll be in the cocktail clear when sperm and egg meet.

- Your general health. Untreated chronic conditions (such as diabetes, lupus, high blood pressure), untreated thyroid problems, and untreated STDs can all increase miscarriage risk. Making sure your body is as healthy as possible before you conceive can help prevent miscarriage, again if there's room for improvement. A complete preconception checkup can screen for any condition that needs treatment.

- Your stress level. Extremely high emotional stress (not everyday stress) has been linked to pregnancy loss. Reducing extreme stress in your life as best you can may help reduce the risk for future miscarriages, as well as boost your fertility while you're TTC.

Chromosomal Defect

"I'm 39, and I just had a second miscarriage. My doctor says there were problems with the baby's chromosomes. Will I ever be able to have a healthy baby?"

It's thought that more than half of all miscarriages are caused by a defect in the chromosomal makeup of the embryo or fetus—so your situation is definitely not unusual. It's even less unusual among women in your age group. That's because as you age, so do your eggs. And older eggs—and possibly your partner's older sperm if he's over 40—are more likely to contain chromosomal abnormalities than younger eggs.

Knowing that your older egg supply might have been responsible for the chromosomal problems in your previous pregnancies can be discouraging—after all, you can't change your age or the age of your eggs. But the happy truth is, the chances that a perfectly healthy egg will pair up spontaneously with a perfectly healthy sperm to create the perfectly healthy baby you're hoping for are excellent. That's what happens most of the time in a case like yours.

But what happens if chromosomal problems keep preventing that happy outcome and that healthy embryo? For a very few couples (particularly older ones), miscarriages caused by chromosomal defects happen again and again. Unfortunately, it's impossible to detect defective chromosomes in an embryo when conception occurs the natural way. But with today's medical technology, physicians are able to screen embryos formed in vitro with PGD/PGS (see the box on page 212). Once an embryo is determined to be free from identifiable chromosomal abnormalities, it can be transferred to your uterus with the hope that it implants and develops into a healthy pregnancy and healthy baby. And for some couples—especially ones who have been suffering from recurrent pregnancy losses—preimplantation testing may help tip the healthy-pregnancy scales in their favor.

Keep in mind, too, that other factors may have contributed to your miscarriages—and those factors might be treatable. After all, just because the last baby had chromosomal problems, it's impossible to determine that the same problem led to your previous pregnancy loss (unless tests were performed on the

Age and Miscarriage Risk

Miscarriage does become some-what more likely to happen as you age. That's because older mothers have older eggs, and older eggs have a greater chance of carrying a chromosomal abnormality. Plus, fewer egg follicles means reduced ovarian hormone production, which may make it more difficult for an older mom-to-be to sustain a pregnancy. Still, the increase in risk may not be as high as you'd think. While a 20-year-old's odds of losing a pregnancy are 15 percent, a 40-year-old has a 40 percent chance of miscarrying—higher, yes, but still with odds in your favor. Though there's nothing you can do about your age or the age of your egg supply, you can definitely maximize your chances of carrying a baby to term by minimizing all the other miscarriage risks that might apply to you.

other fetus as well). So make sure you're screened for all other potential risk factors (including hormonal imbalances that are more common in women over 35) to increase your odds of a successful pregnancy next time around, no matter how you decide to conceive.

Hormonal Imbalance

"I have a thyroid condition, and I'm wondering if that has anything to do with the miscarriage I just had."

It takes an intricate balance of hormones to deliver a pregnancy safely from conception to delivery. Most of the time, nature takes its hormonal course without incident, but sometimes an imbalance can result in a pregnancy loss.

The most common hormonal imbalances associated with miscarriage are:

Hyperprolactinemia. Though the link is not well established, there is a theory that having higher-than-normal levels of prolactin (the hormone responsible for breast milk production) may increase the risk for miscarriage. Signs of hyperprolactinemia can be a milky discharge from your nipples or anovulation (when you have a period but don't ovulate). Blood tests can reveal if you have excess prolactin. While the link between hyperprolactinemia and infertility is stronger than that with miscarriage, your doctor may decide to treat you with medication that decreases the levels of prolactin to increase the chances that your next pregnancy will continue successfully.

Thyroid condition. Thyroid hormone, though not officially a member of the reproductive hormone team, can directly impact reproduction. Very abnormal levels of thyroid hormone can not only reduce fertility, but in cases of severe imbalance, may lead to miscarriage. Thyroid conditions are easily detected through a blood test. In the case of hypothyroidism (the most common thyroid condition, in which your body makes too little thyroid hormone) the treatment is easy, too. Taking thyroid replacement hormone (a daily pill) regulates thyroid hormones and dramatically reduces the risk of miscarriage in future pregnancies. For more on hyperthyroidism, see page 164.

Polycystic ovarian syndrome (PCOS). Women with untreated PCOS are at greater risk of having irregular ovulation and periods because of higher-than-normal levels of testosterone and LH. In some cases, these abnormal hormone levels also increase the risk of miscarriage. Some women with untreated

Luteal Phase Deficiency

Most experts agree that a luteal phase deficiency (LPD)—when the luteal phase (the second half of a menstrual cycle) is shorter than 10 to 12 days—has little clinical significance, and that it doesn't contribute to infertility or miscarriage. Still, the long-circulating theory that it does continues to persist, especially on message boards and blogs, but also among some physicians. The thinking behind it: A short luteal phase doesn't allow enough time in the cycle for progesterone levels to build. Low progesterone levels, the theory goes, can lead to an inadequately prepared uterus (the endometrium can't thicken sufficiently), and the lack of a thick lining in the uterus can make it difficult for an embryo to implant or for a pregnancy to sustain itself.

If your doctor believes that an LPD could be contributing to your miscarriages (or is associated with an underlying condition that may be contributing to your miscarriages), he or she may decide to try treatment that might prevent a repeat loss in future pregnancies. Such treatment may include supplemental natural progesterone taken as an injection, a vaginal suppository, or an oral tablet before conception and continuing through the early stages of pregnancy to help sustain the pregnancy and avoid miscarriage. Clomid (an ovulation inducer; see page 187) can also be used as a treatment, since the medication stimulates more than one follicle to mature, allowing more than one corpus luteum (which produces progesterone) to produce enough of the hormone to sustain the pregnancy. Supplemental hCG can also be used to increase the amount of progesterone secreted by the corpus luteum.

Keep in mind that an LPD is often the by-product of another hormonal imbalance issue (see page 239), and once that other hormonal imbalance is treated, the LPD is also remedied.

PCOS also have insulin resistance (insulin is a hormone, too), and it is thought that this type of hormonal imbalance can prevent the endometrial lining from maturing properly, making it harder for an embryo to implant properly. See page 159 for more on treating PCOS.

Immune System Malfunction

"Is it true that some miscarriages are caused by the mom's body attacking the baby? Is there anything that can be done to prevent that from happening?"

As hard as it is to believe (after all, isn't a mom's body designed to welcome and nurture her developing baby?), what you've heard is true. A very small percentage of miscarriages are thought to be triggered by antibodies in the mom's body. These autoantibodies (antibodies that attack their own) increase the risk of blood clots, decreasing the blood flow to the developing fetus and causing a miscarriage, usually after 10 weeks.

Autoimmune problems in general account for less than 5 percent of recurrent miscarriages. But if you have had multiple miscarriages, blood tests can reveal if you're producing autoantibodies (called antiphospholipid antibodies). Once an immune system malfunction is confirmed, your practitioner may

Preventing a Repeat with CAM

The list of what complementary and alternative medicine (CAM) is purported to do grows longer and longer as more and more of these alternative therapies are being integrated into more and more traditional treatments. And though there aren't any studies to back it up yet, many women and their practitioners maintain that helping prevent recurrent miscarriages makes the list, too. It's believed that the stress-releasing qualities of CAM therapies such as meditation, yoga, tai chi, and acupuncture may explain why they seem to be effective in some cases—particularly when an expectant mom is really stressed about the possibility of another pregnancy loss. Acupuncture may also help promote circulation to the uterus, ensuring a healthier uterine lining and increasing the chances it can sustain and nurture a pregnancy.

What about herbal remedies to prevent pregnancy loss? Herbalists say that herbs such as wild yam, partridge berry, red raspberry leaf, black cohosh, blue cohosh, and others can help (though red raspberry leaf, black cohosh, and blue cohosh, taken in large amounts can actually trigger contractions). But because different herbal practitioners will prescribe different cocktails of favorite herbs purported to prevent miscarriage, because herbal treatments do not undergo testing for safety and effectiveness in this country, and because there are few or no studies to prove whether they work, herbs are best approached with caution. If you do decide to explore herbals, be sure you do so under the supervision of a licensed practitioner and with the knowledge and go-ahead of your traditional medical team.

recommend low-dose aspirin (about ¼ of a regular strength aspirin per day) throughout your pregnancy and/or heparin (a stronger anticoagulant) injections given during the first half of your pregnancy to help stop the formation of blood clots that could be fatal to the fetus. Your pregnancy will be considered high risk, but with excellent prenatal care and continued monitoring, you can look forward to a healthy pregnancy and a healthy baby.

Anatomical Problems of the Uterus

"My doctor mentioned that I have an unusually shaped uterus. Could that be the cause of my miscarriage? Will that mean I'll have another one?"

Possibly, but not necessarily. While experts believe that 10 to 15 percent of all miscarriages result from uterine malformations and other anatomical problems in the uterus and cervix, less than 5 percent of women with a uterine malformation have one that is bad enough to cause a miscarriage. That's because only certain uterine shapes (such as a septum, in which a wall of tissue separates the 2 sides of the uterus) interfere with the healthy implantation of an embryo or make women more prone to miscarriage. Other anatomical obstacles in the uterus, such as large fibroids, may also interfere with implantation and/or the proper growth of a fetus. Tests such as hysterosalpingo-gram (an assessment of the uterus and fallopian tubes using x-ray imaging and dye), hysteroscopy (visualization of the

The Emotional Fallout

Miscarriage can be devastating. The loss of a baby, no matter how early it happens, can leave you with a range of emotions, from grief to denial, anger to sadness—even hopelessness, especially if it has happened more than once. Remember, not only will you need to grieve in your own way and heal at your own pace, but you (and your partner) will need plenty of support as you do. You'll find help coping after a miscarriage in *What to Expect When You're Expecting.*

uterus using a camera), sonohysterogram (visualization using ultrasound), or an MRI can be used to diagnose a uterine problem.

If it turns out that the unusual shape of your uterus is serious enough to have caused your pregnancy loss and may threaten any future conceptions, surgery before you become pregnant again can be a quick and effective fix, making your womb a welcoming space for a baby to grow in. If the issue is fibroids, those can be removed, again making your uterus baby friendly.

If it turns out that the shape of your uterus probably wasn't the cause of your miscarriage, chances are it was a random event that won't repeat—in which case, your risk of miscarrying a second time is just as low as it is for the general pregnant population.

Infections/Fever

"Is it possible the bad cold I had when I conceived caused my miscarriage?"

It takes a lot more than a cold to trigger a pregnancy loss. Though there is a small risk that certain infections may trigger a miscarriage, it applies to much more serious (and much less common) infections such as mumps, measles, CMV, listeria, STDs, Zika virus, and a host of others you've probably never heard of and aren't likely to be exposed to. But it doesn't apply to colds, even bad ones, so it couldn't have been responsible for your miscarriage.

What about a fever? While a brief fever that is promptly brought down isn't cause for concern (and wouldn't be the cause of a loss), a high fever that is prolonged can cause problems in the embryo or fetus, possibly leading to miscarriage. Which is why it's so important to treat any fever you develop while you're TTC or during the early pregnancy period, using pregnancy-safe medication as recommended by your prenatal practitioner.

Prevention should also be part of your preconception MO, and that means staying healthy by practicing healthy hygiene habits (hand washing, avoiding close contact with other people who are infectious, and so on) and making sure you are up-to-date on all your immunizations. Most important on that vaccine list: the flu shot.

Trying Again

If you're like most hopeful parents-to-be, getting pregnant again is the best possible therapy after a pregnancy loss—and it's something you may be aching to do as soon as you can. But it's also possible you'll approach trying to conceive again—like many hopeful parents who have suffered a miscarriage—with a little less excitement and happy anticipation. After all, you now know that a positive pregnancy test doesn't necessarily come with the promise of a healthy baby. The loss of innocence that may follow a pregnancy loss—and the trepidation it can bring when you contemplate conceiving again—is understandable, and very common. Just try to remind yourself that the vast majority of women who have had a miscarriage, or even multiple losses, go on to have healthy pregnancies and healthy babies. Chances are you'll be on your way to starting—or adding to—your family again, just a little later than you'd thought.

When to Try Again

"I just had a miscarriage, and I'm wondering when we can start trying to conceive again. We both want to so badly."

Since there are no definitive rules about when you should start trying to conceive again after a miscarriage, there's no definitive answer to that question. Different practitioners may offer different guidelines—and even the same practitioner may recommend a different waiting period under different circumstances. Many give the go-ahead to start trying again as soon as you feel physically and emotionally up to it after a miscarriage. In fact, some

actually encourage a sooner-than-later approach. That's because reproductive hormones are often elevated and fertility is often at its peak in the 3 months following a miscarriage—meaning that your chances of getting pregnant may be higher than usual during this time. More encouraging news if you're hoping to get an early start: There does not seem to be an increase in the miscarriage rate for women who've conceived immediately after a pregnancy loss.

Still, some practitioners suggest waiting 2 to 3 months before trying to conceive again. That's to allow your cycle to regulate, to give you time to beef up your nutritional reserve (if you hadn't been taking prenatal vitamins before or if your iron stores were depleted due to heavy bleeding), or to give your body time to heal (if the miscarriage was a later one). Other practitioners recommend waiting until you have your first normal period before

Resuming Sex

Even if you're not ready to start trying for a baby right after a miscarriage, it's fine to start having sex again (if you're both up to it emotionally) once the bleeding from the miscarriage (and/or a D&C) stops. Just keep in mind that if you're having sex without birth control, there's a chance you can get pregnant almost immediately— even without getting your period, since ovulation sometimes happens before that. Which, of course, might be exactly what you're hoping for.

Endings and Beginnings

Contemplating beginning a pregnancy when one has just ended can leave your feelings all over the emotional map. Of course, you desperately want that "rainbow" baby (as babies born after a miscarriage are often called)—and a healthy pregnancy that puts that baby in your arms—as soon as possible. But at the same time, trying for another may make you feel almost disloyal to the baby you've lost, even if that loss came very early in the pregnancy.

How to reconcile a fresh beginning with that painful ending? It may help to keep in mind that you're not replacing one pregnancy with another, or one

baby with another. You don't have to stop grieving for your lost pregnancy to start trying to conceive another—and in fact, you can continue remembering the baby you lost for as long as you need to or want to (by commemorating the day of the loss each year, planting a tree in your garden, honoring your baby's memory by giving to organizations that support moms and babies in need).

Of course, also keep in mind that you may not have any feelings of ambivalence when it comes to trying again—in fact, you may be nothing but excited to try again—and that's just as normal and understandable. Your reaction is what's right for you.

actively trying for a baby. The reasoning: so that the next pregnancy will be easier to date (though that's usually less of an issue these days because early ultrasound can provide an accurate date) and to ensure that all the hCG from the previous pregnancy has left your system completely and your hormone levels are back to normal. For most women, that first period will arrive pretty quickly, usually within 4 to 6 weeks after the miscarriage.

Finally, when you'll be given the green light for TTC may also depend on whether or not tests need to be run to rule out conditions that may have caused the miscarriage or whether you have a chronic condition that needs to be better controlled. Either way, taking that extra time—and those extra precautions (if necessary and recommended by your practitioner)—may help ensure that any future conception will develop into a healthy pregnancy.

If your practitioner does give you the immediate go-ahead, go right ahead

and begin your TTC efforts. If he or she recommends waiting, use reliable contraception, preferably of the barrier type (condom, diaphragm) until the waiting time is up. Take advantage of this waiting period—spend it improving your diet and your health habits (if there's any room for improvement) and generally getting your body into tip-top baby-making shape. That way, you'll feel that you're at least doing something constructive while you wait—plus, it'll give you something else to focus on besides the waiting. If your practitioner recommends waiting but you're not sure why, ask—and if you're super eager to start trying again right away, see if there's any wiggle room in that recommendation. Most of the time there is.

Ready . . . or Not

"I just had a miscarriage, and though my doctor told me we could start TTC again, I'm not sure I'm ready, at least emotionally."

For some couples, resuming TTC efforts as soon as possible after a pregnancy loss is just what they need to complete their emotional healing. For them, tracking cervical mucus changes, charting BBT, and actively trying for a baby again can help take their focus off their loss and shift it to something positive. It can also help a woman who's suffered a pregnancy loss recover some of the control over her body that the miscarriage (an experience completely out of her control) took from her.

For others, however, starting to try again right after a loss may not feel right—whether because they're fearful of another miscarriage or because they feel they need more time to grieve. Whichever category you fall into, remember that you need to do what feels right for you. Don't let yourself feel pressured by anyone (your ob, your best friend, your mother-in-law) to pick up where you left off and start trying again right away. Maybe you're ready, maybe you're not—but only you and your partner can make that decision.

Just make sure that you come to that decision together. Though it's your body that has suffered the physical effects of the pregnancy loss, both of you have paid the emotional price. So talk about it. It may help, too, to talk to others who know exactly what you're going through because they're going through it, too—but who are objective in their feedback. In addition to helping you make (or feel better about) your decision, that support can help you heal. If you don't have friends or family who can personally relate, or if you'd just like to get all the support you can, you can also find it on TTC or loss message boards.

If you're still on the fence about whether now's the right time (and keeping in mind that there's no time that's right for everyone), you may want to take into account the physical facts. Since women may be more fertile in the 3 months after a miscarriage, beginning again sooner may bring you success sooner (though it's definitely not a guarantee of success). But don't discount or second-guess your emotions, either. If you feel you need to take a break, and take a breath, before you begin to TTC again, then that's absolutely what you should do. Listen to your heart, and you'll make the decision that's right for you.

Return to a Normal Cycle

"When will I start ovulating and get my period again after my miscarriage?"

Your menstrual cycle can't get up and running until your body realizes you're no longer pregnant—and for that to happen, all of the hCG has to be out of your system. For the hCG to

Keeping Track Again

Since it's hard to know when you've begun ovulating again after a miscarriage (ovulation may begin before your first period or not until you've had 1 or 2), you may be eager to resume charting or keeping track on your app. Probably best not to be too eager. If you begin keeping track immediately after a miscarriage and before you get your first period, you may find those readings all over the place—and largely unreliable. That's normal and to be expected. For better results, wait until after your first normal period and then start fresh with your tracking.

Your Periods After a Loss

Wondering what your periods will be like after you miscarry? Chances are they'll be pretty much the way they were before. So if you were a heavy bleeder before your loss, you should expect the same now. And if your periods were light and quick, they'll resume that way, too. Cycle length also usually returns to the status quo after a miscarriage, though the first couple of cycles may be a little longer than usual.

get out of your system, the developing placenta has to fully detach from the uterine wall (or be removed in a D&C). Once the hCG is completely gone (it takes about 10 days after the placenta detaches for hCG to hit zero), you can expect your period to return within 4 to 6 weeks (if your cycles were regular before conceiving), with ovulation occurring 2 to 4 weeks after your hCG reaches zero.

But don't start counting those weeks from the first day you noticed spotting or bleeding. It could take a week or two (or even longer) from the beginning of the miscarriage until the placenta pulls away and that important hormonal shift takes place (you won't notice these changes, you'll only be aware of continuous bleeding). Which means that if you haven't gotten your period again after 6 weeks from the first day you noticed miscarriage bleeding, there's no need to worry. Wait another week or two before putting in a call to your practitioner. Your period might be just around the corner.

Something else to keep in mind: If your miscarriage occurred late in the first trimester or in the second trimester, you had a lot of hCG in your system (hCG rises as your pregnancy progresses)—and that means it'll take longer to hit that zero mark, and consequently, your period may take a little longer to resume.

Another reason why your period may be late to return: Some women retain tiny fragments of placental tissue after a miscarriage (and more rarely, after a D&C). If that's the case with you, your bleeding may taper off only to resume a few days (or even a week or two) later. This bleeding isn't a period yet—it's the continuation of your pregnancy loss. And that means you can't expect to see a true period until at least 4 weeks after the miscarriage has officially completed (in other words, until 4 weeks after all the placental tissue has pulled away from the uterine wall). Though this scenario is normal (if uncommon), do put in a call to your practitioner just for peace of mind—you might need a D&C to remove all the placental tissue fragments. If your hCG levels are at zero but you still continue spotting, your doctor may give you a prescription for Provera or some other form of progesterone to trick your body into thinking it's time for a period so your cycles can get back to normal. Of course, if at any time the bleeding becomes very heavy again, call your practitioner as soon as you can.

And though the return of your period may indicate that you've begun ovulating, it's not a sure bet. That's because there may be one (or more) anovulatory cycles (in which you get your period without ovulating) after a miscarriage. To figure out whether you're back to ovulation business as usual, you'll need to start up your cycle tracking again.

Of course, the return of your period can also mean that you've already ovulated, as some women ovulate before that first period shows up. Which means that if you're not yet ready to be pregnant again, you should be using birth control even before that first period arrives.

Lingering Pregnancy Symptoms

"We started TTC again right after my miscarriage. I'm still feeling pregnancy symptoms, and I'm wondering if that means I'm pregnant again or if they're leftover symptoms from the pregnancy that I lost."

That's a tough call—and it may be an impossible one to make at this point. The problem is, there are several possible explanations for your symptoms. One is that you're experiencing PMS. As you probably discovered when you were TTC last time, PMS symptoms can be very difficult to distinguish from early pregnancy symptoms (especially tender breasts and bloating), and it might be tricky to figure out if those symptoms might be signaling the return of your period or a new pregnancy—especially if you haven't had a normal period since you miscarried. Also possible: Your body isn't quite ready for the return of your period but is reacting to hormonal fluctuations—which can be substantial after a pregnancy loss.

Another less likely explanation is that what you're feeling are residual pregnancy symptoms—but for that to be the case, you'd still have to have residual hCG in your system. This is possible if your miscarriage was very recent (the hCG is usually out of your system about 10 days after a miscarriage or D&C is complete) or took place later in the first trimester or in the second (in which case the hCG levels might take a little longer than that to hit zero). Until the hCG is completely gone, you can't ovulate, you can't get your period, and you can't get pregnant. You can, however, experience leftover pregnancy symptoms—and even possibly produce a positive pregnancy test, which would further confuse the picture.

Still another explanation—and this is likely the one you're hoping for—is that you might be pregnant again. It is possible to ovulate and conceive before you've had that first post-loss period, though diagnosing that pregnancy might be tricky initially (a home pregnancy test, again, might be responding to residual hCG in your system, rather than newly generated pregnancy hormone).

Sometimes, pregnancy symptoms after a loss can understandably be triggered by emotional causes—you want to be pregnant still (or again), and so your psyche is clinging to the symptoms (which can feel very real even if they're not physically generated).

Check in with your doctor if you're unsure what to think—or if you'd like confirmation of whether you're pregnant. And if you are pregnant, it's time to start seeing your practitioner anyway—so you can get the care you'll need to help you have a healthy pregnancy and that beautiful rainbow baby of your dreams!

PART 4

Keeping Track

Your Fertility Planner

....

Of course you can get pregnant the old-fashioned way—stop using birth control, have sex whenever, wherever, in whatever position, and wait for a missed period. But there's definitely an upside to planning conception—actually many upsides. Taking charge of your fertility planning gives you the opportunity to get your body, your partner's body, and your life in tip-top baby-making shape before your conception campaign begins—and gives you a chance to stack the cards in favor of a speedier conception, a safer and more comfortable pregnancy, and a healthier baby. Plus, it gives you an opportunity to put that multitasking control freak in you (yes, you) to work on one of life's most satisfying projects: baby making. Let the planning begin.

Countdown to Conception

You can never be fully prepared for becoming a parent, or even for becoming pregnant. But when time is on your side (you're just starting to think about taking the baby plunge), it makes sense to put that time to the most productive use possible.

The following schedule is a general guide to conception prep (there may be items to subtract and other items to add to your specific plan). Don't stress too much about keeping to the suggested schedule—just try to get as many items on your to-do list crossed off as you can before you get cracking on conception.

As you count down to conception consider how much to-doing you've got to get done (for instance, if you have a hefty number of pounds to lose, you'll want to get an earlier start on weight loss). Factor in your own time frame for getting pregnant, too. If you want to get busier sooner rather than later, skip right to the 3-month plan.

6 to 12 Months Out

FOR HER

☐ Evaluate your weight and BMI. If you have a lot to lose, start a healthy, balanced weight-loss program now. If you're significantly underweight, start eating with an eye on moving those numbers up (and if you have an eating disorder, get treatment now).

☐ Start taking a daily prenatal vitamin. It's not considered a must-do until 3 months out, but it's never too early to start filling in any nutritional blanks.

☐ If you're on Depo-Provera shots, you'll need to stop them within 6 to 12 months of starting TTC and switch to a short-term birth control method while you're waiting.

☐ If you have substantial problems with your gums and/or teeth, or you think you might, get busy having all necessary dental work done.

☐ If you don't currently have health insurance, make sure you sign up soon for a policy that covers essential health benefits like maternity care, so you're covered when you start TTC.

☐ If you have any chronic medical conditions, take steps to get them under control.

☐ If you're booking future travel now, consider that women are advised to avoid travel to an area with a CDC Zika travel notice at least 8 weeks before TTC.

NOTES: _____

_____

_____

_____

FOR HIM

☐ Evaluate your weight and BMI. If you have a lot of weight to lose, start a healthy, balanced weight-loss program now.

☐ If you have any chronic medical conditions, take steps to get them under control.

☐ If possible, avoid travel to Zika-affected areas in the 6 months before you start TTC. If you must travel to (or if you live in) an area with a Zika travel notice, check with your doctor about preconception precautions you should take.

NOTES: _____

_____

_____

_____

3 Months Out

FOR HER

☐ Evaluate your weight and BMI. If they need a little adjusting (up or down), start a healthy, balanced weight-loss (or weight-gain) program now.

☐ Take a look at your eating habits, and if they're not up to pre-pregnancy par, ease into a healthy eating plan with baby making in mind.

☐ If you normally see a therapist (or think you need to see one) for any mental health issues, a visit for a preconception screening is a good idea.

☐ Start taking a daily prenatal vitamin, if you haven't already.

☐ If you're not up to date on all your immunizations, now's the time to roll up your sleeve for any you're missing.

☐ Cut out smoking. If quitting cold turkey will be too tough, use the next 3 months to cut back slowly until you're nicotine free.

☐ Begin weaning yourself off prescription and over-the-counter medications (under your doctor's guidance) that are not conception compatible and substituting those that are.

☐ Consider undergoing genetic screening. Expanded carrier screening can screen for the carrier genes of more than 300 diseases, giving you the power of knowing whether you and your partner are at risk of passing along any genetic conditions to the baby you conceive together.

☐ Ditch hormonal birth control (the Pill, patch, ring) and use only barrier methods for now (condom, diaphragm, spermicides).

☐ Stop using recreational drugs. If you need help quitting, seek it now.

NOTES: _____

_____

_____

_____

_____

_____

_____

_____

_____

_____

FOR HIM

☐ Evaluate your weight and BMI. If you could drop a few pounds, now's the time to start a healthy, balanced weight-loss program. If you're too thin, consider beefing up a bit.

☐ Take a look at your eating habits. If there's room for improvement, now's a great time to start eating with fertility optimizing in mind.

☐ Take a multivitamin to help ensure your body is well stocked for optimal sperm production.

☐ Cut out smoking. If quitting cold turkey will be too tough, use the next 3 months to cut back slowly until you're nicotine free.

☐ Take stock of your medicine cabinet. With your doctor's help, begin substituting medications that are compatible with baby making for those that aren't.

☐ Stop using recreational drugs. If you need help quitting, seek it now.

☐ Continue taking Zika virus precautions, keeping in mind that men are advised not to TTC for at least 6 months after returning from an area with a CDC Zika travel notice.

☐ Consider undergoing genetic screening. Expanded carrier screening can screen for the carrier genes of more than 300 diseases, giving you the power of knowing whether you and your partner are at risk of passing along any genetic conditions to the baby you conceive together.

NOTES: _____

_____

_____

_____

_____

_____

_____

_____

_____

_____

_____

_____

_____

_____

2 Months Out

FOR HER

☐ Make an appointment with your gynecologist or chosen prenatal practitioner for a complete top-to-bottom preconception checkup to make sure all baby-making systems are go.

☐ Get a dental checkup and cleaning, if you haven't recently.

☐ Begin (or continue) a moderate exercise program (aim for 30 minutes each day).

☐ Start to limit the amount of caffeine you get each day (goal: no more than 200 mg, or about 2 small cups, of coffee a day).

☐ Stop dieting for significant weight loss and continue eating balanced healthy foods that will maintain your loss.

☐ Take a good look at your workplace environment. If any occupational hazards might be a problem when trying to conceive (or during pregnancy), find ways to limit your exposure.

☐ Avoid travel to areas with a CDC Zika travel notice for at least 8 weeks before you actively start to TTC. If you live in a Zika-affected area, check with your doctor about precautions you should take and visit cdc.gov/zika.

☐ Reduce your exposure to BPA and phthalates by choosing BPA-free and phthalate-free products, opting for cloth bags instead of plastic, and using glass food and drink containers instead of plastic ones.

☐ Begin keeping track of your basal body temperature (BBT) and your cervical mucus (CM) changes. Also track any other cycle changes and ovulation signs you notice so you'll be able to pinpoint ovulation.

NOTES: _____

_____

_____

_____

_____

_____

_____

_____

_____

_____

_____

FOR HIM

☐ See your doctor for a full-body checkup. Be sure to let him or her know you and your partner are about to start trying to conceive and ask if any special tests or exams might be important now.

☐ Evaluate your work environment. If you're exposed to any hazards that may harm your fertility or the health of your sperm, find ways to limit exposure for now.

☐ Reduce your exposure to BPA and phthalates by choosing BPA-free and phthalate-free products, opting for cloth bags instead of plastic, and using glass food and drink containers instead of plastic ones.

☐ Keep cool by staying out of hot tubs, hot baths, and saunas. Treat your laptop as a desktop and keep your cell phone out of your pants pocket.

☐ Continue taking precautions to avoid exposure to Zika virus.

NOTES: _____

_____

_____

_____

_____

_____

_____

_____

_____

_____

_____

_____

_____

_____

_____

_____

_____

_____

1 Month Out

FOR HER

☐ Start reducing your alcohol intake with the aim of cutting it out altogether once you start trying to conceive.

☐ Make sure your finances are in order, including your insurance policies and will.

☐ Learn ways to relax and try to avoid stressful situations starting now (as best you can).

☐ Create regular sleep and wake patterns, with the goal of catching 6 to 9 hours of shut-eye per night.

☐ Continue tracking your BBT, your CM changes, and other ovulation signs.

☐ Don't forget that daily vitamin.

☐ Continue taking precautions to avoid exposure to Zika virus.

☐ Think happy baby thoughts!

NOTES: _____

_____

_____

_____

FOR HIM

☐ Cut back on alcohol for now to keep your sperm production high and in good baby-making shape.

☐ Cut back on overly strenuous exercise routines (especially heavy-duty bicycling).

☐ Make sure your finances are in order, including your insurance policies and will.

☐ Learn ways to relax and try to avoid stressful situations starting now (as best you can).

☐ Create regular sleep and wake patterns, with the goal of catching 7 to 8 hours of sleep a night.

☐ Continue to take precautions to avoid exposure to Zika virus.

NOTES: _____

_____

_____

_____

Ready? Set? Now GO TTC!

Your Fertility Charts

You know there's an app for that, but you'd prefer to keep track of your fertility on paper? This all-in-one fertility chart will let you keep track of all your ovulation and fertility signs, enabling you to better pinpoint when ovulation is happening (and when you should start getting busy in bed). Begin a few months before you start TTC so you can get a head start. Here's how to put it all together:

1. Using a digital basal body thermometer, take your temperature each morning before you get out of bed and mark each daily reading on the graph. Connect the dots to help pinpoint ovulation.

2. In the row marked "Cervical Mucus (CM) Consistency," note the consistency of your CM (dry, sticky, creamy, or slippery), as detailed on page 100, to help identify when you're most fertile.

3. You can mark down whether your cervix is opened or closed in the row marked "Cervical Position."

4. Fill in the appropriate boxes and corresponding dates in the rows marked "Period/Spotting," "Miscellaneous," and "Sex."

5. Finally, if you're using any fertility monitors, OPKs, saliva tests, or chloride-ion (fertility watch) tests, you can input the results on this chart as well in the appropriate spaces.

6. If you've figured out your ovulation day, circle it.

7. If you're taking a home pregnancy test (HPT) this month, input the results in the appropriate boxes.

8. Record your thoughts and feelings during the charting cycle, and keep track of the time you spend each month relaxing (important when you're in the baby-making mode).

Not a Charter?

Charting is a great way to keep track of your fertility, but it's definitely not a requirement of TTC. If you're just not into charting, or you'd rather play your cycle by ear—or instinct—skip this section. Or just fill in as much—or as little—of each chart as you'd like (just a few rows each month). Don't feel obligated to keep it up, either, if the charting gets old after a while. Rather chart electronically? Check out the many fertility tracking apps available.

2

5

8

KEEPING TRACK

Example

Fertility Chart

Month October - November Year_____ Last month's cycle length 28 This cycle length 29

Cycle Day	1	2	3	4	5	6	7	8	9	10	11	12	13	14	15
Date	17	18	19	20	21	22	23	24	25	26	27	28	29	30	31
Time Temp Taken	7:00	~~	~~	~~	~~	8:00	9:30	7:00	~~	~~	~~	~~	~~	8:15	~~

Basal Body Waking Temperature (°F): values 99 down to 97.9 as grid.

Cycle Day		2		4		6		8		10		12		14	
Period/Spotting	P	P	P	P	P										
Cervical Mucus (CM) Consistency*						D	D	D	S	S	C	C	C	E	E
Cervical Position**									C	C	C	O	O	O	
OPK/LH Surge										-	-	-	+		
Fertility Monitor										Low	Low	High	High	Peak	Peak
Saliva Test										-	-	-	+	+	
Chloride-ion Surge								~	~	-	+	+			
Miscellaneous (travel, illness, stress, medication, change in schedule, late night, etc.)			Ibuprofen		Late Night										
Sex						x								x	x
HPT (pregnancy test)															

*Cervical Fluid Consistency: **D:** Dry **E:** Egg White/Slippery **S:** Sticky **C:** Creamy

Thoughts and feelings _____ **Ways I relaxed this month** _____

16	17	18	19	20	21	22	23	24	25	26	27	28	29	30	31	32	33	34	35
1	2	3	4	5	6	7	8	9	10	11	12	13	14	15	16	17	18	19	20
7:00	~~	~~	~~	~~	8:00	9:30	7:00	~~	~~	~~	~~	8:15	~~	7:00	~~	~~	9:00	~~	
99	99	99	99	99	99	99	99	99	99	99	99	99	99	99	99	99	99	99	99
.9	.9	.9	.9	.9	.9	.9	.9	.9	.9	.9	.9	.9	.9	.9	.9	.9	.9	.9	.9
.8	.8	.8	.8	.8	.8	.8	.8	.8	.8	.8	.8	.8	.8	.8	.8	.8	.8	.8	.8
.7	.7	.7	.7	.7	.7	.7	.7	.7	.7	.7	.7	.7	.7	.7	.7	.7	.7	.7	.7
.6	.6	.6	.6	.6	.6	.6	.6	.6	.6	.6	.6	.6	.6	.6	.6	.6	.6	.6	.6
.5	.5	.5	.5	.5	.5	.5	.5	.5	.5	.5	.5	.5	.5	.5	.5	.5	.5	.5	.5
.4	.4	.4	.4	.4	4	.4	.4	.4	.4	.4	.4	.4	.4	.4	.4	.4	.4	.4	.4
.3	.3	.3	.3	.3	.3	.3	.3	.3	.3	.3	.3	.3	.3	.3	.3	.3	.3	.3	.3
.2	.2	.2	.2	.2	.2	.2	.2	.2	.2	.2	.2	.2	.2	.2	.2	.2	.2	.2	.2
.1	.1	.1	.1	.1	.1	.1	.1	.1	.1	.1	.1	.1	.1	.1	.1	.1	.1	.1	.1
98	98	98	98	98	98	98	98	98	98	98	98	98	98	98	98	98	98	98	98
.9	.9	.9	.9	.9	.9	.9	.9	.9	.9	.9	.9	.9	.9	.9	.9	.9	.9	.9	.9
.8	.8	.8	.8	.8	.8	.8	.8	.8	.8	.8	.8	.8	.8	.8	.8	.8	.8	.8	.8
.7	.7	.7	.7	.7	.7	.7	.7	.7	.7	.7	.7	.7	.7	.7	.7	.7	.7	.7	.7
.6	.6	.6	.6	.6	.6	.6	.6	.6	.6	.6	.6	.6	.6	.6	.6	.6	.6	.6	.6
.5	.5	.5	.5	.5	.5	.5	.5	.5	.5	.5	.5	.5	.5	.5	.5	.5	.5	.5	.5
.4	.4	.4	.4	.4	.4	.4	.4	.4	.4	.4	.4	.4	.4	.4	.4	.4	.4	.4	.4
.3	.3	.3	.3	.3	.3	.3	.3	.3	.3	.3	.3	.3	.3	.3	.3	.3	.3	.3	.3
.2	.2	.2	.2	.2	.2	.2	.2	.2	.2	.2	.2	.2	.2	.2	.2	.2	.2	.2	.2
.1	.1	.1	.1	.1	.1	.1	.1	.1	.1	.1	.1	.1	.1	.1	.1	.1	.1	.1	.1
97	97	97	97	97	97	97	97	97	97	97	97	97	97	97	97	97	97	97	97
.9	.9	.9	.9	.9	.9	.9	.9	.9	.9	.9	.9	.9	.9	.9	.9	.9	.9	.9	.9
	17		19		21		23		25		27		29		31		33		35
E	C	C	S	D	D	D													
O	C	C																	
High	Low																		

Stomach bug

| x | x | | x | | | | | | | | | | | | | | | | |
| | | | | | | | | | | Neg | Neg | Pos | | | | | | | |

**Cervical Position: O: Open/Soft C: Closed/Firm

Fertility Chart

Month_____ Year_____ Last month's cycle length_____ This cycle length_____

Cycle Day	1	2	3	4	5	6	7	8	9	10	11	12	13	14	15
Date															
Time Temp Taken															
	99	99	99	99	99	99	99	99	99	99	99	99	99	99	99
	.9	.9	.9	.9	.9	.9	.9	.9	.9	.9	.9	.9	.9	.9	.9
	.8	.8	.8	.8	.8	.8	.8	.8	.8	.8	.8	.8	.8	.8	.8
	.7	.7	.7	.7	.7	.7	.7	.7	.7	.7	.7	.7	.7	.7	.7
	.6	.6	.6	.6	.6	.6	.6	.6	.6	.6	.6	.6	.6	.6	.6
	.5	.5	.5	.5	.5	.5	.5	.5	.5	.5	.5	.5	.5	.5	.5
	.4	.4	.4	.4	.4	.4	.4	.4	.4	.4	.4	.4	.4	.4	.4
	.3	.3	.3	.3	.3	.3	.3	.3	.3	.3	.3	.3	.3	.3	.3
Basal Body	.2	.2	.2	.2	.2	.2	.2	.2	.2	.2	.2	.2	.2	.2	.2
Waking	.1	.1	.1	.1	.1	.1	.1	.1	.1	.1	.1	.1	.1	.1	.1
Temperature (°F)	98	98	98	98	98	98	98	98	98	98	98	98	98	98	98
	.9	.9	.9	.9	.9	.9	.9	.9	.9	.9	.9	.9	.9	.9	.9
	.8	.8	.8	.8	.8	.8	.8	.8	.8	.8	.8	.8	.8	.8	.8
	.7	.7	.7	.7	.7	.7	.7	.7	.7	.7	.7	.7	.7	.7	.7
	.6	.6	.6	.6	.6	.6	.6	.6	.6	.6	.6	.6	.6	.6	.6
	.5	.5	.5	.5	.5	.5	.5	.5	.5	.5	.5	.5	.5	.5	.5
	.4	.4	.4	.4	.4	.4	.4	.4	.4	.4	.4	.4	.4	.4	.4
	.3	.3	.3	.3	.3	.3	.3	.3	.3	.3	.3	.3	.3	.3	.3
	.2	.2	.2	.2	.2	.2	.2	.2	.2	.2	.2	.2	.2	.2	.2
	.1	.1	.1	.1	.1	.1	.1	.1	.1	.1	.1	.1	.1	.1	.1
	97	97	97	97	97	97	97	97	97	97	97	97	97	97	97
	.9	.9	.9	.9	.9	.9	.9	.9	.9	.9	.9	.9	.9	.9	.9
Cycle Day	1	2	3	4	5	6	7	8	9	10	11	12	13	14	15
Period/Spotting															
Cervical Mucus (CM) Consistency*															
Cervical Position**															
OPK/LH Surge															
Fertility Monitor															
Saliva Test															
Chloride-ion Surge															
Miscellaneous (travel, illness, stress, medication, change in schedule, late night, etc.)															
Sex															
HPT (pregnancy test)															

*Cervical Fluid Consistency: **D:** Dry **E:** Egg White/Slippery **S:** Sticky **C:** Creamy

Thoughts and feelings _____ | **Ways I relaxed this month** _____

_____ | _____

_____ | _____

16	17	18	19	20	21	22	23	24	25	26	27	28	29	30	31	32	33	34	35
99	99	99	99	99	99	99	99	99	99	99	99	99	99	99	99	99	99	99	99
.9	.9	.9	.9	.9	.9	.9	.9	.9	.9	.9	.9	.9	.9	.9	.9	.9	.9	.9	.9
.8	.8	.8	.8	.8	.8	.8	.8	.8	.8	.8	.8	.8	.8	.8	.8	.8	.8	.8	.8
.7	.7	.7	.7	.7	.7	.7	.7	.7	.7	.7	.7	.7	.7	.7	.7	.7	.7	.7	.7
.6	.6	.6	.6	.6	.6	.6	.6	.6	.6	.6	.6	.6	.6	.6	.6	.6	.6	.6	.6
.5	.5	.5	.5	.5	.5	.5	.5	.5	.5	.5	.5	.5	.5	.5	.5	.5	.5	.5	.5
.4	.4	.4	.4	.4	.4	.4	.4	.4	.4	.4	.4	.4	.4	.4	.4	.4	.4	.4	.4
.3	.3	.3	.3	.3	.3	.3	.3	.3	.3	.3	.3	.3	.3	.3	.3	.3	.3	.3	.3
.2	.2	.2	.2	.2	.2	.2	.2	.2	.2	.2	.2	.2	.2	.2	.2	.2	.2	.2	.2
.1	.1	.1	.1	.1	.1	.1	.1	.1	.1	.1	.1	.1	.1	.1	.1	.1	.1	.1	.1
98	98	98	98	98	98	98	98	98	98	98	98	98	98	98	98	98	98	98	98
.9	.9	.9	.9	.9	.9	.9	.9	.9	.9	.9	.9	.9	.9	.9	.9	.9	.9	.9	.9
.8	.8	.8	.8	.8	.8	.8	.8	.8	.8	.8	.8	.8	.8	.8	.8	.8	.8	.8	.8
.7	.7	.7	.7	.7	.7	.7	.7	.7	.7	.7	.7	.7	.7	.7	.7	.7	.7	.7	.7
.6	.6	.6	.6	.6	.6	.6	.6	.6	.6	.6	.6	.6	.6	.6	.6	.6	.6	.6	.6
.5	.5	.5	.5	.5	.5	.5	.5	.5	.5	.5	.5	.5	.5	.5	.5	.5	.5	.5	.5
.4	.4	.4	.4	.4	.4	.4	.4	.4	.4	.4	.4	.4	.4	.4	.4	.4	.4	.4	.4
.3	.3	.3	.3	.3	.3	.3	.3	.3	.3	.3	.3	.3	.3	.3	.3	.3	.3	.3	.3
.2	.2	.2	.2	.2	.2	.2	.2	.2	.2	.2	.2	.2	.2	.2	.2	.2	.2	.2	.2
.1	.1	.1	.1	.1	.1	.1	.1	.1	.1	.1	.1	.1	.1	.1	.1	.1	.1	.1	.1
97	97	97	97	97	97	97	97	97	97	97	97	97	97	97	97	97	97	97	97
.9	.9	.9	.9	.9	.9	.9	.9	.9	.9	.9	.9	.9	.9	.9	.9	.9	.9	.9	.9
16	17	18	19	20	21	22	23	24	25	26	27	28	29	30	31	32	33	34	35

Cervical Position: O: Open/Soft **C:** Closed/Firm

Fertility Chart

Month_____ Year_____ Last month's cycle length_____ This cycle length_____

Cycle Day	1	2	3	4	5	6	7	8	9	10	11	12	13	14	15
Date															
Time Temp Taken															
Basal Body Waking Temperature (°F)	99 .9 .8 .7 .6 .5 .4 .3 .2 .1 98 .9 .8 .7 .6 .5 .4 .3 .2 .1 97 .9														
Cycle Day	1	2	3	4	5	6	7	8	9	10	11	12	13	14	15
Period/Spotting															
Cervical Mucus (CM) Consistency*															
Cervical Position**															
OPK/LH Surge															
Fertility Monitor															
Saliva Test															
Chloride-ion Surge															
Miscellaneous (travel, illness, stress, medication, change in schedule, late night, etc.)															
Sex															
HPT (pregnancy test)															

*Cervical Fluid Consistency: **D:** Dry **E:** Egg White/Slippery **S:** Sticky **C:** Creamy

Thoughts and feelings _____ | **Ways I relaxed this month** _____

16	17	18	19	20	21	22	23	24	25	26	27	28	29	30	31	32	33	34	35
99	99	99	99	99	99	99	99	99	99	99	99	99	99	99	99	99	99	99	99
.9	.9	.9	.9	.9	.9	.9	.9	.9	.9	.9	.9	.9	.9	.9	.9	.9	.9	.9	.9
.8	.8	.8	.8	.8	.8	.8	.8	.8	.8	.8	.8	.8	.8	.8	.8	.8	.8	.8	.8
.7	.7	.7	.7	.7	.7	.7	.7	.7	.7	.7	.7	.7	.7	.7	.7	.7	.7	.7	.7
.6	.6	.6	.6	.6	.6	.6	.6	.6	.6	.6	.6	.6	.6	.6	.6	.6	.6	.6	.6
.5	.5	.5	.5	.5	.5	.5	.5	.5	.5	.5	.5	.5	.5	.5	.5	.5	.5	.5	.5
.4	.4	.4	.4	.4	.4	.4	.4	.4	.4	.4	.4	.4	.4	.4	.4	.4	.4	.4	.4
.3	.3	.3	.3	.3	.3	.3	.3	.3	.3	.3	.3	.3	.3	.3	.3	.3	.3	.3	.3
.2	.2	.2	.2	.2	.2	.2	.2	.2	.2	.2	.2	.2	.2	.2	.2	.2	.2	.2	.2
.1	.1	.1	.1	.1	.1	.1	.1	.1	.1	.1	.1	.1	.1	.1	.1	.1	.1	.1	.1
98	98	98	98	98	98	98	98	98	98	98	98	98	98	98	98	98	98	98	98
.9	.9	.9	.9	.9	.9	.9	.9	.9	.9	.9	.9	.9	.9	.9	.9	.9	.9	.9	.9
.8	.8	.8	.8	.8	.8	.8	.8	.8	.8	.8	.8	.8	.8	.8	.8	.8	.8	.8	.8
.7	.7	.7	.7	.7	.7	.7	.7	.7	.7	.7	.7	.7	.7	.7	.7	.7	.7	.7	.7
.6	.6	.6	.6	.6	.6	.6	.6	.6	.6	.6	.6	.6	.6	.6	.6	.6	.6	.6	.6
.5	.5	.5	.5	.5	.5	.5	.5	.5	.5	.5	.5	.5	.5	.5	.5	.5	.5	.5	.5
.4	.4	.4	.4	.4	.4	.4	.4	.4	.4	.4	.4	.4	.4	.4	.4	.4	.4	.4	.4
.3	.3	.3	.3	.3	.3	.3	.3	.3	.3	.3	.3	.3	.3	.3	.3	.3	.3	.3	.3
.2	.2	.2	.2	.2	.2	.2	.2	.2	.2	.2	.2	.2	.2	.2	.2	.2	.2	.2	.2
.1	.1	.1	.1	.1	.1	.1	.1	.1	.1	.1	.1	.1	.1	.1	.1	.1	.1	.1	.1
97	97	97	97	97	97	97	97	97	97	97	97	97	97	97	97	97	97	97	97
.9	.9	.9	.9	.9	.9	.9	.9	.9	.9	.9	.9	.9	.9	.9	.9	.9	.9	.9	.9
16	17	18	19	20	21	22	23	24	25	26	27	28	29	30	31	32	33	34	35

Cervical Position: O: Open/Soft **C:** Closed/Firm

Fertility Chart

Month_____ Year_____ Last month's cycle length_____ This cycle length_____

Cycle Day	1	2	3	4	5	6	7	8	9	10	11	12	13	14	15
Date															
Time Temp Taken															
Basal Body Waking Temperature (°F)	99–97.9 scale														
Cycle Day	1	2	3	4	5	6	7	8	9	10	11	12	13	14	15
Period/Spotting															
Cervical Mucus (CM) Consistency*															
Cervical Position**															
OPK/LH Surge															
Fertility Monitor															
Saliva Test															
Chloride-ion Surge															
Miscellaneous (travel, illness, stress, medication, change in schedule, late night, etc.)															
Sex															
HPT(pregnancy test)															

*Cervical Fluid Consistency: **D:** Dry **E:** Egg White/Slippery **S:** Sticky **C:** Creamy

Thoughts and feelings _____ | **Ways I relaxed this month** _____

16	17	18	19	20	21	22	23	24	25	26	27	28	29	30	31	32	33	34	35
99	99	99	99	99	99	99	99	99	99	99	99	99	99	99	99	99	99	99	99
.9	.9	.9	.9	.9	.9	.9	.9	.9	.9	.9	.9	.9	.9	.9	.9	.9	.9	.9	.9
.8	.8	.8	.8	.8	.8	.8	.8	.8	.8	.8	.8	.8	.8	.8	.8	.8	.8	.8	.8
.7	.7	.7	.7	.7	.7	.7	.7	.7	.7	.7	.7	.7	.7	.7	.7	.7	.7	.7	.7
.6	.6	.6	.6	.6	.6	.6	.6	.6	.6	.6	.6	.6	.6	.6	.6	.6	.6	.6	.6
.5	.5	.5	.5	.5	.5	.5	.5	.5	.5	.5	.5	.5	.5	.5	.5	.5	.5	.5	.5
.4	.4	.4	.4	.4	.4	.4	.4	.4	.4	.4	.4	.4	.4	.4	.4	.4	.4	.4	.4
.3	.3	.3	.3	.3	.3	.3	.3	.3	.3	.3	.3	.3	.3	.3	.3	.3	.3	.3	.3
.2	.2	.2	.2	.2	.2	.2	.2	.2	.2	.2	.2	.2	.2	.2	.2	.2	.2	.2	.2
.1	.1	.1	.1	.1	.1	.1	.1	.1	.1	.1	.1	.1	.1	.1	.1	.1	.1	.1	.1
98	98	98	98	98	98	98	98	98	98	98	98	98	98	98	98	98	98	98	98
.9	.9	.9	.9	.9	.9	.9	.9	.9	.9	.9	.9	.9	.9	.9	.9	.9	.9	.9	.9
.8	.8	.8	.8	.8	.8	.8	.8	.8	.8	.8	.8	.8	.8	.8	.8	.8	.8	.8	.8
.7	.7	.7	.7	.7	.7	.7	.7	.7	.7	.7	.7	.7	.7	.7	.7	.7	.7	.7	.7
.6	.6	.6	.6	.6	.6	.6	.6	.6	.6	.6	.6	.6	.6	.6	.6	.6	.6	.6	.6
.5	.5	.5	.5	.5	.5	.5	.5	.5	.5	.5	.5	.5	.5	.5	.5	.5	.5	.5	.5
.4	.4	.4	.4	.4	.4	.4	.4	.4	.4	.4	.4	.4	.4	.4	.4	.4	.4	.4	.4
.3	.3	.3	.3	.3	.3	.3	.3	.3	.3	.3	.3	.3	.3	.3	.3	.3	.3	.3	.3
.2	.2	.2	.2	.2	.2	.2	.2	.2	.2	.2	.2	.2	.2	.2	.2	.2	.2	.2	.2
.1	.1	.1	.1	.1	.1	.1	.1	.1	.1	.1	.1	.1	.1	.1	.1	.1	.1	.1	.1
97	97	97	97	97	97	97	97	97	97	97	97	97	97	97	97	97	97	97	97
.9	.9	.9	.9	.9	.9	.9	.9	.9	.9	.9	.9	.9	.9	.9	.9	.9	.9	.9	.9
16	17	18	19	20	21	22	23	24	25	26	27	28	29	30	31	32	33	34	35

Cervical Position: O: Open/Soft **C:** Closed/Firm

Fertility Chart

Month_____ Year_____ Last month's cycle length_____ This cycle length_____

Cycle Day	1	2	3	4	5	6	7	8	9	10	11	12	13	14	15
Date															
Time Temp Taken															
	99	99	99	99	99	99	99	99	99	99	99	99	99	99	99
	.9	.9	.9	.9	.9	.9	.9	.9	.9	.9	.9	.9	.9	.9	.9
	.8	.8	.8	.8	.8	.8	.8	.8	.8	.8	.8	.8	.8	.8	.8
	.7	.7	.7	.7	.7	.7	.7	.7	.7	.7	.7	.7	.7	.7	.7
	.6	.6	.6	.6	.6	.6	.6	.6	.6	.6	.6	.6	.6	.6	.6
	.5	.5	.5	.5	.5	.5	.5	.5	.5	.5	.5	.5	.5	.5	.5
	.4	.4	.4	.4	.4	.4	.4	.4	.4	.4	.4	.4	.4	.4	.4
	.3	.3	.3	.3	.3	.3	.3	.3	.3	.3	.3	.3	.3	.3	.3
Basal Body	.2	.2	.2	.2	.2	.2	.2	.2	.2	.2	.2	.2	.2	.2	.2
Waking	.1	.1	.1	.1	.1	.1	.1	.1	.1	.1	.1	.1	.1	.1	.1
Temperature (°F)	98	98	98	98	98	98	98	98	98	98	98	98	98	98	98
	.9	.9	.9	.9	.9	.9	.9	.9	.9	.9	.9	.9	.9	.9	.9
	.8	.8	.8	.8	.8	.8	.8	.8	.8	.8	.8	.8	.8	.8	.8
	.7	.7	.7	.7	.7	.7	.7	.7	.7	.7	.7	.7	.7	.7	.7
	.6	.6	.6	.6	.6	.6	.6	.6	.6	.6	.6	.6	.6	.6	.6
	.5	.5	.5	.5	.5	.5	.5	.5	.5	.5	.5	.5	.5	.5	.5
	.4	.4	.4	.4	.4	.4	.4	.4	.4	.4	.4	.4	.4	.4	.4
	.3	.3	.3	.3	.3	.3	.3	.3	.3	.3	.3	.3	.3	.3	.3
	.2	.2	.2	.2	.2	.2	.2	.2	.2	.2	.2	.2	.2	.2	.2
	.1	.1	.1	.1	.1	.1	.1	.1	.1	.1	.1	.1	.1	.1	.1
	97	97	97	97	97	97	97	97	97	97	97	97	97	97	97
	.9	.9	.9	.9	.9	.9	.9	.9	.9	.9	.9	.9	.9	.9	.9
Cycle Day	1	2	3	4	5	6	7	8	9	10	11	12	13	14	15
Period/Spotting															
Cervical Mucus (CM) Consistency*															
Cervical Position**															
OPK/LH Surge															
Fertility Monitor															
Saliva Test															
Chloride-ion Surge															
Miscellaneous (travel, illness, stress, medication, change in schedule, late night, etc.)															
Sex															
HPT (pregnancy test)															

*Cervical Fluid Consistency: **D:** Dry **E:** Egg White/Slippery **S:** Sticky **C:** Creamy

Thoughts and feelings _____ | **Ways I relaxed this month** _____

_____ | _____

_____ | _____

16	17	18	19	20	21	22	23	24	25	26	27	28	29	30	31	32	33	34	35
99	99	99	99	99	99	99	99	99	99	99	99	99	99	99	99	99	99	99	99
.9	.9	.9	.9	.9	.9	.9	.9	.9	.9	.9	.9	.9	.9	.9	.9	.9	.9	.9	.9
.8	.8	.8	.8	.8	.8	.8	.8	.8	.8	.8	.8	.8	.8	.8	.8	.8	.8	.8	.8
.7	.7	.7	.7	.7	.7	.7	.7	.7	.7	.7	.7	.7	.7	.7	.7	.7	.7	.7	.7
.6	.6	.6	.6	.6	.6	.6	.6	.6	.6	.6	.6	.6	.6	.6	.6	.6	.6	.6	.6
.5	.5	.5	.5	.5	.5	.5	.5	.5	.5	.5	.5	.5	.5	.5	.5	.5	.5	.5	.5
.4	.4	.4	.4	.4	.4	.4	.4	.4	.4	.4	.4	.4	.4	.4	.4	.4	.4	.4	.4
.3	.3	.3	.3	.3	.3	.3	.3	.3	.3	.3	.3	.3	.3	.3	.3	.3	.3	.3	.3
.2	.2	.2	.2	.2	.2	.2	.2	.2	.2	.2	.2	.2	.2	.2	.2	.2	.2	.2	.2
.1	.1	.1	.1	.1	.1	.1	.1	.1	.1	.1	.1	.1	.1	.1	.1	.1	.1	.1	.1
98	98	98	98	98	98	98	98	98	98	98	98	98	98	98	98	98	98	98	98
.9	.9	.9	.9	.9	.9	.9	.9	.9	.9	.9	.9	.9	.9	.9	.9	.9	.9	.9	.9
.8	.8	.8	.8	.8	.8	.8	.8	.8	.8	.8	.8	.8	.8	.8	.8	.8	.8	.8	.8
.7	.7	.7	.7	.7	.7	.7	.7	.7	.7	.7	.7	.7	.7	.7	.7	.7	.7	.7	.7
.6	.6	.6	.6	.6	.6	.6	.6	.6	.6	.6	.6	.6	.6	.6	.6	.6	.6	.6	.6
.5	.5	.5	.5	.5	.5	.5	.5	.5	.5	.5	.5	.5	.5	.5	.5	.5	.5	.5	.5
.4	.4	.4	.4	.4	.4	.4	.4	.4	.4	.4	.4	.4	.4	.4	.4	.4	.4	.4	.4
.3	.3	.3	.3	.3	.3	.3	.3	.3	.3	.3	.3	.3	.3	.3	.3	.3	.3	.3	.3
.2	.2	.2	.2	.2	.2	.2	.2	.2	.2	.2	.2	.2	.2	.2	.2	.2	.2	.2	.2
.1	.1	.1	.1	.1	.1	.1	.1	.1	.1	.1	.1	.1	.1	.1	.1	.1	.1	.1	.1
97	97	97	97	97	97	97	97	97	97	97	97	97	97	97	97	97	97	97	97
.9	.9	.9	.9	.9	.9	.9	.9	.9	.9	.9	.9	.9	.9	.9	.9	.9	.9	.9	.9
16	17	18	19	20	21	22	23	24	25	26	27	28	29	30	31	32	33	34	35

Cervical Position: O: Open/Soft **C:** Closed/Firm

Fertility Chart

Month_____ Year_____ Last month's cycle length_____ This cycle length_____

Cycle Day	1	2	3	4	5	6	7	8	9	10	11	12	13	14	15
Date															
Time Temp Taken															
Basal Body Waking Temperature (°F)	99.9–98.1 / 98.9–97.9 scale														
Cycle Day	1	2	3	4	5	6	7	8	9	10	11	12	13	14	15
Period/Spotting															
Cervical Mucus (CM) Consistency*															
Cervical Position**															
OPK/LH Surge															
Fertility Monitor															
Saliva Test															
Chloride-ion Surge															
Miscellaneous (travel, illness, stress, medication, change in schedule, late night, etc.)															
Sex															
HPT (pregnancy test)															

*Cervical Fluid Consistency: **D:** Dry **E:** Egg White/Slippery **S:** Sticky **C:** Creamy

Thoughts and feelings _____ | **Ways I relaxed this month** _____

16	17	18	19	20	21	22	23	24	25	26	27	28	29	30	31	32	33	34	35
99	99	99	99	99	99	99	99	99	99	99	99	99	99	99	99	99	99	99	99
.9	.9	.9	.9	.9	.9	.9	.9	.9	.9	.9	.9	.9	.9	.9	.9	.9	.9	.9	.9
.8	.8	.8	.8	.8	.8	.8	.8	.8	.8	.8	.8	.8	.8	.8	.8	.8	.8	.8	.8
.7	.7	.7	.7	.7	.7	.7	.7	.7	.7	.7	.7	.7	.7	.7	.7	.7	.7	.7	.7
.6	.6	.6	.6	.6	.6	.6	.6	.6	.6	.6	.6	.6	.6	.6	.6	.6	.6	.6	.6
.5	.5	.5	.5	.5	.5	.5	.5	.5	.5	.5	.5	.5	.5	.5	.5	.5	.5	.5	.5
.4	.4	.4	.4	.4	.4	.4	.4	.4	.4	.4	.4	.4	.4	.4	.4	.4	.4	.4	.4
.3	.3	.3	.3	.3	.3	.3	.3	.3	.3	.3	.3	.3	.3	.3	.3	.3	.3	.3	.3
.2	.2	.2	.2	.2	.2	.2	.2	.2	.2	.2	.2	.2	.2	.2	.2	.2	.2	.2	.2
.1	.1	.1	.1	.1	.1	.1	.1	.1	.1	.1	.1	.1	.1	.1	.1	.1	.1	.1	.1
98	98	98	98	98	98	98	98	98	98	98	98	98	98	98	98	98	98	98	98
.9	.9	.9	.9	.9	.9	.9	.9	.9	.9	.9	.9	.9	.9	.9	.9	.9	.9	.9	.9
.8	.8	.8	.8	.8	.8	.8	.8	.8	.8	.8	.8	.8	.8	.8	.8	.8	.8	.8	.8
.7	.7	.7	.7	.7	.7	.7	.7	.7	.7	.7	.7	.7	.7	.7	.7	.7	.7	.7	.7
.6	.6	.6	.6	.6	.6	.6	.6	.6	.6	.6	.6	.6	.6	.6	.6	.6	.6	.6	.6
.5	.5	.5	.5	.5	.5	.5	.5	.5	.5	.5	.5	.5	.5	.5	.5	.5	.5	.5	.5
.4	.4	.4	.4	.4	.4	.4	.4	.4	.4	.4	.4	.4	.4	.4	.4	.4	.4	.4	.4
.3	.3	.3	.3	.3	.3	.3	.3	.3	.3	.3	.3	.3	.3	.3	.3	.3	.3	.3	.3
.2	.2	.2	.2	.2	.2	.2	.2	.2	.2	.2	.2	.2	.2	.2	.2	.2	.2	.2	.2
.1	.1	.1	.1	.1	.1	.1	.1	.1	.1	.1	.1	.1	.1	.1	.1	.1	.1	.1	.1
97	97	97	97	97	97	97	97	97	97	97	97	97	97	97	97	97	97	97	97
.9	.9	.9	.9	.9	.9	.9	.9	.9	.9	.9	.9	.9	.9	.9	.9	.9	.9	.9	.9
16	**17**	**18**	**19**	**20**	**21**	**22**	**23**	**24**	**25**	**26**	**27**	**28**	**29**	**30**	**31**	**32**	**33**	**34**	**35**

Cervical Position: O: Open/Soft **C: Closed/Firm

Fertility Chart

Month_____ Year_____ Last month's cycle length_____ This cycle length_____

Cycle Day	1	2	3	4	5	6	7	8	9	10	11	12	13	14	15
Date															
Time Temp Taken															
Basal Body Waking Temperature (°F)	99	99	99	99	99	99	99	99	99	99	99	99	99	99	99
	.9	.9	.9	.9	.9	.9	.9	.9	.9	.9	.9	.9	.9	.9	.9
	.8	.8	.8	.8	.8	.8	.8	.8	.8	.8	.8	.8	.8	.8	.8
	.7	.7	.7	.7	.7	.7	.7	.7	.7	.7	.7	.7	.7	.7	.7
	.6	.6	.6	.6	.6	.6	.6	.6	.6	.6	.6	.6	.6	.6	.6
	.5	.5	.5	.5	.5	.5	.5	.5	.5	.5	.5	.5	.5	.5	.5
	.4	.4	.4	.4	.4	.4	.4	.4	.4	.4	.4	.4	.4	.4	.4
	.3	.3	.3	.3	.3	.3	.3	.3	.3	.3	.3	.3	.3	.3	.3
	.2	.2	.2	.2	.2	.2	.2	.2	.2	.2	.2	.2	.2	.2	.2
	.1	.1	.1	.1	.1	.1	.1	.1	.1	.1	.1	.1	.1	.1	.1
	98	98	98	98	98	98	98	98	98	98	98	98	98	98	98
	.9	.9	.9	.9	.9	.9	.9	.9	.9	.9	.9	.9	.9	.9	.9
	.8	.8	.8	.8	.8	.8	.8	.8	.8	.8	.8	.8	.8	.8	.8
	.7	.7	.7	.7	.7	.7	.7	.7	.7	.7	.7	.7	.7	.7	.7
	.6	.6	.6	.6	.6	.6	.6	.6	.6	.6	.6	.6	.6	.6	.6
	.5	.5	.5	.5	.5	.5	.5	.5	.5	.5	.5	.5	.5	.5	.5
	.4	.4	.4	.4	.4	.4	.4	.4	.4	.4	.4	.4	.4	.4	.4
	.3	.3	.3	.3	.3	.3	.3	.3	.3	.3	.3	.3	.3	.3	.3
	.2	.2	.2	.2	.2	.2	.2	.2	.2	.2	.2	.2	.2	.2	.2
	.1	.1	.1	.1	.1	.1	.1	.1	.1	.1	.1	.1	.1	.1	.1
	97	97	97	97	97	97	97	97	97	97	97	97	97	97	97
	.9	.9	.9	.9	.9	.9	.9	.9	.9	.9	.9	.9	.9	.9	.9
Cycle Day	1	2	3	4	5	6	7	8	9	10	11	12	13	14	15
Period/Spotting															
Cervical Mucus (CM) Consistency*															
Cervical Position**															
OPK/LH Surge															
Fertility Monitor															
Saliva Test															
Chloride-ion Surge															
Miscellaneous (travel, illness, stress, medication, change in schedule, late night, etc.)															
Sex															
HPT (pregnancy test)															

*Cervical Fluid Consistency: **D:** Dry **E:** Egg White/Slippery **S:** Sticky **C:** Creamy

Thoughts and feelings _____ | **Ways I relaxed this month** _____

16	17	18	19	20	21	22	23	24	25	26	27	28	29	30	31	32	33	34	35
99	99	99	99	99	99	99	99	99	99	99	99	99	99	99	99	99	99	99	99
.9	.9	.9	.9	.9	.9	.9	.9	.9	.9	.9	.9	.9	.9	.9	.9	.9	.9	.9	.9
.8	.8	.8	.8	.8	.8	.8	.8	.8	.8	.8	.8	.8	.8	.8	.8	.8	.8	.8	.8
.7	.7	.7	.7	.7	.7	.7	.7	.7	.7	.7	.7	.7	.7	.7	.7	.7	.7	.7	.7
.6	.6	.6	.6	.6	.6	.6	.6	.6	.6	.6	.6	.6	.6	.6	.6	.6	.6	.6	.6
.5	.5	.5	.5	.5	.5	.5	.5	.5	.5	.5	.5	.5	.5	.5	.5	.5	.5	.5	.5
.4	.4	.4	.4	.4	.4	.4	.4	.4	.4	.4	.4	.4	.4	.4	.4	.4	.4	.4	.4
.3	.3	.3	.3	.3	.3	.3	.3	.3	.3	.3	.3	.3	.3	.3	.3	.3	.3	.3	.3
.2	.2	.2	.2	.2	.2	.2	.2	.2	.2	.2	.2	.2	.2	.2	.2	.2	.2	.2	.2
.1	.1	.1	.1	.1	.1	.1	.1	.1	.1	.1	.1	.1	.1	.1	.1	.1	.1	.1	.1
98	98	98	98	98	98	98	98	98	98	98	98	98	98	98	98	98	98	98	98
.9	.9	.9	.9	.9	.9	.9	.9	.9	.9	.9	.9	.9	.9	.9	.9	.9	.9	.9	.9
.8	.8	.8	.8	.8	.8	.8	.8	.8	.8	.8	.8	.8	.8	.8	.8	.8	.8	.8	.8
.7	.7	.7	.7	.7	.7	.7	.7	.7	.7	.7	.7	.7	.7	.7	.7	.7	.7	.7	.7
.6	.6	.6	.6	.6	.6	.6	.6	.6	.6	.6	.6	.6	.6	.6	.6	.6	.6	.6	.6
.5	.5	.5	.5	.5	.5	.5	.5	.5	.5	.5	.5	.5	.5	.5	.5	.5	.5	.5	.5
.4	.4	.4	.4	.4	.4	.4	.4	.4	.4	.4	.4	.4	.4	.4	.4	.4	.4	.4	.4
.3	.3	.3	.3	.3	.3	.3	.3	.3	.3	.3	.3	.3	.3	.3	.3	.3	.3	.3	.3
.2	.2	.2	.2	.2	.2	.2	.2	.2	.2	.2	.2	.2	.2	.2	.2	.2	.2	.2	.2
.1	.1	.1	.1	.1	.1	.1	.1	.1	.1	.1	.1	.1	.1	.1	.1	.1	.1	.1	.1
97	97	97	97	97	97	97	97	97	97	97	97	97	97	97	97	97	97	97	97
.9	.9	.9	.9	.9	.9	.9	.9	.9	.9	.9	.9	.9	.9	.9	.9	.9	.9	.9	.9
16	**17**	**18**	**19**	**20**	**21**	**22**	**23**	**24**	**25**	**26**	**27**	**28**	**29**	**30**	**31**	**32**	**33**	**34**	**35**

Cervical Position: O: Open/Soft **C:** Closed/Firm

Fertility Chart

Month_____ Year_____ Last month's cycle length_____ This cycle length_____

Cycle Day	1	2	3	4	5	6	7	8	9	10	11	12	13	14	15
Date															
Time Temp Taken															
Basal Body Waking Temperature (°F)	99	99	99	99	99	99	99	99	99	99	99	99	99	99	99
	.9	.9	.9	.9	.9	.9	.9	.9	.9	.9	.9	.9	.9	.9	.9
	.8	.8	.8	.8	.8	.8	.8	.8	.8	.8	.8	.8	.8	.8	.8
	.7	.7	.7	.7	.7	.7	.7	.7	.7	.7	.7	.7	.7	.7	.7
	.6	.6	.6	.6	.6	.6	.6	.6	.6	.6	.6	.6	.6	.6	.6
	.5	.5	.5	.5	.5	.5	.5	.5	.5	.5	.5	.5	.5	.5	.5
	.4	.4	.4	.4	.4	.4	.4	.4	.4	.4	.4	.4	.4	.4	.4
	.3	.3	.3	.3	.3	.3	.3	.3	.3	.3	.3	.3	.3	.3	.3
	.2	.2	.2	.2	.2	.2	.2	.2	.2	.2	.2	.2	.2	.2	.2
	.1	.1	.1	.1	.1	.1	.1	.1	.1	.1	.1	.1	.1	.1	.1
	98	98	98	98	98	98	98	98	98	98	98	98	98	98	98
	.9	.9	.9	.9	.9	.9	.9	.9	.9	.9	.9	.9	.9	.9	.9
	.8	.8	.8	.8	.8	.8	.8	.8	.8	.8	.8	.8	.8	.8	.8
	.7	.7	.7	.7	.7	.7	.7	.7	.7	.7	.7	.7	.7	.7	.7
	.6	.6	.6	.6	.6	.6	.6	.6	.6	.6	.6	.6	.6	.6	.6
	.5	.5	.5	.5	.5	.5	.5	.5	.5	.5	.5	.5	.5	.5	.5
	.4	.4	.4	.4	.4	.4	.4	.4	.4	.4	.4	.4	.4	.4	.4
	.3	.3	.3	.3	.3	.3	.3	.3	.3	.3	.3	.3	.3	.3	.3
	.2	.2	.2	.2	.2	.2	.2	.2	.2	.2	.2	.2	.2	.2	.2
	.1	.1	.1	.1	.1	.1	.1	.1	.1	.1	.1	.1	.1	.1	.1
	97	97	97	97	97	97	97	97	97	97	97	97	97	97	97
	.9	.9	.9	.9	.9	.9	.9	.9	.9	.9	.9	.9	.9	.9	.9
Cycle Day	1	2	3	4	5	6	7	8	9	10	11	12	13	14	15
Period/Spotting															
Cervical Mucus (CM) Consistency*															
Cervical Position**															
OPK/LH Surge															
Fertility Monitor															
Saliva Test															
Chloride-ion Surge															
Miscellaneous (travel, illness, stress, medication, change in schedule, late night, etc.)															
Sex															
HPT (pregnancy test)															

*Cervical Fluid Consistency: **D:** Dry **E:** Egg White/Slippery **S:** Sticky **C:** Creamy

Thoughts and feelings _____ | **Ways I relaxed this month** _____

16	17	18	19	20	21	22	23	24	25	26	27	28	29	30	31	32	33	34	35
99	99	99	99	99	99	99	99	99	99	99	99	99	99	99	99	99	99	99	99
.9	.9	.9	.9	.9	.9	.9	.9	.9	.9	.9	.9	.9	.9	.9	.9	.9	.9	.9	.9
.8	.8	.8	.8	.8	.8	.8	.8	.8	.8	.8	.8	.8	.8	.8	.8	.8	.8	.8	.8
.7	.7	.7	.7	.7	.7	.7	.7	.7	.7	.7	.7	.7	.7	.7	.7	.7	.7	.7	.7
.6	.6	.6	.6	.6	.6	.6	.6	.6	.6	.6	.6	.6	.6	.6	.6	.6	.6	.6	.6
.5	.5	.5	.5	.5	.5	.5	.5	.5	.5	.5	.5	.5	.5	.5	.5	.5	.5	.5	.5
.4	.4	.4	.4	.4	.4	.4	.4	.4	.4	.4	.4	.4	.4	.4	.4	.4	.4	.4	.4
.3	.3	.3	.3	.3	.3	.3	.3	.3	.3	.3	.3	.3	.3	.3	.3	.3	.3	.3	.3
.2	.2	.2	.2	.2	.2	.2	.2	.2	.2	.2	.2	.2	.2	.2	.2	.2	.2	.2	.2
.1	.1	.1	.1	.1	.1	.1	.1	.1	.1	.1	.1	.1	.1	.1	.1	.1	.1	.1	.1
98	98	98	98	98	98	98	98	98	98	98	98	98	98	98	98	98	98	98	98
.9	.9	.9	.9	.9	.9	.9	.9	.9	.9	.9	.9	.9	.9	.9	.9	.9	.9	.9	.9
.8	.8	.8	.8	.8	.8	.8	.8	.8	.8	.8	.8	.8	.8	.8	.8	.8	.8	.8	.8
.7	.7	.7	.7	.7	.7	.7	.7	.7	.7	.7	.7	.7	.7	.7	.7	.7	.7	.7	.7
.6	.6	.6	.6	.6	.6	.6	.6	.6	.6	.6	.6	.6	.6	.6	.6	.6	.6	.6	.6
.5	.5	.5	.5	.5	.5	.5	.5	.5	.5	.5	.5	.5	.5	.5	.5	.5	.5	.5	.5
.4	.4	.4	.4	.4	.4	.4	.4	.4	.4	.4	.4	.4	.4	.4	.4	.4	.4	.4	.4
.3	.3	.3	.3	.3	.3	.3	.3	.3	.3	.3	.3	.3	.3	.3	.3	.3	.3	.3	.3
.2	.2	.2	.2	.2	.2	.2	.2	.2	.2	.2	.2	.2	.2	.2	.2	.2	.2	.2	.2
.1	.1	.1	.1	.1	.1	.1	.1	.1	.1	.1	.1	.1	.1	.1	.1	.1	.1	.1	.1
97	97	97	97	97	97	97	97	97	97	97	97	97	97	97	97	97	97	97	97
.9	.9	.9	.9	.9	.9	.9	.9	.9	.9	.9	.9	.9	.9	.9	.9	.9	.9	.9	.9
16	17	18	19	20	21	22	23	24	25	26	27	28	29	30	31	32	33	34	35

Cervical Position: O: Open/Soft **C:** Closed/Firm

Fertility Chart

Month_____ Year_____ Last month's cycle length_____ This cycle length_____

Cycle Day	1	2	3	4	5	6	7	8	9	10	11	12	13	14	15
Date															
Time Temp Taken															
Basal Body Waking Temperature (°F)	99	99	99	99	99	99	99	99	99	99	99	99	99	99	99
	.9	.9	.9	.9	.9	.9	.9	.9	.9	.9	.9	.9	.9	.9	.9
	.8	.8	.8	.8	.8	.8	.8	.8	.8	.8	.8	.8	.8	.8	.8
	.7	.7	.7	.7	.7	.7	.7	.7	.7	.7	.7	.7	.7	.7	.7
	.6	.6	.6	.6	.6	.6	.6	.6	.6	.6	.6	.6	.6	.6	.6
	.5	.5	.5	.5	.5	.5	.5	.5	.5	.5	.5	.5	.5	.5	.5
	.4	.4	.4	.4	.4	.4	.4	.4	.4	.4	.4	.4	.4	.4	.4
	.3	.3	.3	.3	.3	.3	.3	.3	.3	.3	.3	.3	.3	.3	.3
	.2	.2	.2	.2	.2	.2	.2	.2	.2	.2	.2	.2	.2	.2	.2
	.1	.1	.1	.1	.1	.1	.1	.1	.1	.1	.1	.1	.1	.1	.1
	98	98	98	98	98	98	98	98	98	98	98	98	98	98	98
	.9	.9	.9	.9	.9	.9	.9	.9	.9	.9	.9	.9	.9	.9	.9
	.8	.8	.8	.8	.8	.8	.8	.8	.8	.8	.8	.8	.8	.8	.8
	.7	.7	.7	.7	.7	.7	.7	.7	.7	.7	.7	.7	.7	.7	.7
	.6	.6	.6	.6	.6	.6	.6	.6	.6	.6	.6	.6	.6	.6	.6
	.5	.5	.5	.5	.5	.5	.5	.5	.5	.5	.5	.5	.5	.5	.5
	.4	.4	.4	.4	.4	.4	.4	.4	.4	.4	.4	.4	.4	.4	.4
	.3	.3	.3	.3	.3	.3	.3	.3	.3	.3	.3	.3	.3	.3	.3
	.2	.2	.2	.2	.2	.2	.2	.2	.2	.2	.2	.2	.2	.2	.2
	.1	.1	.1	.1	.1	.1	.1	.1	.1	.1	.1	.1	.1	.1	.1
	97	97	97	97	97	97	97	97	97	97	97	97	97	97	97
	.9	.9	.9	.9	.9	.9	.9	.9	.9	.9	.9	.9	.9	.9	.9
Cycle Day	1	2	3	4	5	6	7	8	9	10	11	12	13	14	15
Period/Spotting															
Cervical Mucus (CM) Consistency*															
Cervical Position**															
OPK/LH Surge															
Fertility Monitor															
Saliva Test															
Chloride-ion Surge															
Miscellaneous (travel, illness, stress, medication, change in schedule, late night, etc.)															
Sex															
HPT (pregnancy test)															

*Cervical Fluid Consistency: **D:** Dry **E:** Egg White/Slippery **S:** Sticky **C:** Creamy

Thoughts and feelings _____ | **Ways I relaxed this month** _____

16	17	18	19	20	21	22	23	24	25	26	27	28	29	30	31	32	33	34	35
99	99	99	99	99	99	99	99	99	99	99	99	99	99	99	99	99	99	99	99
.9	.9	.9	.9	.9	.9	.9	.9	.9	.9	.9	.9	.9	.9	.9	.9	.9	.9	.9	.9
.8	.8	.8	.8	.8	.8	.8	.8	.8	.8	.8	.8	.8	.8	.8	.8	.8	.8	.8	.8
.7	.7	.7	.7	.7	.7	.7	.7	.7	.7	.7	.7	.7	.7	.7	.7	.7	.7	.7	.7
.6	.6	.6	.6	.6	.6	.6	.6	.6	.6	.6	.6	.6	.6	.6	.6	.6	.6	.6	.6
.5	.5	.5	.5	.5	.5	.5	.5	.5	.5	.5	.5	.5	.5	.5	.5	.5	.5	.5	.5
.4	.4	.4	.4	.4	.4	.4	.4	.4	.4	.4	.4	.4	.4	.4	.4	.4	.4	.4	.4
.3	.3	.3	.3	.3	.3	.3	.3	.3	.3	.3	.3	.3	.3	.3	.3	.3	.3	.3	.3
.2	.2	.2	.2	.2	.2	.2	.2	.2	.2	.2	.2	.2	.2	.2	.2	.2	.2	.2	.2
.1	.1	.1	.1	.1	.1	.1	.1	.1	.1	.1	.1	.1	.1	.1	.1	.1	.1	.1	.1
98	98	98	98	98	98	98	98	98	98	98	98	98	98	98	98	98	98	98	98
.9	.9	.9	.9	.9	.9	.9	.9	.9	.9	.9	.9	.9	.9	.9	.9	.9	.9	.9	.9
.8	.8	.8	.8	.8	.8	.8	.8	.8	.8	.8	.8	.8	.8	.8	.8	.8	.8	.8	.8
.7	.7	.7	.7	.7	.7	.7	.7	.7	.7	.7	.7	.7	.7	.7	.7	.7	.7	.7	.7
.6	.6	.6	.6	.6	.6	.6	.6	.6	.6	.6	.6	.6	.6	.6	.6	.6	.6	.6	.6
.5	.5	.5	.5	.5	.5	.5	.5	.5	.5	.5	.5	.5	.5	.5	.5	.5	.5	.5	.5
.4	.4	.4	.4	.4	.4	.4	.4	.4	.4	.4	.4	.4	.4	.4	.4	.4	.4	.4	.4
.3	.3	.3	.3	.3	.3	.3	.3	.3	.3	.3	.3	.3	.3	.3	.3	.3	.3	.3	.3
.2	.2	.2	.2	.2	.2	.2	.2	.2	.2	.2	.2	.2	.2	.2	.2	.2	.2	.2	.2
.1	.1	.1	.1	.1	.1	.1	.1	.1	.1	.1	.1	.1	.1	.1	.1	.1	.1	.1	.1
97	97	97	97	97	97	97	97	97	97	97	97	97	97	97	97	97	97	97	97
.9	.9	.9	.9	.9	.9	.9	.9	.9	.9	.9	.9	.9	.9	.9	.9	.9	.9	.9	.9
16	17	18	19	20	21	22	23	24	25	26	27	28	29	30	31	32	33	34	35

Cervical Position: O: Open/Soft **C:** Closed/Firm

Index

F

Faint line, on pregnancy test, 147–148
Fallopian sperm transfer insemination, 185
Fallopian tubes, 85
  blockages in, and IUI, 185
  blockages in, and IVF, 202
  conception and, 93, 95
  endometriosis in, 156
  healthy, and IVF success, 211
  infection of, 155, 156
  ovulation and, 92, 93
  pregnancy in. See Ectopic pregnancy
  scar tissue in, 157–158, 177
  surgery for, 158, 199–201
  transfer of egg and sperm into, in GIFT, 216–218
  transfer of zygote into, in ZIFT, 218
  untying, 200
FAM. See Fertility awareness method
Familial dysautonomia, genetic screening for, 15
Family
  telling about fertility treatments, 228
  telling about TTC plans, 129
Family and Medical Leave Act, 42
  fertility treatments and, 173
Family health history, 7
  check of, during preconception checkup, 7
  fertility and, 109–110
FAST technique, 185
Fat, body, 45–47. See also Overweight, Underweight
  male fertility and, 48, 52, 167
  estrogen and, 45, 47, 48
Fat, dietary, 62, 74–76
  dairy and, 62
  monounsaturated, 76
  omega-3. See Omega-3 fatty acids
  polyunsaturated, 76
  saturated, 75
  trans, 76
Fathers. See Male
Fatigue
  as early pregnancy sign, 143
  Femara and, 189
FDA
  -approved lubricants, 119
  herbal supplements and, 134
  on donor eggs, 222
  on fish, 73

on trans fats, 75–76
sperm banks, 225
Female
  anatomy, 84–87
  reproductive system, 84–87
Femara, 162, 189
  male use of, 188
  PCOS and, 159, 189
Feminine hygiene sprays and wipes, 123
Fern, saliva ovulation test and, 105
Fertile foods, 62–73
  for males, 66–67
Fertile window, 91, 92, 96, 98, 105
Fertility. See also Fertility, male
  after miscarriage, 243, 245–247
  age and, 90, 110–113
  alcohol and, 18, 167
  apps, 98, 99
  awareness, birth control method, 117
  BPA and, 33–34
  bracelet, to detect ovulation, 106
  busters, foods, 73–77
  caffeine and, 16–17
  CAM and, 131–136
  challenges to, 154–169
  charts, 257
  chemical exposure and, 33–34, 36, 79
  clinics, rankings of, 214
  diet and, 58–81
  drugs. See Clomid; Hormone injections
  exam, female, 174–178
  exercise and, 23–25
  family history and, 109–110
  figuring out your, 107–113
  foods that harm, 73–77
  foods that help, 62–73
  full-fat dairy and, 62
  genetics and, 109–110
  herbs and, 133–136
  kit, 135
  lifestyle and, 15–37
  marijuana and, 22–23
  medications and, 10–12
  mercury and, 73, 77
  monitors, to detect ovulation, 105
  phthlalates and, 33–34
  planner, 250–286
  screening, at home, 174
  signs, 96–106
  smoking and, 19–22
  stress and, 28–32
  subtle signs of, 116, 212, 122
  supplements and, 133–136
  tracker bracelet, 106

vitamins and, 69–71
watch, 105
weight and, 44–57
workplace and, 35–37
workup, 170–178
Fertility, male
  age and, 112, 167
  alcohol and, 18, 167
  BPA and, 33
  caffeine and, 16
  challenges to, 166–167
  chemical exposure and, 167
  exercise and, 25, 167
  foods that help, 66–67, 72
  foods that hurt, 73
  heat and, 25, 26, 127, 167
  herbs and, 134
  marijuana and, 22–23
  medications that affect, 14
  phthlalates and, 33
  screening, at home, 174
  smoking and, 19
  supplements and, 134
  underwear choice and, 127
  vitamins and, 66–67
  workplace and, 36
  workup, 176–177
Fertility awareness method, 117
Fertility clinics, 211, 214
Fertility medications
  injectable, 190–198
  male, 188
  oral, 187–189
Fertility specialist
  finding a, 173
  when to see one for help, 113, 171–173
Fertility treatments, 181–232.
  See also individual treatments
  at home, 183–187
  CAM and, 217
  chances of multiples and, 162, 188–189, 190
  health insurance and, 172–173, 230
  male, 188, 201
  paying for, 172–173, 230–231
  pregnancy testing and, 148, 198, 209
  same sex couples and, 183, 186, 202, 220–221
  telling friends and family about, 228
  using an HPT and, 148, 192, 198
Fertilization, 92–95. See also Conception
  in ICSI, 213
  in IUI, 184–185
  in IVF cycle, 205
  time it takes from sex, 92
FET. See Frozen embryo transfers